Psychobiology of Reproductive Behavior

An Evolutionary Perspective

Psychobiology of Reproductive Behavior
An Evolutionary Perspective

David Crews, *Editor*

Prentice-Hall, Inc., *Englewood Cliffs, NJ 07632*

Library of Congress Cataloging-in-Publication Data

Psychobiology of reproductive behavior.

   Bibliography: p.
   Includes index.
   1. Sexual behavior in animals. 2. Reproduction.
3. Psychobiology. I. Crews, David.
QL761.P76 1987   599.56   86–25185
ISBN 0–13–732090–6

Editorial/production supervision
and interior design: PATRICK WALSH
Cover design: WANDA LUBELSKA DESIGN
Manufacturing buyer: ED O'DOUGHERTY
Chapter-opening illustrations: L. LASZLO MESZOLY

Printed in the United States of America

10 9 8 7 6 5 4 3 2

ISBN 0-13-732090-6   025

Prentice-Hall International (UK) Limited, *London*
Prentice-Hall of Australia Pty. Limited, *Sydney*
Prentice-Hall Canada Inc., *Toronto*
Prentice-Hall Hispanoamericana, S.A., *Mexico*
Prentice-Hall of India Private Limited, *New Delhi*
Prentice-Hall of Japan, Inc., *Tokyo*
Prentice-Hall of Southeast Asia Pte. Ltd., *Singapore*
Editora Prentice-Hall do Brasil, Ltda., *Rio de Janeiro*

Contents

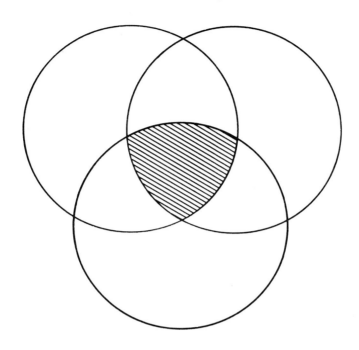

Preface

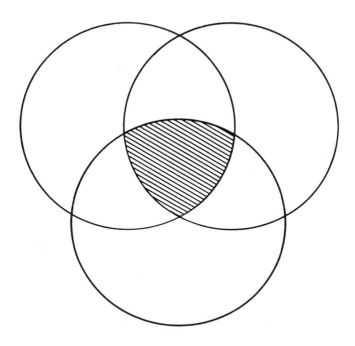

The biological bases of behavior are among the most fascinating, and useful, topics in the behavioral sciences today. However, almost all of our knowledge regarding this subject has been gathered on only a small number of species of domesticated animals observed under controlled laboratory conditions. While this has been, and will continue to be, a fruitful and rewarding approach for learning about the physiological bases of behavior, it can lead to an unrealistic and overly narrow conceptual framework about organisms living under natural conditions. Both the underlying mechanisms and the functional outcomes of behavior are products of natural selection. Since the mechanisms controlling behavior arose in response to a specific set of environmental conditions, the physical and social environments of the animal must be considered and, if possible, incorporated into any investigation. In this way we gain added insight into how physiology, behavior, and the environment are functionally interrelated.

This volume is designed as an introduction to the psychobiology of reproductive behavior from an evolutionary perspective. The intended audience is the upper-division undergraduate and first-year graduate student in zoology, psychology, or anthropology. Both animal and human studies are included. To understand human behavior, one must first understand the fundamental principles governing complex biological processes. Comparative animal studies instruct us in this complex interplay between the physical and social environment, the organism's behavior, and its physiology.

The comparative approach, the traditional method of biological investigation, continues to be the most powerful tool we have for investigations of the biological bases of behavior. Although the comparative approach has its greatest power when specific phenomena are compared among closely related species, considerable knowledge is also gained when the organisms used are distantly related. The generality, but not necessarily the validity, of a principle increases with the phyletic scope of the species examined. Atypical organisms can be especially informative, as their unusual adaptations illustrate alternative solutions to particular problems. As George A. Bartolomew has pointed out, they "often force one to abandon standard methods and standard points of view," with the result that, "in trying to comprehend their special and often unusual adaptations, one often serendipitously stumbles on new insights."

Our knowledge of the biological bases of behavior has come largely from study of the physiological mechanisms and functional outcomes of behavior. These studies have produced considerable information on the immediate, or proximal, causes of behavior. It is important to appreciate that this is only one side of the coin. An individual's survival depends upon the ability of the nervous system to respond in an adaptive manner to the changing environment. Knowledge of diversity and adaptations complete our understanding of the biological bases of behavior. We obtain this information from comparison of carefully selected species. Such comparisons yield clues about both evolutionary history and present adaptations. This phylogenetic perspective probes not only into the past, but also into the potential of the mechanisms that control behavior.

Reproductive behaviors are often the most striking displays of social signals. This is probably because beyond survival, reproduction is the most important event in the life of an organism. Quite simply, if the individual or a close relative does not reproduce, its genes will not be represented in subsequent generations. The importance of these behaviors is reflected in their marked stereotypy characteristic of each species. This quality makes them particularly well suited for quantification and has resulted in a large and rich literature on reproductive behavior and its endocrinological and neurophysiological correlates.

Behavioral biologists have long noted that the behaviors associated with reproduction tend to be characteristic of each species and each sex. These behaviors are crucial to both reproductive function at a physiological level as well as at a social level. A large body of research has shown how successful reproduction depends on the precise coordination and synchronization of myriad factors: The individual's reproductive capacity is influenced by the physical, biotic, and social cues in its immediate environment as well as by its developmental and evolutionary history. Behavior is controlled by the neural and endocrine processes occurring within the individual as well as the individual's interaction with other individuals. Thus you often find that species-typical behaviors are embedded in a chain of complementary stimulus-response interactions, each stage of which depends upon the preceding events and, at the same time, sets the stage for those to follow.

The diversity of reproductive behaviors can tell us much about the mechanisms that underlie such behaviors. This is now being addressed by studies of the psychobiology of behavior. There are three elements characteristic of this body of research (see cover illustration). They often involve the study of diverse species under both laboratory and field conditions. They integrate different levels of biological organization from the molecule to the population. Finally they utilize a variety of state-of-the-art techniques, thereby enabling one to illuminate the relations between the different levels of biological organization.

This book is unlike any other that is presently available. It attempts to present evolutionary or comparative aspects of the causal mechanisms and functional outcomes of reproductive behavior in a systematic and thorough manner, while dealing extensively with the hormonal and ecological factors that play a role in the control of reproductive behavior. The authors were selected because their research is comparative, naturalistic, and multidisciplinary. Thus, each chapter is centered around one or more research programs to convey one or more concepts. In this manner the reader gains an up-to-date overview of many fundamental issues from an established investigator. By summarizing the state of our knowledge in the area of the psychobiology of reproductive behavior in the various vertebrate classes, the reader also will gain an understanding of the intricate web of cause and effect that underlies the reproductive process.

As will become immediately apparent, the chapters deal with animals many people have had at least some contact with. This approach should appeal to a larger audience than do more traditional texts concerned with this subject but concentrating on domesticated and/or laboratory animals. The volume is organized roughly according to vertebrate class. With the exception of the jawless fishes and the cartilaginous fishes, all vertebrate classes are represented. Depending upon the structure of the course, the instructor may choose a phylogenetic approach or a topical approach.

As a whole, the volume considers the problem of what the similarities and differences among species mean. Some of the chapters document variation in reproductive strategies and in the mechanisms that underlie reproductive behaviors. Here the lesson to be learned is that there are multiple pathways by which a particular adaptive response is mediated. Indeed, it appears that the diversity of mechanisms activating reproductive behavior is correlated with the diversity in reproductive strategies. Other chapters document the "model system" approach in which extensive study of a particular biological phenomenon in a single species is detailed. Here the lesson is that atypical species can be used profitably to approach relatively old problems in new ways, providing new insights.

I wish to single out a few of the many friends and colleagues who, knowingly or not, were so helpful in the creation of this volume: Jenneatte Blanchette, Mark Grassman, Neil Greenberg, Jonathan Lindzey, Elizabeth Lester, Robert Mason, Yuki Morris, and Joan Whittier. I wish to give particular thanks to Hillary Miller, who has been a constant source of support and good advice.

David Crews
Austin, Texas

Psychobiology
of Reproductive Behavior

An Evolutionary Perspective

ONE
Diversity in Reproductive Patterns and Behavior in Teleost Fishes

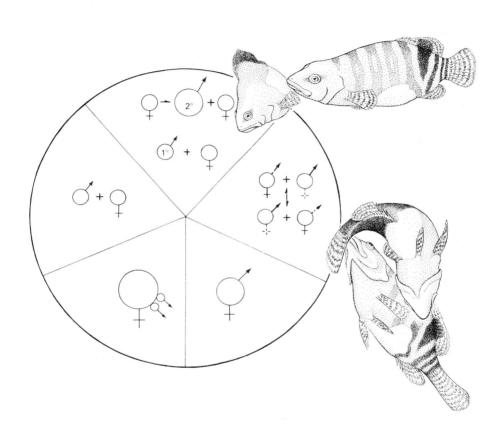

Leo S. Demski
School of Biological Sciences
University of Kentucky
Lexington, Kentucky

The teleosts or modern bony fishes exhibit the greatest diversity in reproductive patterns among vertebrates. The patterns range from: (1) gonochoristic species having testis-bearing (male) and ovary-bearing (female) individuals which form typical monogamous pairs; (2) deep-sea anglerfish in which the male attaches himself to the female, possibly relinquishing control over his own testis; (3) sequentially hermaphroditic species in which individuals change from one sex to another; (4) simultaneously hermaphroditic species in which individuals trade eggs and sperm during mating, frequently reversing their sexual roles; and (5) simultaneously hermaphroditic species in which individuals self-fertilize under natural conditions.

Differences in evolutionary strategies have been suggested to account for this diversity, especially as it compares to the almost complete pervasiveness of gonochorism of terrestrial animals (see Warner, 1984). Some ultimate causes have been suggested. Sex switching usually occurs where size is an advantage to the sexual production of one sex versus the other and/or individuals are widely separated. For instance, it becomes adaptive when an individual can produce more eggs or fertilize more eggs throughout its adult life by being one sex while small and then changing to the other after attaining a certain "relative" size.

Protogyny (first female, then male) is favored where dominance of males is a major factor. This reproductive pattern is observed in species where a male guards a number of females (harem) or protects a territory (lek) which females enter to mate. In many of these instances, smaller males mate only infrequently, if at all, and it is certainly an advantage to be a female at this time in the life cycle. Protandry (first male, then female), on the other hand, occurs in small stable groups with essentially a monogamous relationship between one pair that reproduces. The largest males change sex, becoming females; large females produce the greatest number of eggs. Protandry is common in instances where small males can fertilize the eggs of the larger females and, for one reason or the other, large males cannot sexually monopolize groups of females.

Simultaneous hermaphroditism is obviously advantageous to animals existing in low population densities (Charnov et al., 1976), since the condition assures that any two adults can form a pair. However, this argument cannot account for its occurrence in abundant species unless one postulates that these fish in their evolutionary history have experienced such low population densities and have retained the hermaphroditism related to it.

Because of the great diversity in reproductive patterns and behaviors found in the bony fishes, they provide the comparative reproductive biologist with a wealth of "natural experiments" from which basic control processes can be studied to advantage. This paper deals primarily with "how" questions and will outline behavioral and neuroendocrine mechanisms underlying several of these reproductive patterns. The gonochores will not be covered in any detail, as this is the topic of other chapters in this volume.

ACQUIRED HERMAPHRODITISM

Based on examination of gonadal tissue, certain deep-sea fishes which lack means for bioluminescence are thought to be simultaneous hermaphrodites. This may be an adaptation to the low population densities and conditions of darkness, which make finding mates difficult. The ceratioid anglers, whose light organs are probably used only for luring prey, have evolved an unusual mode of reproduction that can be considered intermediate between gonochronism and hermaphroditism. In certain species, the males become parasites, permanently attaching themselves to females (see Figure 1.1A and review by Pietsch, 1976). Indeed, in some forms males probably never feed on their own. A male that finds a female attaches to her body by biting and retaining this hold. This becomes a permanent bond, as the tissues of the male's head become fused with those of the female's body (Figure 1.1B). Figures 1.1B and C show that part of the cranial skeleton and surface features are distorted in the attached males (Regan and Trewavas, 1932; Demski and Rosenblatt, unpublished observations). A confluence of blood systems of the two fish has been suggested based on histology (see Figure 1.1C and Pietsch, 1976). This would certainly be adaptive in providing a source of nutriment and blood gas exchange to the male, as well as a means through which the female could control endocrine functions in the male via hormones secreted by her brain, pituitary, and ovaries (see below). The latter would be most important to synchronize sperm maturation and discharge with egg production and release.

Several other equally drastic sexual dimorphisms are evident in these animals. Males are described as "progenetic," which indicates precocious maturity in animals retaining many larval or juvenile characteristics (Marshall, 1984). Males mature early and are small, while females mature over much longer periods and attain a far greater size. The olfactory bulb or area of the brain involved with smell, the peripheral olfactory organs, and the eyes are more elaborate in free-swimming males.

These sexual dimorphisms can be considered with regard to the peculiar reproductive patterns of this group. The progenesis of the male may have evolved to permit rapid sexual development at the expense of body growth and differentiation of most other adult systems. Pheromones or chemical sex attractants given off by mature females (see Chapters 2, 4, 10) are probably the most important sensory stimuli that permit the males to find the females, hence the elaboration of the olfactory systems in males, but not in females. Visual cues such as bioluminescence could potentially also be

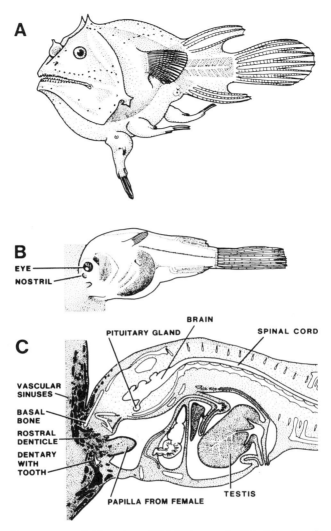

Figure 1.1. Deep-sea ceratioid anglers, *Edriolychnus schmidti*, Linophrynidae. (A) Adult female with attached parasitic males. Actual size of the female is about 50 mm standard length (nose to beginning of the caudal fin). (B) Enlargement of the left side of an attached male (ca. 12 mm standard length). In this case, the eye and nares appear to be intact. Fusion of the jaw apparatus with the female's body is apparent. (C) Sagittal section of attached male (ca. 13 mm standard length) with the same orientation as in B. Numerous blood sinuses are associated with the area of attachment and the extension of the female tissue as a papilla into the mouth. Portions of the rostral denticle, which is a specialized dermal denticle used to anchor into the female's body, can also be recognized. A typical tooth is also present. The telencephalon, optic lobes or midbrain tectum, and cerebellum of the brain are clearly visible, although they may be rather undifferentiated (see text for discussion). The spinal cord and pituitary or hypophysis are indicated, but further details such as functional state are not available. Connections between the brain and the eye and olfactory organs are not illustrated; they may well have been omitted to simplify the drawing. The testis and sperm duct (not labeled) are well developed. (A–C redrawn after Regan and Trewavas, *Dana Report* Vol. 1 No. 2, (1932) Oxford University Press)

used. The greater size and later maturation of the female are probably necessary to insure adequate egg production or fecundity.

It may someday be feasible to carry out physiological studies on these fishes, but for the present we must be satisfied with speculations based on anatomical studies. For example, if it is assumed that parasitic males do not waste sperm but produce and release it only when the female's eggs are ripe, then one must also assume that either (1) the male is responding to the same proximate stimuli the female is responding to, (2) the male is controlling its own testis in response to cues generated by the female, or (3) the female is directly regulating the male's gonads via hormone secretion into a common circulation. Research in other vertebrates demonstrating potent hormonal effects when there is a vascular anastomosis (see Chapters 6 and 10) indicates it is possible that the maintenance of sperm production is controlled by the secretion of the female's gonadotropin-releasing hormone (GnRH). The effects could be mediated by gonadotropin release from pituitary glands in either the female, the male, or both. The problem of how sperm release is synchronized with egg discharge may be even more difficult to determine.

Neural pathways have been identified that trigger both sperm and egg release in goldfish (*Carassius auratus*) and other teleosts. They originate in the preoptic area (POA) of the telencephalon and extend to the spinal cord (Demski and Sloan, 1985). The system can be activated by olfactory tract stimulation, which is thought to relate to pheromonal modulation of sexual reflexes (see Chapter 2). Experiments have shown that administration of gonadotropin-releasing hormone (GnRH), a hypothalamic peptide known to be involved in reproduction (see Chapters 2, 5) directly into the POA will facilitate sperm release (see discussion in Demski and Dulka, 1984). Hence, if in the attached male anglerfish the olfactory system is intact, pheromones from the female might be able to trigger sperm release (SR), provided the SR system is similar to that of goldfish. Alternatively, secretion of GnRH in high quantities by the female could possibly trigger the SR system more directly by causing activation of cells in the POA. This presumes that the GnRH is not rapidly degraded by enzymes in the blood plasma. It is also possible that pressure changes on the female's body wall caused by ovulated eggs could be used as a signal. This seems unlikely, because they would be difficult to detect against a background of noise generated by swimming movements, etc. Perhaps a combination of these and/or other factors are used to synchronize gamete production and delivery.

SEQUENTIAL SEX CHANGERS

Most teleost hermaphrodites develop and function as one sex and change to the other at some later time, depending on their size, age, individual dominance status, and/or the sex ratio in their social group. Protogynous hermaphrodites change from female to male, while the reverse occurs in protandrous species. Protogny seems to be more prevalent, being common in wrasses (Labridae), sea bass and groupers (Serranidae), and parrotfish (Scaridae). It frequently occurs when dominance by large males significantly increases the number of females with which they can mate. Typical situations include male defense of favored spawning areas and maintenance of harems.

In certain protogynous labroid fishes (wrasses and parrotfish), two types of males are present, a situation referred to as diandry. Primary males develop initially as males and have testes and sperm ducts typical of gonochoristic males. They are small and resemble the females in their somewhat drab or initial-phase color pattern. They do not have individual territories and mate either in large spawning aggregations of a female with many males or by "sneaking" in on the paired matings of the terminal males (see below). Secondary males are sex-inverted females and have testes containing remnants of ovaries and oviducts. They are large, maintain individual territories, have a bright coloration referred to as the terminal-phase pattern, and mate individually with females (Figure 1.2). In some species, primary males as well as females can develop into terminal-phase

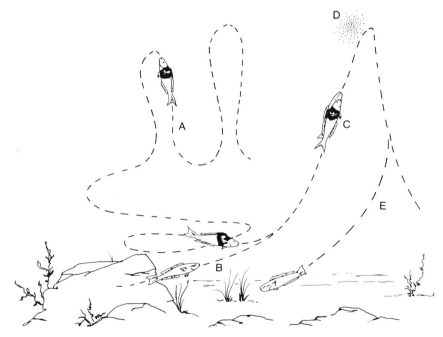

Figure 1.2. Courtship and spawning in the bluehead wrasse, *Thalassoma bifasciatum*. Terminal-phase males advertise by performing a looping movement (A). At the approach of a female, the male swims vigorously back and forth above her (B) while vibrating his pectoral fins. If the female is ready, she ascends, and the pair move quickly up off the bottom (C) and release gametes (D). Afterward, the female moves away (E), while the male returns to courtship behavior. (Reproduced from Thresher, 1984)

males (see Warner, 1982). The opposite of diandry is monoandry, which refers to protogynous mating systems with only secondary or reversed males.

Protandry represents a mating strategy which takes advantage of a direct relationship between female size and fecundity and the ability of small males to produce sufficient sperm to fertilize the eggs of larger females. For the system to be stable, male dominance must be restricted so that they cannot gain a reproductive advantage by mating with a number of females (Warner, 1984).

Sex change in sequential hermaphrodites can be triggered by social factors (see reviews by Shapiro, 1979, and Warner, 1984). Indeed, such factors have been identified and controlled in both field and laboratory experiments. These behavioral systems hold great potential for identification of psychoneuroendocrine mechanisms underlying sex change. A few of the better-studied examples are discussed in some detail (for descriptions of additional systems, see Chan and Yeung, 1983; Thresher, 1984; Warner, 1984).

Labridae

Wrasses are common coral-reef fishes with similar species found in the Atlantic and Pacific oceans. The fish are small and adaptable to experimentation. Robertson (1972) studied the Pacific cleaner wrasse, *Labroides dimidiatus*, which lives in groups of 1 male, 3 to 6 mature females, and several juveniles. The male defends the harem against intruders and mates with each female once a day. Removal of the male triggers a sex change in the largest female, provided she can prevent other neighboring males from taking over the group. The sex reversal is evident within 1.5 hours, beginning with the development of aggressive responses and territorial behavior typical of the male. Full development of male courtship and spawning behavior can be completed within 2 to 4 days and sperm released by 14 to 18 days. The testis develops from spermatogenic tissue in the ovarian lamellae. There are apparently no primary males in this species.

Sex change in the dominant female appears to be inhibited by male aggression, while sex reversal in lower-ranking females is prevented by repeated aggressive encounters with more dominant females. Removal of a male suddenly eliminates aggression on the dominant female, and this presumably triggers the behavioral and physiological responses that cause sex changes.

Concerning mechanisms, several reasonable working hypotheses can be suggested. One possibility is that aggression functions as a stressor, causing production of adrenal steroids, which in turn inhibit brain pathways for male behavior. Such dominance-related stress reactions are known in other vertebrates (see Brain and Benton, 1983; and Chapter 11). Another possibility is that prostaglandins are produced in response to the attacks and that these hormones, which are known to preferentially activate female behavior in male goldfish and other teleosts (see Chapters 2 and 5), may inhibit the expression of male characteristics. Experimentation is needed to identify the psychoneuroendocrine mechanisms involved.

Wrasses of the genus *Thalassama* have been especially well studied. These fishes are typically diandric, although the percentage of primary to secondary males can vary considerably, depending on the spawning environment (Warner, 1984). Primary males and females are small to moderate size and exhibit a similar initial-phase coloration which in the bluehead wrasse, *T. bifasciatum*, is yellow with a brown stripe. Large females and, in some species, primary males can change into terminal-phase males. In blueheads, terminal males have a bright blue head followed by a series of black, white, and black bands and a green body (see Figure 1.2 and color photographs in Thresher, 1984, and Warner, 1984).

Studies by several investigators have revealed that social signals initiate the sex change. Warner (1982) carried out experiments using the rainbow wrasse, *T. lucasanum*, of the eastern tropical Pacific. Ten experimental groups of females and primary males in the initial phase were placed together in outdoor pens and monitored for development of terminal-phase color patterns. Control groups had a terminal-phase male placed with the other fish. The largest animal in each of the experimental groups changed into a terminal-phase male; four were females and six were primary males. Nine of the 10 transformations were completed within 7 weeks. None of the animals in the control groups became terminal-phase males. These results establish that social stimuli, specifically the presence of a terminal-phase male, can inhibit the tendency of the largest fish to change color and/or sex.

Ross and co-workers (1983) performed a more detailed analysis of the factors triggering change of females into terminal-phase males in the saddleback wrasse, *T. duperrey*. Groups of up to 4 adult fish were placed in open pens in a lagoon; in some cases a barrier was used to separate the fish. The barrier could prevent individuals either from touching one another (tactile isolation) or from touching and seeing one another (tactile and visual isolation). Channels for olfactory, acoustic, and lateral line communication were still available. Fish of different size groups, sexes, and/or color phase were placed together in each pen. The largest female was monitored for change to terminal-phase coloration. Each experiment ran for 3 months, at which time the fish were killed and the gonads examined histologically. In this species, the gonads of individuals that have undergone a sex change lack intact oocytes and have abundant sperm in advanced stages of development.

Single fish did not change, while those in the presence of a smaller female did, regardless of their absolute size. Changes did not occur when fish were paired with a smaller female of a different species of *Thalassoma*. Placement with either a smaller initial-phase or a smaller terminal-phase male *T. duperrey* still resulted in change. The presence of a smaller conspecific of either sex or color phase was sufficient to trigger the sex reversal. The larger member of a pair of fish separated from each other by a simple barrier (screen) that allowed visual contact changed sex, while placement of an additional barrier to visual communication blocked the response. Visual estimation of relative size appeared to be the critical parameter being assessed. A few groups were also tested in which small, medium, and large females were separated from each other but remained in visual contact. Although the medium-sized fish were well in the range of animals that sex-reverse, only the largest of the three changed, indicating that the presence of a larger fish can exert an inhibitory influence on sex reversal.

A few attempts have been made to identify the physiological mechanisms of sex and color change in the wrasses. A single injection of 1 to 2.5 mg of testosterone given to primary males and females in the initial phase can trigger development of the terminal phase in *T. bifasciatum* and other protogynous wrasses (Stoll, 1955; Reinboth, 1975; Chan and Yeung, 1983). The color change can occur within several weeks, while, in the females, change in the gonads may require 6–7 weeks or longer if it occurs at all. It is not known if under natural conditions increased production of testosterone or other androgens normally triggers these changes. It does appear that coloration and gonadal development are controlled by somewhat separate mechanisms.

Serranidae

Anthias squamipinnis is a small anthiine sea bass found on Pacific coral reefs. The fish are protogynus hermaphrodites in which production of males depends on the make-up of social groups. Males have longer fins and are more brightly colored than females and hence easy to identify (see color figures in Thresher, 1984). Fishelson (1970) originally noted that individuals in captive groups with 10 to 20 females and 1 or 2 males did not change sex, whereas in similar groups without males one of the females developed into a male within 2 weeks. If this new male was removed, one of the remaining females changed, and the process could be continued until 19 females in the original group were converted into males; fish housed singly do not change.

Shapiro (1980) performed a series of more detailed experiments on this problem, both in the field and laboratory. He demonstrated that color changes in a sex-changing female begin within 3–9 days of male removal, with the full male color pattern being developed by the 7th to the 16th day. Unlike the wrasses, color-changed *A. squamipinnis* all have functional testes. The number of fish that change sex is dependent on the number removed. Social groups can exist in several forms ranging from all females, to small single-male aggregations, to larger groups with 50 males and approximately 300 females. Working on coral reefs in the Philippines, Shapiro removed 3–9 males from 15 experimental groups and single males from another 11 control groups. He then monitored the groups for alterations in the color pattern of the females. The results were remarkable in that 57 females changed sex to replace 58 males removed from the experimental groups. As expected, in most control groups, a single female reversed. In the experimental groups, fish changed sex in a sequential fashion with a delay of about 1.5–2 days between each initiation of color change.

The precision of the system could not be explained by existing models for initiation of sex change based on size, maturity, or male dominance. Hence, Shapiro postulated that the sex reversal in this species is controlled by complex behavioral interactions within subgroups of females which maintain clearly defined dominance relationships. He predicted that male removal would result in changes in behavioral profiles (quantitative assessments of several responses) of each individual based on responses given to or received from others, and that these changes might trigger the sex reversals.

Indeed, detailed observations revealed that male and female *A. squamipinnis* of different levels in the dominance hierarchy each have their own characteristic behavior profiles (Shapiro, 1981a, b). Following male removal in single male groups in the laboratory, one of the females begins to perform in a fashion typical of males. Three responses were most dramatically increased: rushes toward another fish, U-swims (Figure 1.3), and third-dorsal-spine erections. Rushes performed increased by day 2 but did not reach male-typical levels until 3–4 weeks. In contrast, U-swims and third-dorsal-spine erections began to increase later (4–5 and 10–11 days, respectively) and took more than 14 days to reach male levels. Reception rates of U-swims and rushes by the sex-changing fish fell to virtually zero (a pattern typical of males) on the day after removal of the male and remained at zero for the duration of the observations. The reception rate of bent approaches, a possible appeasement gesture by the females toward more dominant fish (especially the males), increased toward the reversing fish; this began at about day 3 following removal of the male. The immediate causes of the behavioral changes are unknown. The fact that the changes have different latency periods suggests mediation by somewhat different behavioral triggers and/or neural and endocrine systems.

From the above data, one might assume that sex change of the dominant female is normally inhibited by male aggression, as in the cleaner wrasse. For *A. squamipinnis* this cannot be the case, since there are all-female groups in which sex reversals do not occur over weeks of observations. In other words, in this species there is a difference between male absence and male removal. Shapiro was thus forced to search for additional factors that could explain the sex changes.

When the percentage of rushes given was calculated (rushes given divided by rushes given and received) for several groups, it became apparent that the males were near 100%, low-level subordinates near zero, with others in between (Figure 1.4, top). Because of heavy male aggression on the dominant female, her score was lower than the second- and third-ranking females. Following male removal, she suddenly began displaying rushes without any rushes being directed toward her (100%). Other females also increased their percentages of rushes, since the male had directed some aggression toward them as well, but only the dominant female experienced

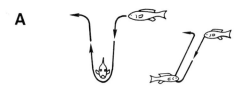

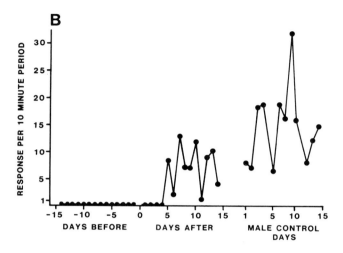

Figure 1.3. (A) Variations in the U-swim response typical of male *Anthias squamipinnis*. The response is directed toward subordinate females. The fish turns on its side throughout the movement and makes large and rapid lateral motions of its body and tail. The response also includes a characteristic set of fin postures. (B) The daily rate of U-swims performed by sex-reversing female *A. squamipinnis* (left side) both before and after removal of the male (day 0) in its group and rates shown by this male in the 15 days before its removal (male control days on right side). Medians are for 7 females, and the differences before and after male removal are highly significant, as the graph suggests. (A and B redrawn from Shapiro, 1981a)

a large change (Figure 1.4, bottom). Therefore, this change in the ratio of rushes given to total rushes may be a critical factor responsible for triggering the sex reversal in only the dominant female of the group.

Shapiro and Boulon (1982) studied the role of other females in initiation of sex change. They observed that in groups of less than 4 females the chances of male removal's triggering a sex reversal were greatly diminished. The result may be due to alteration in the rushes-given ratio and/or behavior-received profile of the dominant female because of limited interactions with other females. They also removed the largest female in all-female groups and did not observe sex change, illustrating that these females are not the behavioral equivalent of a male in the heterosexual groups.

A few experiments have questioned whether the loss of close contact rather than simple visual cues from the male can induce sex change (Shapiro,

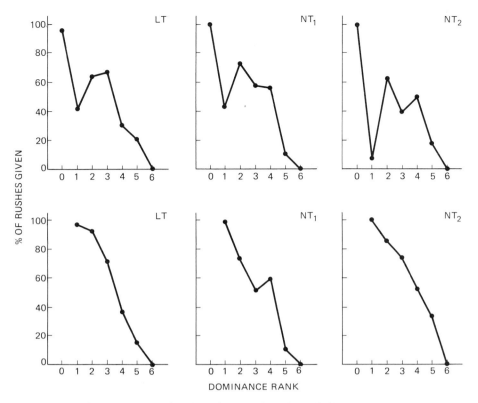

Figure 1.4. The percentage of rushes given (rushes given divided by number given plus number received) of the male and six subordinate females in three groups (LT, NT_1, and NT_2) before (top row) and following (bottom row) removal of the male. The females are listed in order of decreasing dominance rank. Note that the dominant female (#1) had a lower score than females 2 and 3 before removal. This is because the male directs most of the rushes toward the dominant female. Following male removal, this individual suddenly changes to a 100% score, since she typically receives no rushes from the other females. The behavioral change is thought to be a factor which triggers sex reversal in this fish (see text for details). (Redrawn from Shapiro, 1981b)

1983). In single-male groups in laboratory aquaria, the male was placed in a centrally located small cylinder which was either transparent or opaque. Water flow was permitted between the cylinder and females in the larger tank. At least one female changed sex in each group regardless of treatment, indicating that the loss of behavioral interaction rather than visual stimuli from the male is the important factor triggering the sex change. Acoustic and chemical cues were presumably still available to the females and can thus be excluded as the major factors that inhibit sex change.

It was still possible that if females could see male-female interactions, they might be prevented from changing sex. To test this idea, a male and a female were placed in a small aquarium inside the large tank with the other females. Water flow occurred through a screen top on the smaller tank, but the fish on the outside could not interact with the pair. In half the groups, the male and female were separated by a transparent barrier inside the smaller container. Only the males given free access to a female demonstrated all of the "normal" interactions characteristic of males in social groups. Regardless of condition, at least one female changed sex in each group and none of the females enclosed with the male reversed. The results support the hypothesis that behavioral interaction with the male can prevent sex reversal. They also indicate that female interactions with other females are necessary for sex change to occur, since females placed near the males but separated from them as well as other females did not reverse.

Shapiro concludes that changes in the behavior-received profile, which includes an individual's interactions with all members of its group, are the most likely factor(s) initiating and sustaining the sex change. This hypothesis explains how equal numbers of females change to replace males removed from large groups. Assuming that each male interacts only with a specific subpopulation of females, then removal of that male would result in change of the dominant female in that subgroup alone. Seeing the effects of removal of males in adjacent subgroups would have no effect on females outside the group, as indicated by the above experiments.

Little is known of the physiological mechanisms controlling sex reversal in *A. squamipinnis*. Treatment of females by addition of testosterone (1.5 mg/l; 3.0 mg/l; 5.0 mg/l) to their tanks results in the development of male coloration, increases in male-type behavior patterns, and change in the gonad. The highest concentrations used were most effective (Fishelson, 1975). After 12 days in the medium with the testosterone, some of the fish were transferred to a seminatural habitat with other females; the remaining fish were killed for examination of the gonads. The animals given the low dose began to lose their only poorly developed male coloration after day 3 and by two weeks later had reverted to female color and behavior patterns; the gonads of fish in this treatment group had degenerated oogenic tissue but no development of sperm. In contrast, the largest of the fish receiving the highest dose maintained their male coloration, aggressive behavior, and territoriality until the end of the experiment three weeks later; the gonads of fish receiving the high dose had typical spermatogenic tissue.

In another experiment, sex-reversing females from which sperm could be stripped were placed in aquaria with treatments of either 1.0 mg/l or 2.0 mg/l of estradiol added on five successive days. After six days, the fish began to lose their male coloration patterns. At ten days, the gonads of some of the fish were examined, revealing atretic or degenerated oocytes, dense testicular tissue but no sperm. Other fish were placed in a community tank and behaved like other untreated females. After an additional 10–12 days, they began to demonstrate male patterns of aggressive behavior. By 18–20 days, they were again performing the U-swim and had regained the coloration typical of sex-reversing females, suggesting that the effects of estrogen treatment were transitory. The condition of the gonads of these individuals was not reported.

These results suggest that androgens initiate sex reversal and that estrogens can at least temporarily inhibit the process. They point to a need for additional experiments in which the hormones are given directly as intramuscular injections or subcutaneous implants (testosterone, for example, is not very soluble in water) and detailed behavioral observation conducted. Several additional lines of experimentation can be suggested. Studies on castrates given systemic hormone replacement therapy or hormone implantation directly into brain areas known to have steroid-concentrating cells would likely provide important information (see Chapter 4). Other necessary steps in defining basic mechanisms of behavioral control of reproductive development and physiology include detection of changes in steroidogenic pathways in gonadal tissue under natural and hormone-induced sex reversal and measurement of circulating sex steroids in male, female, and sex-reversing animals (such as have been carried out in other species, see Chan and Yeung, 1983).

EGG TRADERS

With few exceptions, simultaneous hermaphrodites belong to a single subfamily of sea basses (Serraninae). These are small (usually only 3–4 inches) fish that typically inhabit coral reefs or rocky coastal areas in the Mediterranean, Pacific, and Atlantic oceans. Two genera, *Serranus* and *Hypoplectrus*, include all of the species studied in detail. The former is widespread and the latter more localized to Atlantic tropical reef environments.

These sea bass have functional ovotestis and, during a daily spawning period, will form pairs or sometimes larger mating groups. Each individual will perform as both male and female, reversing its sex role with its partner several times until the eggs of both have been shed. This reciprocal parcellation of small units of eggs has been termed *Egg Trading* (Fischer, 1980). Fischer provides convincing evidence that Egg Trading stabilizes simultaneous hermaphroditism by preventing cheating or nonreciprocation from the partner in the male phase.

Hermaphroditic sea bass expend more reproductive effort in female functions (Fischer, 1980). For example, courtship displays emphasize the swollen abdomen of individuals with ovulated eggs, and the more gravid individual initiates spawning. Similarly, in terms of bioenergetic cost, more energy is invested in the female part of the gonad. This is predicted from theoretical models (Fischer, 1981), which also suggest how the simultaneous hermaphroditism can exist as an *evolutionarily stable strategy* (*ESS*). As defined by Parker (1984), "a strategy is simply one of a series of alternative courses of action" and it "is an ESS, if when adopted by most members of a population, it cannot be invaded by the spread of any rare alternative strategy."

Not all of the serranines trade eggs. In those species where stable pair bonds and pair-defended territoriality have evolved, such as in the harlequin

TABLE 1.1 Mating-system characteristics of several species of simultaneously hermaphroditic serranids (modified after Fischer, 1984). See text for additional details.

Species	Egg Trading	Spawning Displays	Conspicuous Egg Patch	Pair Shares Territory	Streaking
Hypoplectrus nigricans	yes	yes	no	no	no
Serranus baldwini	no	yes	no	yes	low
S. scriba	yes	yes	yes	no	yes
S. subligarius	yes	yes	yes	no*	low*
S. tigrinus	no	yes	yes	yes	low
S. tortugarium	yes	no	no	no	high

*Demski and Dulka, 1983 and unpublished observations.

bass (*S. tigrinus*), individuals of a pair only mate once each day as each sex (Pressley, 1981); that is, they perform once as a male and once as a female. In the barred serrano (*S. fasciatus*), large males guard territories with up to eight smaller hermaphrodites and mate with each of them individually while the latter are in the female phase (Petersen, 1983). These species appear to be exceptions to the basic pattern found in serranines and represent alternative reproductive strategies that may lead in the direction of gonochorism and protogyny, respectively.

Within the *Serranus* species, there is also sperm competition from individuals that join a pair at the point of spawning climax or *Snap*. These fish are called *streakers* and are individuals in the male phase that move in and release sperm, attempting to fertilize the eggs as they are released. Streakers can succeed by coordinating their behavior with visual signals mostly from the female-phase partner. The pair will attempt to prevent streaking by chasing away nearby unpaired fish. Fischer (1984) indicates that species with high rates of streaking tend to have more subtle signals concerning the readiness of the female to Snap (see Table 1.1). Also, the speed of the spawning response appears to be directly proportional to the likelihood of interference by streakers. Thus the elaborateness of the sexual communication system can be predicted based on distribution patterns (streaking is greatest in closely aggregated species).

In summary, the serranine fishes provide the richest source among vertebrates for study of simultaneous hermaphroditism. Although interesting variations exist, the Egg Trading strategy seems to be basic to maintenance of these patterns. The following is a brief account of some possible endocrine and neurobehavioral mechanisms that underlie the reproductive development and behavior of certain Egg Trading species.

Gonadal morphology has been described in many sea bass including both simultaneous and successive (protogynous) hermaphrodites (see Smith, 1965; Hastings and Bortone, 1980; Chan and Yeung, 1983). In the serranines, the testicular tissue is separate from the ovarian tissue, with the minor exception of occasional oocytes in the testicular portion. The testis forms either a narrow band on the ventral and lateral aspects of the ovary in *S. tigrinus* (Figure 1.5) or a broader flattened band that encircles the posterior aspect of the gonad as in *S. subligarius* (Hastings and Bortone, 1980). Each tissue also has its own duct system (sperm duct and oviduct). This anatomical separation leaves little possibility of internal fertilization as occurs in certain killifish (see later section). Behavioral observations of spawning in laboratory aquaria (Clark, 1959; 1965) and the results of brain-stimulation experiments suggest that egg and sperm release are controlled independently, thus preventing accidental self-fertilization during pair-spawning.

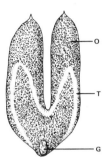

Figure 1.5. Drawing of the ventral aspect of the gonad of *Serranus tigrinus*. Note that the testicular tissue (T) forms a continuous band on the underside of the ovarian tissue (O), fusing anteriorly to form a loop on either side. The two types of tissue have separate openings in the region of the genital mound or papilla (G). (Redrawn after Smith, 1965; courtesy of American Museum of Natural History)

I have been studying the psychobiology of *Serranus subligarius* with several students, both in the field (Panama City, Florida) and in the laboratory. Our aim is a better understanding of how brain mechanisms control the alternation of sex roles during spawning. We have concentrated on the color patterns associated with the release of different gametes. These responses were chosen because they have distinct relationships to the sexual roles and have control mechanisms that are amenable to neurophysiological study (Bauer and Demski, 1980; Demski, 1983).

In field studies we use an underwater video system which permits recording of the sexual behavior for later analysis. We have taped 52 spawnings in 29 pairs and are now analyzing these tapes with particular emphasis on the possible role of color patterns as signals between the partners. This information provides essential baseline data against which we will compare animals in our brain-stimulation experiments. Of the six different color patterns recorded, five relate to the female role. When a fish is obviously bloated with eggs, it accentuates a white abdominal marking which Fischer (1984) calls an *Egg Patch*. It also exhibits a color pattern which we call *Dark Posterior* (*DP*) in which the caudal part of the fish is almost black (Figure 1.6B). The fish perform courtship by swimming in a confined area and *S-curving* (Figure 1.6B) with the belly directed at the nose of the other fish. Presumably this advertises the presence of eggs. Other behaviors include a *Tail-up* posture and a jerky *Half Turn* with a flip. After numerous exchanges of these displays, one of the fish begins to *Follow* and discontinues the other responses. The latter individual also begins to change color pattern to a barred or *Banded* phase (*Bd*) which is characteristic of the male role. Bands are most intense on the posterior part of the fish but also extend to the head. The more rostral ones typically have light interspaces (Figure 1.6C). Both the DP and Bd patterns include a dark spot on the dorsal fin at about its mid-rostrocaudal position.

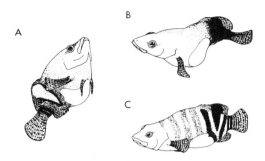

Figure 1.6. Color patterns typical of the male and female roles of the sea bass, *Serranus subligarius*. (A) The Head-Up posture with Reverse Banding is given by the female-phase animal just before shooting toward the surface to spawn or Snap. It is thought to serve as a signal to the male-phase fish to follow. The pattern of bands on the fish's posterior is the inverse or complement of those seen in the male-phase. (B) The Dark Posterior color pattern is shown on a female-phase fish performing the S-curve response. The white Egg Patch on the abdomen is emphasized by the posture which is characteristic of courtship activity. As the intensity of the behavior increases, the dark spot on the dorsal fin will begin to fade. (C) A male-phase animal has a Banding coloration characterized by vertical bars on the body from head to caudal fin. The anterior stripes are lighter with distinct white intraband markings while the posterior ones are very dark and solid throughout. The dorsal fin spot is continuous ventrally with a V-shaped marking and forms an ice-cream-cone-shaped structure. The area is white in the Reverse V in A. The drawings were made from videotapes. (Demski, Dulka and Hornby, unpublished observations)

As courtship proceeds, the individual performing the female role swims rapidly and circles the spawning area, giving S-curves. This fish then thrusts its belly at the other fish, which begins using its nose to *Nudge* (See figure on p. 1) at the ventral area of the displayed abdomen. As the intensity of this activity increases, the individual assuming the male role becomes maximally banded and the fish performing as the female begins to show a clear fading of the dorsal fin spot. As spawning climax nears, the fading increases ventrally into the dark area of the body wall. The animal in the female role then suddenly stops and takes a *Head-up* posture, *Quivers*, and demonstrates a *Reverse V* (RV) color pattern which forms an ice-cream-cone-like figure on the side of the fish. In addition to a continued fading of the ventrum, there is a relative darkening of the normal light spaces between the dark posterior bars in the Bd pattern (Figure 1.6A). In other words, the RV is a partial reverse image of Bd (cf. Figure 1.6A and C). The pair usually then shoot toward the surface and quickly release gametes, with the fish shedding eggs curved in front of the nose of the animal releasing sperm in a behavior termed the *Snap* (See figure on p. 1). The RV is only displayed for several seconds. Following the Snap, the pair typically sit on the bottom for a few minutes and then begin courtship again, usually with roles and color patterns reversed. Thus, *S. subligarius* has an elaborate set of visual signals which synchronize reproductive behavior of the pair. These include complex color patterns generated by neurally controlled chromatophores.

In some cases, streakers joined the pair in the Snap. Their speed precludes analysis of color pattern but presumably they are attempting to release sperm (see discussion in Fischer, 1984). It appears as if the streakers are keying on the Head-up posture and RV. The fact that streaking is infrequent is probably due to relatively distant spacing of individuals (usually at least several feet) and frequent low visibility in the area.

Experiments to distinguish neural mechanisms underlying the control of the color patterns and other aspects of sex behavior in this species are underway (Demski et al., 1984; Demski and Dulka, 1986). Pathways for color changes and sperm release had been identified in studies on freshwater fishes (see Demski, 1983, for details). Therefore, it seemed likely that the analogous systems might be similarly localized in sea bass. The brain of *S. subligarius* was mapped for sites from which the three main sex-related color patterns and/or gamete release could be evoked by electrical stimulation in fish anesthetized in 2% urethane and held in a surgical apparatus. A small container of seawater is placed under the fish for monitoring gamete discharge. The animals are maintained with seawater perfusing their gills. Electrodes made of insect pins are lowered into the brain while small electrical currents are passed (10–150 μA). If a color change and/or sperm or egg release is evoked, the site is marked with a stain (Prussian blue) for later histological identification. All sessions were videotaped so that color patterns could be correlated with the electrophysiological studies.

Color responses have been evoked from 15 brain sites identified in 10 of the animals (Figure 1.7). The Bd pattern characteristic of the male phase was evoked most frequently. The typical response was a change from a slight banding before to an intense pattern during stimulation. Following the stimulation, the fish would return to its prestimulation condition in several minutes. The slow recovery is mainly due to chromatophores, which aggregate or disperse pigment granules in response to nerve activity. The typical DP or pattern characteristic of the female role was observed in only a few animals. In order to obtain the response at all, we had to either test fish in the field within several hours of ovulation or, for fish that had been in the laboratory, give intracranial injections of prostaglandins, hormones associated with ovulation (see Chapter 2). These procedures are necessary because the response appears to be dependent on ovulation, and animals in the laboratory for periods longer than about 2–3 days stop ovulating and show male coloration (Clark, 1969; Demski and Dulka, unpublished observations). The RV, typical of the female role in spawning, was most often observed as an after-response at the termination of the stimulation, sometimes in cases where either Bd or DP was triggered during the test. The RV pattern occurred only infrequently during stimulation.

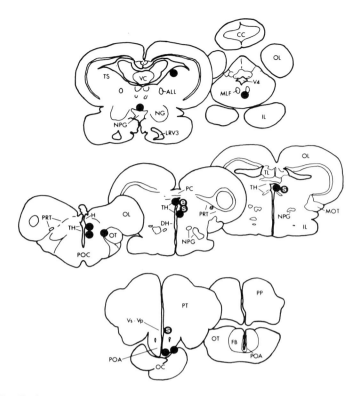

Figure 1.7. Brain sites from which electrical stimulation in lightly anesthetized sea bass, *Serranus subligarius*, evoked sex-color patterns with gamete discharge (solid dots with *s* for sperm and *e* for eggs) or without the latter response (unlabeled solid dots). Points are plotted on representative transverse sections starting at the level of the optic chiasma (bottom left) and running to the rostral medulla (top right). Stimulation areas from both sides of the brain are indicated together on the right side. See text for a description of the responses. Abbreviations: ALL, acoustico-lateral lemniscus; CC, corpus or body of the cerebellum; DH, dorsal hypothalamus; FB, forebrain bundles; H, habenula; IL, inferior lobe of the hypothalamus; LRV3, lateral recess of the third ventricle; MLF, medial longitudinal fasciculus; MOT, marginal optic tract; NG, nucleus glomerulosus; NPG, nucleus preglomerulosus; OC, optic chiasma; OL, optic lobe; OT, optic tract; PC, posterior commissure; POA, preoptic area; POC, postoptic commissures; PP, posterior pole of the telencephalon; PRT, pretectal area; PT, posterior telencephalon; TH, thalamus; TL, torus longitudinalis; TS, torus semicircularis; VC, valvula of the cerebellum; Vs, area telencephali ventralis, pars supracommissuralis; Vp, area telencephali ventralis, pars posterioris; V4, fourth ventricle.

Gamete discharge was elicited from four of the points positive for color change (Figure 1.7). Sperm release was evoked by stimulation of three points with thresholds of 20, 50, and 50 μA, and egg discharge occurred during testing of one site (80–100 μA) in a recently ovulated fish. Many eggs were found in the water following stimulation; however, the animal gave strong swimming movements in response to the stimulation and we could not directly observe their release. It is possible that they were discharged by the rapid body movement rather than through natural mechanisms used in spawning. This seems unlikely, because normal ovulated fish can be handled and swim rapidly without loss of eggs, and it takes considerable pressure to strip them from the fish. In addition, the stimulation in this case also evoked the DP color pattern, which suggests that pathways involved in the female reproduction were activated.

Darkening (a response similar to the female DP color phase) and the RV were elicited from sites in the ventral forebrain, more specifically the preoptic area (POA) and the area ventralis telencephali pars supracommissuralis (Vs), a probable homolog of part of the amygdaloid nucleus of tetrapod vertebrates (Northcutt and Davis, 1983). Sperm release was also evoked from the Vs, while Bd resulted from stimulation in the POA (see bottom row of sections in Figure 1.7). Both of the regions have cells that concentrate sex-steroid hormones and contain either GnRH-containing cells and/or fibers in other fishes (see references below). Furthermore, lesion and brain-stimulation experiments with freshwater teleosts have implicated these areas in the control of sexual behavior (Demski, 1983, 1984). There is also evidence that the POA may be involved in triggering sexual behavior in response to pheromones, at least in goldfish (Demski, 1984; see Chapter 2). In this regard, it is interesting that *S. subligarius* seem to be attracted when sperm is manually expressed from individuals in the male phase (Demski, unpublished observations). The stimulation data indicate that forebrain areas controlling sexual responses in simultaneous hermaphrodites are basically similar to those of gonochores.

All three color patterns as well as sperm and egg release were elicited from the thalamus, which is the major part of the dorsal diencephalon (see middle sections in Figure 1.7). In teleosts, this region receives a strong input from visual areas including the retina and optic lobes or midbrain tectum (see Braford and Northcutt, 1983). The visual connections are consistent with thalamic control of color patterns which serve as visual signals and appear to change in response to visual cues from a partner. Hormonal modulation of thalamic activity is also suggested by the identification of sex steroid-concentrating nerve cells in the area in several species (see review by Demski and Hornby, 1982). In addition, GnRH-containing neurons have been located in the thalamus of sticklebacks (Borg et al., 1982), a species with well-known visually and hormonally controlled male and female color patterns (Hoar, 1962). Nerve axons containing the neuropeptide have also been observed in the area in sticklebacks (Borg et al., 1982) as well as other teleosts (Münz et al., 1981). Thus, the same steroids and peptide hormones implicated in the control of sexual behavior in a wide variety of vertebrates (see Demski, 1984, and chapters in this volume) have representation in the teleost thalamus. Presumably they regulate the responsiveness of the thalamus and, through this, the reaction of the fish to various socially related visual signals (Figure 1.8).

Neurophysiological studies are needed to further determine thalamic involvement in the sexual behavior of *S. subligarius*. Recording from single nerve cells that respond to specific aspects of the color patterns would be

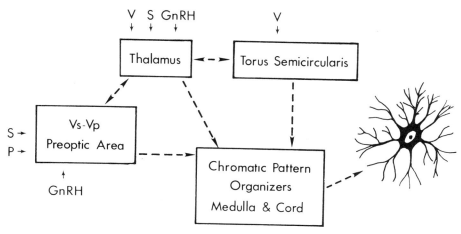

Figure 1.8. Tentative model of pathways involved in color-pattern control in *Serranus subligarius*. The model stresses the complex interaction of sex hormones and sensory inputs working at different levels in the CNS in determining the color pattern during different sexual roles. Brain areas from which color responses can be evoked by electrical stimulation are indicated, and hypothetical interconnections between these areas and suggested pathways to the lower chromatophore-motor systems are represented by the dashed lines. Presumed sensory and hormonal modulation of the color-control system(s) is indicated by the abbreviations and small arrows. See text for additional details. Abbreviations: GnRH, gonadotropin-releasing hormone; P, prostaglandins; S, sex-steroid hormones (i.e., androgens or estrogens); V, visual input; Vs-Vp, the supracommissural and posterior parts of the area ventralis telencephali.

especially significant for beginning to construct the neuronal circuitry mediating the change in sex roles. Modulation of the responsiveness of such units by hormonal manipulation should also provide important information concerning the role of sex hormones in sensorimotor integration. Brain-behavioral studies are called for to test specific hypotheses (e.g., bilateral thalamic lesions will interfere with intrapair communication during courtship and spawning).

The other positive sites associated with Bd have a distribution consistent with pathways for vertical banding in sunfish, which is an agonistic or defensive response (Bauer and Demski, 1980). Electrodes eliciting the Bd pattern in *S. subligarius* were located in the torus semicircularis of the midbrain and central areas of the midbrain and medulla (see top row of sections in Figure 1.7). In this regard, the regions stimulated probably identify the motor pathway controlling the bands rather than centers performing complex integration of sensory and hormonal information (Figure 1.8).

Our results support the idea that sea bass can release each gamete independently. Most notably, sperm and eggs were not released together in the one ovulated fish that was stimulated. This is somewhat analogous to findings in male goldfish, where there are separate neural pathways for testis and spermduct contractions (Dulka and Demski, 1986). It would not be surprising to find that hermaphrodites have independent neural control of the oviducts and spermducts.

SELF-FERTILIZING HERMAPHRODITES

Self-fertilization is a rare phenomenon among vertebrates, occurring in a few simultaneous hermaphrodites. Among fishes, it has only been well documented as a natural reproductive pattern in *Rivulus marmoratus*, a small killifish (Harrington, 1961, 1975). This animal occurs in southern Florida, Cuba, the Bahamas, and Netherlands Antilles and is generally neotropical in its distribution. Descendants of fish caught in the wild have been maintained for numerous generations in the laboratory, where they reproduce readily. Eggs are fertilized internally and retained within the parent for periods ranging from one hour (single-cell stage) to as long as 2.5 days (stage of pectoral fin development). The fish deposits the eggs and continues the incubation externally for two weeks or longer.

Three clones of homozygous, isogenetic individuals have been developed from three individual animals. Under laboratory conditions of moderate temperatures (26 ± 1°C), all of the offspring develop into hermaphrodites with functional ovotestis. If fertilized eggs are exposed to temperatures at or below 19 ± 0.08°C during a critical period of development (between the stage of neural and hemal arch formation and hatching), approximately two-thirds will become *primary* males instead of hermaphrodites. A primary male will never develop ovarian tissue and is readily distinguished from the hermaphrodite by its color pattern. Hermaphrodites have a caudal eye spot or ocellus and have prominent body markings with barred fins, while primary males lack these features and are uniformly bright orange with a black margin on the caudal fin. This period of temperature sensitivity may represent a normal mechanism through which external influences produce males that can mate with hermaphrodites and thus reduce the occurrences of homozygous clones. This in fact appears to be the case in the Antilles, where primary males are common. On the other hand, in Florida only one primary male has been found, presumably because temperatures remain high during the breeding period.

A third phenotype has been created in the laboratory. If hermaphrodites are exposed to high temperatures early in life, some will develop into males at first sexual maturity, while shortening the day length can induce the response in others as adults. Males created by these methods are called *secondary* males as opposed to the primary males (also see discussion above of sequential sex-changers). The secondary males can be easily distinguished histologically by virtue of their vestigial oviducts. They have a distinctive color pattern that seems intermediate to those of the hermaphrodite and the primary male. Secondary males lack the ocellus but retain the body markings and barred fins present in juveniles and hermaphrodites while acquiring orange spots and an orange background pigmentation. The latter is presumably related to orange coloration of the primary male and may be under similar hormonal control. Secondary males have not been found in the wild.

Unfortunately, little is known of the behavior of these sexual phenotypes except that the hermaphrodites perform the S-curving typically associated with spawning in cyprinodonts. Presumably the color patterns associated with the different phenotypes are, or at least were in the past, important for sexual identification. Descriptions of the mating of primary and secondary males with hermaphrodites are lacking. If indeed this occurs, there must be some mechanism by which hermaphrodites can stop sperm release and thus discharge at least some unfertilized eggs. The control system would probably require stimuli from the male to inhibit the sperm release or production via either hormonal and/or neural pathways. It may be possible to test this idea by pairing males created in the laboratory with hermaphrodites available from the clones.

What lessons can we expect to learn from this unique fish? The killifish demonstrate dramatic reproductive adaptations to environmental factors. The natural self-fertilization of the hermaphrodite is most likely a response to conditions of alternate dryness and flooding. The resulting short mating seasons undoubtedly make production of offspring without the necessity of finding a mate advantageous. The occasional development of males under conditions of temperature extremes or perhaps other environmental influences may be a means to somewhat limit the inbreeding process. In this regard, the laboratory results suggest that secondary males may also be present in the wild, although they have yet to be found. The studies have demonstrated that *R. marmoratus* has at least the capability under certain conditions to produce sexual phenotypes similar to non-self-fertilizing hermaphrodites.

CONCLUSIONS

Functional hermaphroditism is a normal mode of reproduction in teleost fishes and is common in certain families. Hermaphroditism, in one form or the other, offers the reproductive biologist unique opportunities to study interactions between male and female systems in the same fish, either simultaneously or through successive developmental stages. Examples discussed in this chapter cover a broad range of representative types.

Acquired hermaphroditism occurs in deep-sea anglerfish in which males become parasites attached to females, which appear to gain control of their testis. The fish demonstrate extreme sexual dimorphism, perhaps the greatest among all vertebrates. Sequential sex change is common in wrasses and sea bass. In the former, the most complex systems have two types of males (diandry) and two different color phases. Sex-changed females (secondary males) are produced in response to the particular needs of their social group. Absence of a male and the presence of a smaller fish are the critical cues that trigger sex reversal in female wrasses of the genus *Thalassama*. In the sea bass *Anthias squamipinnis*, changes in complex behavioral interactions within a social group following removal of its male rapidly result in male-typical behavior in the largest female. Later she develops a male color pattern and functional testes.

Most simultaneous hermaphrodites are sea bass in the subfamily Serraninae. Individuals have functional ovotestes and typically occur in pairs that mate several times in succession with alternate reversals of sex role. The behavior is called Egg Trading and presumably helps to prevent male cheating. Some of the species have developed elaborate visual signals for sex-role identification. The ultimate in hermaphroditism is a small self-fertilizing killifish. This species normally produces homozygous, isogenetic clones. Males can develop under specific environmental conditions, and pairing of males and hermaphrodites may serve to limit the genetic uniformity.

Few experimental studies have been carried out with the aim of identifying the neurological and endocrine substrates underlying reproductive behavior in hermaphroditic fishes. Anatomical observations of deep-sea anglers are consistent with the hypothesis that the female controls the male's testes through hormones circulated in a common vascular system. This control may entail secretion of GnRH by the female, with subsequent release of gonadotropins by either one or both of the animals. Sperm and egg release may be synchronized by female hormones and/or male detection of cues from the female. In sequential sex-changers, testosterone administration can trigger sex-color, behavior, and gonadal reversal in female wrasses. Androgens can also initiate sex change in the protogynous sea bass *A. squamipinnis*, while estrogens appear to at least temporarily inhibit the response.

Considerable information is available on gonadal development and function in Egg Trading sea bass, but little is known of their psychobiology. We have identified several areas of the brain from which sex-color changes and/or gamete release can be evoked by artificial electrical stimulation. Telencephalic regions include the area ventralis telencephali pars supracommissuralis (a homolog of the amygdala of tetrapods) and the preoptic area. These are regions which control sexual development and behavior in gonochores and are thought to be substrates for sex-steroid and perhaps GnRH modulation of the activities. In the diencephalon, stimulation of the thalamus resulted in sex-color change and both sperm and egg release. The area may regulate sexual activity in response to visual signals and circulating levels of sex steroids and GnRH. Neurophysiological studies are needed to further test these hypotheses.

Unfortunately, almost nothing is known concerning the mechanisms of behavior in the self-fertilizing killifish. Determination of how normal internal fertilization is regulated and possibly suspended if and when hermaphrodites mate with males could provide insight into gamete control systems in general.

The systems outlined demonstrate some of the variation in reproductive patterns in the vertebrates. In this regard, fishes, like reptiles (see Chapter 4), are ideal subjects for comparative reproductive studies. For teleosts, the work of describing and understanding the patterns has only begun, with most of the 20–30 thousand species yet to be observed. Surely there are some great surprises remaining to be discovered.

ACKNOWLEDGMENTS

Financial support for the author's work has been provided by NIH grant NS19431, BioMedical Research Support Funds, and a grant from the University of Kentucky Research Foundation. Use of facilities at Gulf Coast Research Laboratory and St. Andrews State Park, Florida, is greatly appreciated. The assistance of Mary Demski, Joseph Dulka, and Pamela Hornby has been invaluable in carrying out studies on sea bass. I also wish to thank David Crews for providing many insightful suggestions and helpful editorial advising.

REFERENCES

BAUER, D.H., and L.S. DEMSKI (1980) Vertical banding evoked by electrical stimulation of the brain in anesthetized green sunfish, *Lepomis cyanellus*, and bluegills, *Lepomis macrochirus*. J. Exp. Biol. *84*:149–160.

BORG, B., H.J.TH. GOOS, and M. TERLOU (1982) LHRH-immunoreactive cells in the brain of the three-spined stickleback, *Gasterosteus aculeatus* L. (Gasterosteidae). Cell Tissue Res. *226*:695–699.

BRAFORD, M.R., JR., and R.G. NORTHCUTT (1983) Organization of the diencephalon and pretectum of the ray-finned fishes. In *Fish Neurobiology*, Vol. 2. R.E. Davis and R.G. Northcutt, eds., pp. 117–163, Univ. of Michigan Press, Ann Arbor.

BRAIN, P.F., and D. BENTON (1983) Conditions of housing, hormones, and aggressive behavior. In *Hormones And Aggressive Behavior*. B.B. Svare, ed., pp. 351–372, Plenum Press, New York.

CHAN, S.T.H., and W.S.B. YEUNG (1983) Sex control and sex reversal in fish under natural conditions. In *Fish Physiology*, Vol. IX. W.S. Hoar, D.J. Randall, and E.M. Donaldson, eds., pp. 171–222, Academic Press, New York.

CHARNOV, E.L., J.M. SMITH, and J.J. BULL (1976) Why be an hermaphrodite? Nature *263*:125–126.

CLARK, E. (1959) Functional hermaphroditism and self-fertilization in a serranid fish. Science *129*:215–216.

CLARK, E. (1965) Mating of groupers. Natural History *74*:22–26.

CLARK, E. (1969) *The Lady And The Sharks*. pp. 57–71, Harper and Row, New York.

DEMSKI, L.S. (1983) Behavioral effects of electrical stimulation of the brain. In *Fish Neurobiology*, Vol. 2. R.E. Davis and R.G. Northcutt, eds., pp. 317–359, Univ. of Michigan Press, Ann Arbor.

DEMSKI, L.S. (1984) The evolution of neuroanatomical substrates of reproductive behavior: Sex steroid and LHRH-specific pathways including the terminal nerve. Amer. Zool. *24*:809–830.

DEMSKI, L.S., and J.G. DULKA (1983) Underwater observations on color patterns and spawning in a synchronous hermaphroditic sea bass. Amer. Zool. *23*:881.

DEMSKI, L.S., and J.G. DULKA (1984) Functional-anatomical studies on sperm release evoked by electrical stimulation of the olfactory tract in goldfish. Brain Res. *291*:241–247.

DEMSKI, L.S., and J.G. DULKA (1986) Thalamic stimulation evokes sex-color change and gamete release in a vertebrate hermaphrodite. Experientia (in press).

DEMSKI, L.S., J.G. DULKA, and P.J. HORNBY (1984) Sex-color changes evoked by brain stimulation in fishes. Society for Neuroscience, Abstract 122.10-404.

DEMSKI, L.S., and P.J. HORNBY (1982) Hormonal control of fish reproductive behavior: Brain-gonadal steroid interactions. Can. J. Fish. Aquat. Sci. *39*:36–47.

DEMSKI, L.S., and H.E. SLOAN (1985) A direct magnocellular-preopticospinal pathway in goldfish: Implications for control of sex behavior. Neurosci. Lett. *55*:283–288.

DULKA, J.G., and L.S. DEMSKI (1986) Sperm duct contractions mediate centrally evoked sperm release in goldfish. J. Exp. Zool. *237*:271–279.

FISCHER, E.A. (1980) The relationship between mating system and simultaneous hermaphroditism in the coral reef fish, *Hypoplectrus nigricans* (Serranidae). Anim. Behav. *28*:620–633.

FISCHER, E.A. (1981) Sexual allocation in a simultaneously hermaphroditic coral reef fish. Amer. Nat. *117*:64–82.

FISCHER, E.A. (1984) Egg trading in the chalk bass, *Serranus tortugarum*, a simultaneous hermaphrodite. Z. Tierpsychol. *66*:143–151.

FISHELSON, L. (1970) Protogynous sex reversal in the fish *Anthias squamipinnis* (Teleostei, Anthiidae) regulated by the presence or absence of a male fish. Nature *227*:90–91.

FISHELSON, L. (1975) Ecology and physiology of sex reversal in *Anthias squamipinnis* (Peters), (Teleostei, Anthiidae). In *Intersexuality In The Animal Kingdom*. R. Reinboth, ed., pp. 284–294, Springer-Verlag, New York.

HARRINGTON, R.W., JR. (1961) Oviparous hermaphroditic fish with internal self-fertilization. Science *134*:1749–1750.

HARRINGTON, R.W., JR. (1975) Sex determination and differentiation among uniparental homozygotes of the hermaphroditic fish *Rivulus marmoratus* (Cyprinodontidae: Atheriniformes). In *Intersexuality In The Animal Kingdom*. R. Reinboth, ed., pp. 249–262, Springer-Verlag, New York.

HASTINGS, P.A., and S.A. BORTONE (1980) Observations on the life history of the belted sandfish, *Serranus subligarius* (Serranidae). Env. Biol. Fish. *5*:365–374.

HOAR, W.S. (1962) Reproductive behavior of fish. Gen. Comp. Endocrinol., *Suppl. 1*:206–216.

MARSHALL, N.B. (1984) Progenetic tendencies in deep-sea fishes. In *Fish Reproduction: Strategies and Tactics*. G.W. Potts and R.J. Wootton, eds., pp. 91–101, Academic Press, New York.

Münz, H., W.E. Stumpf, and L. Jennes (1981) LHRH systems in the brain of platyfish. Brain Res. *221*:1–13.

Northcutt, R.G., and R.E. Davis (1983) Telencephalic organization in ray-finned fishes. In *Fish Neurobiology*, Vol. 2. R.E. Davis and R.G. Northcutt, eds., pp. 203–236, Univ. of Michigan Press, Ann Arbor.

Parker, G.A. (1984) Evolutionarily stable strategies. In *Behavioural Ecology: An Evolutionary Approach*. J.R. Krebs and N.B. Davies, eds., pp. 30–61, Sinauer Assoc., Sunderland, Mass.

Petersen, C.W. (1983) Reproductive strategies in a simultaneously hermaphroditic reef fish, *Serranus fasciatus*. Amer. Zool. *23*:880.

Pietsch, T.W. (1976) Dimorphism, parasitism and sex: Reproductive strategies among deepsea ceratioid anglerfishes. Copeia *1976*:781–793.

Pressley, P.H. (1981) Pair formation and joint territoriality in a simultaneous hermaphrodite: The coral reef fish *Serranus tigrinus*. Z. Tierpsychol. *56*:33–46.

Regan, C.T., and E. Trewavas (1932) Deep-sea angler-fishes (Ceratioidea). Dana Rep. 2, pp. 1–122.

Reinboth, R. (1975) Spontaneous and hormone-induced sex-inversion in wrasses (Labridae). Pubbl. Staz. Zool. Napoli *39 Suppl*:550–573.

Robertson, D.R. (1972) Social control of sex reversal in a coral-reef fish. Science *177*:1007–1009.

Ross, R.M., G.S. Losey, and M. Diamond. (1983) Sex change in a coral-reef fish: Dependence of stimulation and inhibition on relative size. Science *221*:574–575.

Shapiro, D.Y. (1980) Serial female sex changes after simultaneous removal of males from social groups of a coral reef fish. Science *209*:1136–1137.

Shapiro, D.Y. (1981a) Behavioural changes of protogynous sex reversal in a coral reef fish in the laboratory. Anim. Behav. *29*:1185–1198.

Shapiro, D.Y. (1981b) Intragroup behavioural changes and the initiation of sex reversal in a coral reef fish in the laboratory. Anim. Behav. *29*:1199–1212.

Shapiro, D.Y. (1983) Distinguishing behavioral interactions from visual cues as causes of adult sex change in a coral reef fish. Horm. Behav. *17*:424–432.

Shapiro, D.Y., and R.H. Boulon, Jr. (1982) The influence of females on the initiation of female-to-male sex change in a coral reef fish. Horm. Behav. *16*:66–75.

Smith, C.L. (1965) The patterns of sexuality and the classification of serranid fishes. Amer. Mus. Novitates *2207*:1–20.

Stoll, L.M. (1955) Hormonal control of the sexually dimorphic pigmentation of *Thalassoma bifasciatum*. Zoologica *40*:125–135.

Thresher, R.E. (1984) *Reproduction In Reef Fishes*. T.F.H. Publications, Neptune City, NJ. 339 pp.

Warner, R.R. (1982) Mating systems, sex change and sexual demography in the rainbow wrasse, *Thalassoma lucasanum*. Copeia *1982*:653–661.

Warner, R.R. (1982) Mating behavior and hermaphroditism in coral reef fishes. Amer. Sci. *72*:128–136.

TWO
Roles of Hormones and Pheromones in Fish Reproductive Behavior

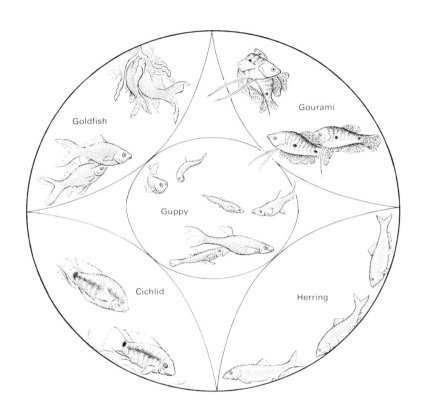

Goldfish

Gourami

Guppy

Cichlid

Herring

N. E. Stacey
Department of Zoology
The University of Alberta
Edmonton, Alberta, Canada

Reproduction of any vertebrate species cannot succeed unless the sexual behaviors of the individual are exhibited at the correct time: i.e., correctly synchronized with its own gonadal development and with the activities of potential mates. Both within and between individuals, chemical signals play important roles in ensuring that the correct timing of sexual behavior *is* achieved. *Within* the individuals of many species (see Chapters 5, 6, 10, 11), hormones are released into the blood in amounts related to gonadal condition; they also function as a common internal chemical signal which stimulates sexual behaviors at the appropriate stage of gonadal development. Reproductive pheromones perform functions analogous to those of hormones but transmit chemical information *between* individuals to alter reproductive behavior or physiology.

The teleost fishes comprise a tremendously diverse range of species for those interested in exploring the roles of hormones and pheromones in controlling reproductive behavior in aquatic vertebrates. For the endocrinologist and physiologist are the challenges of identifying the hormones and pheromones produced, determining how their production is related to reproductive activity, and where they might act to induce behavioral change. For those whose focus is more behavioral, the teleosts present a range of behavioral repertoires. At one extreme are species whose sexual behaviors are restricted to a brief and evidently promiscuous shedding of the gametes, while at the other extreme are species that form pair bonds, prepare and defend a spawning site, and care for the young. Finally, from an evolutionary perspective, teleosts provide an instructive example of how a major change in reproductive strategy—the shift from external to internal fertilization—has been accompanied by an equally dramatic change in the regulation of female reproductive behavior. The roles of hormones and pheromones in fish reproductive behavior have recently been reviewed in detail (Liley and Stacey, 1983; Stacey et al., 1986). In this brief overview, I will emphasize several areas where investigations have been most fruitful and will suggest promising lines of future enquiry.

HORMONES AND FEMALE REPRODUCTIVE BEHAVIOR

In all vertebrate groups including the fish, there are species in which the sexual behaviors of the female are controlled by the gonadal steroid hormones. However, among the fish species so far examined, it is clear that the relative importance of steroid hormones in regulating female sex behavior is dependent on the mode of reproduction employed (Liley and

Stacey, 1983). That is, in a species which utilizes internal fertilization, ovarian estrogen plays a primary role in stimulating sexual behavior of the female. In marked contrast, female sexual behaviors of several externally fertilizing fishes are stimulated by prostaglandins.

The Guppy: An Internally Fertilizing Fish

Anyone who has had the opportunity to observe the persistent courtship behaviors and frequent mating attempts of male guppies (*Poecilia reticulata*) in a pet shop or home aquarium might easily conclude that sexual behavior in this species is essentially continuous. While for the male this may well be true, closer examination reveals that the female usually ignores or avoids the male's advances. When sexually receptive, however, the female responds with a series of stereotyped behaviors culminating in copulation. The female first *glides* slowly toward the male, *arches* her body briefly in the vertical plane, and then performs a *wheeling* behavior in which she swims in a tight circle. It is at this stage that the male, swimming below and beside the female, is able to insert his gonopodium—an intromittent organ formed from the modified anal fin—into the female's gonopore and deposit spermatophores.

Sexual receptivity in the female guppy is cyclical and is synchronized with the cycle of ovarian activity. The birth (parturition) of a brood is followed within several days by copulation. If fertilization is successful, a pregnancy results which lasts approximately three weeks, depending on the temperature of the water. Experiments involving removal of the ovary (ovariectomy) or the pituitary gland (hypophysectomy) and injection of exogenous steroid hormones strongly suggest that ovarian estrogen stimulates the onset of female receptivity in the early postpartum period (Liley and Stacey, 1983).

Before considering the evidence that estrogen stimulates receptivity in the female guppy, it is important to understand that the female's responsiveness to the male is not determined solely by endocrine activity, but also by recent sexual experience. This has been shown clearly in sexually naive virgin females which have never been exposed to male courtship (Liley and Wishlow, 1974).

When first courted by a male, these naive virgins are highly receptive, but rapidly become less receptive with repeated exposure to male courtship. This loss of sexual responsiveness is not due to any changes resulting from intromission or pregnancy, as intact and gonopodectomized males are equally effective in modifying the female's behavior. Neither is ovarian estrogen responsible either for the initially high levels of receptive behavior in virgins or for the decline in receptivity resulting from exposure to male courtship. Virgins ovariectomized almost a month before being placed with males are initially as responsive as intact females, and show a similar decline in receptivity in further sexual encounters (Figure 2.1). However, whereas intact females show a transient recovery of sexual responsiveness during

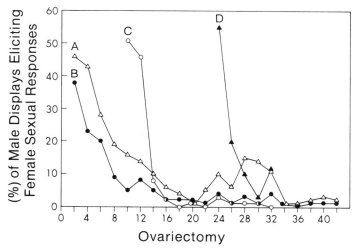

Figure 2.1. Initial receptivity of sexually naive, virgin female guppies (*Poecilia reticulata*) is not affected by ovariectomy. Groups of 10–12 females were placed with gonopodectomized males for 15 minutes on alternate days beginning either 2 days after a sham operation (Group A), or 2 days (Group B), 10 days (Group C), or 24 days (Group D) after ovariectomy. Receptivity was measured as the proportion of male courtship displays which evoked sexual responses (*glide, arch, wheel*) in the female. (Redrawn from Liley and Wishlow, 1974)

several weeks of repeated testing, ovariectomized females remain completely unresponsive.

There is good evidence that ovarian estrogen is responsible for the transient episodes of receptivity displayed by intact virgin females during repeated courtship sessions with gonopodectomized males. If ovariectomized females are injected with estradiol after becoming unresponsive to male courtship, their receptivity increases dramatically; ovariectomized females receiving control saline injections remain unresponsive.

These studies of the regulation of sexual behavior in the female guppy clearly demonstrate the stimulatory effect of estrogen and the inhibitory effect of sexual experience. However, as the experiments have used only virgin females, it remains to be shown that this interaction of endocrine and experiential factors functions to determine the timing and duration of sexual behavior in nonvirgin fish.

The Goldfish: An Externally Fertilizing Fish

Much of the evidence supporting a role for prostaglandins in regulating sexual behavior of female fish comes from studies of the goldfish (*Carassius auratus*) (Stacey and Goetz, 1982; Liley and Stacey, 1983). In this temperate species, ovarian growth begins during the winter months, with vitellogenesis (yolk formation) being completed by late spring. Ovulation (release of oocytes from the follicles into the ovarian cavity) and spawning are reported to occur when temperatures reach about 20°C. Laboratory studies have shown that the tendency of mature goldfish to ovulate is influenced by at least two factors—water temperature and aquatic vegetation. If females are held in aquaria without vegetation they never ovulate in cold water (12°C), while a small proportion may do so if the temperature is increased to 20°C. If vegetation is present, however, some females will ovulate at 12°C, although the proportion doing so increases dramatically at 20°C, often reaching 100 percent. There are good reasons why goldfish have evolved an ovulatory mechanism responsive to these two environmental cues. Vegetation is the preferred substrate on which to deposit the eggs, while increasing water temperature serves as a good predictor of increasing food supplies for the fry.

In nature, goldfish are group or gang spawners. This means that a number of males will compete vigorously for a position beside the female at the moment she oviposits. The energetic courtship activities of the males are a result of intrasexual competition for the female and are not required to trigger female spawning activity. Provided that a single male is present, the female commences spawning very soon after ovulation—likely within a matter of minutes, although this is difficult to determine precisely. The female initiates each spawning or oviposition act by leading the male(s) into aquatic vegetation. In floating vegetation, where observation is easiest, the pair first turn on their side, the male beneath and slightly behind the female, and then swim rapidly through a short arc, usually breaking the water surface. Some gametes are shed at this point and the eggs, which rapidly become adhesive on exposure to water, stick to the vegetation. After a few hours and as many as several hundred spawning acts, the supply of ovulated eggs is exhausted and spawning ceases. The female goldfish will not become sexually active again until the next ovulation. Depending on the developmental state of her remaining ovarian follicles, this can occur later in the spawning season or not until the following spring.

In their natural habitat, goldfish are reported to spawn in the early morning hours, a temporal pattern of behavior which is now known to be a direct result of the way in which ovulation is regulated (Stacey et al., 1979). For example, if mature female goldfish are placed in aquaria with aquatic vegetation on day 1 and the water temperature is increased to 20°C, many will ovulate on day 3 (Figure 2.2), even though they are handled one or more times to obtain blood samples. The time of ovulation for each female can easily be determined by *stripping*, in which gentle pressure is applied to the abdomen to release a stream of eggs from the ovipore. Clearly, ovulation is restricted to a small portion of the day—in this case the latter portion of the 8-hour dark phase—and is preceded by a dramatic surge in the blood of pituitary gonadotropin (GtH). This elevation in circulating GtH acts on the ovary to trigger a series of events culminating in follicular rupture (Goetz, 1983). The synchronization of ovulation with the daily photoperiod (Figure 2.2) is not simply due to the fact that all the females were placed in stimulatory conditions at the same time. Females which do not ovulate on day 3 may do so on day 4 or 5, but always in the latter half of the dark phase.

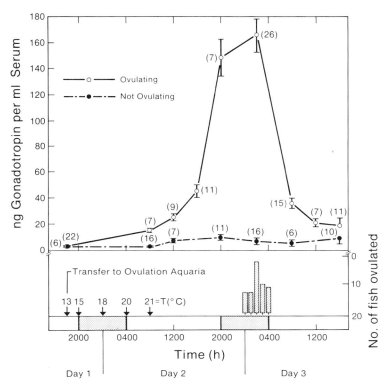

Figure 2.2. Spontaneous ovulation in goldfish (*Carassius auratus*) is synchronized by the daily photoperiod. Ovulation in mature goldfish was triggered by placing them in aquaria containing aquatic vegetation and increasing the water temperature. Females which ovulated in response to this treatment exhibited a dramatic preovulatory "surge" of blood gonadotropin. (Redrawn from Stacey et al., 1979, courtesy of Academic Press for Gen. Comp. Endocrinol)

Judging by the way ovulation is timed in the laboratory, it seems very likely that early morning spawning of wild goldfish is simply the result of nocturnal ovulation. Certainly there is no evidence that in the female goldfish sexual responsiveness per se varies throughout the day. Indeed, if mature females are injected with GtH, they spawn normally soon after ovulation regardless of when this occurs.

It makes sense that in externally fertilizing fish the females should become sexually active only when they have ovulated eggs to release. However, the possibility that there is a causal relationship between the presence of ovulated eggs and the onset of spawning activity apparently was not formally recognized until 1965, when Yamazaki found that spawning of goldfish could be prematurely terminated by stripping out the ovulated eggs, and suggested that ovulated eggs stimulated spawning "via some pathway" (see Liley and Stacey, 1983). A series of subsequent experiments have delineated this pathway.

If stripped eggs are injected through the ovipore and into the ovarian

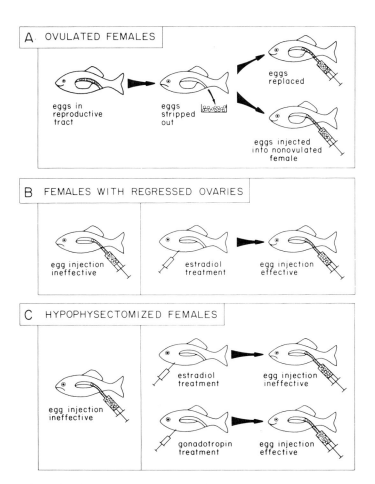

Figure 2.3. Spawning behavior in female goldfish (*Carassius auratus*) is stimulated by ovulated eggs in the reproductive tract. (A) Spawning behavior of ovulated females stops when the eggs are removed and resumes when eggs are replaced. Mature, nonovulated females also spawn in response to egg injection. (B) Females with regressed ovaries do not respond to egg injection unless they are pretreated with estradiol. (C) Spawning response of hypophysectomized females can be restored by gonadotropin treatment, but not by estradiol.

lumen, the female goldfish will quickly resume normal spawning behavior (Stacey and Liley, 1974) (Figure 2.3). More importantly, such an egg injection also will rapidly induce spawning behavior in females which have not recently ovulated. What these results imply is that while ovulation must normally precede spawning behavior, the physiological and endocrine events leading to ovulation are not required for spawning behavior. All that appears to be required to trigger spawning behavior in a mature, nonovulated female goldfish is the presence of ovulated eggs in the ovarian lumen or oviduct.

Perhaps not surprisingly, the mechanism coordinating sex behavior with ovulation in the goldfish turns out to be more complicated than the first egg-injection experiments might have suggested. First, it seems clear that the reproductive endocrine system is somehow involved in determining whether the female will respond to ovulated eggs. For example, if females are kept in warm water to promote ovarian regression—atresia and resorption of the yolky oocytes—they show very little spawning behavior when injected with eggs. However, if these females are injected with estradiol or other steroids before receiving eggs, their spawning responses improve significantly (Stacey and Liley, 1974; Stacey, 1977). Females also fail to respond to injected eggs after hypophysectomy, an operation which would drastically reduce endogenous sex steroid hormone production (Figure 2.3). However, if hypophysectomized females are injected with gonadotropin, thereby stimulating steroid hormone synthesis, their response to eggs is increased (Stacey, 1977). All these results would suggest that some action of estrogen is required in order for eggs to stimulate spawning behavior. The problem is that injections of estradiol or other sex steroid hormones are completely ineffective in restoring responsiveness to eggs in hypophysecto-mized fish; in contrast, estradiol does restore sexual behaviors of hypophysectomized female guppies (Liley and Stacey, 1983).

At present, all that can be concluded from these findings is that while there is evidence that activity of the pituitary-ovarian axis somehow primes responsiveness to ovulated eggs, nothing is really known of the hormone(s) responsible. A more important point to emerge from these studies is that, whatever the hormonal priming involved, it is not restricted to the few days when the female ovulates and is sexually active, but is exerted for a period of months outside the spawning season. This is strikingly different from that seen in females of many internally fertilizing terrestrial vertebrate species, where sexual activity is very closely linked to increased estrogen production at a discrete stage of the ovarian cycle.

Unlike the attempts to determine the nature of pituitary-ovarian involvement in the response to ovulated eggs, attempts to answer the more important question of how eggs stimulate behavior have been very rewarding. Theoretically, spawning behavior of female goldfish could be initiated in the postovulatory period either by a neural mechanism (i.e., through the action of ovulated eggs on mechanoreceptors or chemoreceptors in the ovarian lumen or oviduct) or by a hormonal mechanism (i.e., through release into the bloodstream of some ovarian or oviducal product). Although the former possibility has not yet been investigated, there is evidence that the latter mechanism exists and that prostaglandins (PGs) are the blood-borne factors involved.

Prostaglandins are involved in many reproductive functions of vertebrates including gonadotropin release, ovulation, and sexual behavior in the female (Behrman, 1979; Stacey and Goetz, 1982). Prostaglandins are not stored preformed, but are produced rapidly when required for a specific function and then rapidly metabolized. Precursors to PGs are stored as fatty acids (e.g., arachidonic acid) incorporated in the lipids of cell membranes. Stimuli as diverse as steroid hormones and mechanical agitation can release the fatty acid precursors, which then are quickly converted into a variety of compounds including the PGs. Generally, PGs are not regarded to function as classical blood-borne hormones but rather as local intra- and intercellular regulators. However, one of the well-known exceptions is the effect of uterine PGs in suppressing the function of corpora lutea in the ovaries of several mammalian species.

The widespread and volatile nature of PG synthesis presents problems for the study of PG function. In particular, it often is difficult to determine which of the many PGs is involved in a particular function. Further, it is difficult to determine when PGs are synthesized, since anesthesia, blood sampling, tissue extraction, and in vitro conditions all can affect both the rate of PG synthesis and the types of PG produced. A great boost to research on PGs has been provided by the fairly recent discovery that some nonsteroidal antiinflammatory drugs (e.g., aspirin, indomethacin) act primarily by inhibiting the enzymes which convert free fatty acid precursors to PGs. Use of these drugs in studying PG function is really analogous to the use of gonadectomy in studying sex-steroid hormone function, except that drugs remove the endogenous factor pharmacologically rather than surgically.

The first evidence that PGs mediate the effect of ovulated eggs on spawning behavior in goldfish was the finding that injection of the PG synthesis inhibitor, indomethacin, would block spawning behavior both in ovulated females and in nonovulated females which had been injected with ovulated eggs (Liley and Stacey, 1983). If PGs were then injected into the indomethacin-treated females, they resumed spawning behavior. Of the three PGs tested (PGE_1, PGE_2, and $PGF_{2\alpha}$), $PGF_{2\alpha}$ was the most effective. Importantly, ovulated eggs do not have to be present in the reproductive tract in order for PGs to exert their effect on sexual behavior. Simply injecting PGs into nonovulated and otherwise untreated females rapidly induces a period of sexual activity during which spawning behavior appears indistinguishable from that of ovulated fish, with the obvious exception that egg release does not occur.

Prostaglandins thus appear to play an indispensable role in the process whereby sexual behavior in the female goldfish is temporally synchronized with ovulation. However, before proceeding further with this story, it is important to appreciate the role of PGs in the normal chain of events leading to spawning. Spawning in the female goldfish is not the inevitable consequence of completed ovarian growth and development, but instead depends on the occurrence of ovulation, which in turn is stimulated by the photoperiodically synchronized gonadotropin surge. Viewed from this perspective, it is the neuroendocrine signal—triggered by temperature and vegetation cues and in turn triggering ovulatory gonadotropin release—which ultimately determines the time of spawning.

If we accept that the behavioral responses to injection of PG or indomethacin are indicative of a physiological role for PG in goldfish spawning, we might expect the temporal features of the behavioral response to PGs to be consistent with what is observed during natural spawning: that is, the rapid onset of spawning after ovulation and the rapid termination of spawning with depletion of the ovulated eggs. Indeed, the latency to respond to exogenous PG is very short, as spawning can begin within several *minutes* of injection. The termination of the spawning response is more difficult to interpret, as nothing is yet known about metabolism and clearance of injected PGs in fish. However, since duration of the responsive period increases with PG dosage, it would appear that PG metabolism is rapid; that is, responsiveness persists only as long as PG levels are sufficiently elevated. If true, the rapid termination of spawning normally observed when ovulated eggs are depleted could result from a reduction of PG synthesis combined with rapid metabolism of the PG already synthesized.

It could be hypothesized that the period of normal spawning behavior in ovulated females is terminated either by a decline in responsiveness to PGs, or by some inhibitory feedback effect of performing spawning behavior. There is no evidence for either mechanism. For example, if the responsiveness to PGs declines with duration of exposure to PGs, then the response to one injection should be greater than responses to subsequent injections; however, this is not the case (Figure 2.4; groups A and D). Also, engaging in spawning behavior does not appear to reduce further spawning activity, since spawning with a male in the first hour after PG injection does not affect the number of spawning acts performed in the second hour (Figure 2.4; groups A and B). In summary, the available evidence suggests that an ovulated goldfish stops spawning activity because PG synthesis falls when the supply of ovulated eggs is exhausted.

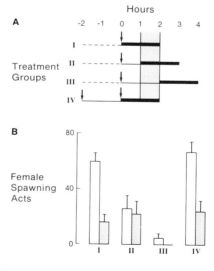

Figure 2.4. Effect of delay between prostaglandin $F_{2\alpha}$ (PGF$_{2\alpha}$) injection and behavioral testing, and of a second PGF$_{2a}$ injection on spawning behavior in female goldfish (*Carassius auratus*). (A) Arrows indicate times of PGF$_{2\alpha}$ injections (0.1 μg/g; intramuscular) and horizontal bars indicate time of the 2-hour behavioral test. (B) Female spawning acts performed during the 2-hour test (clear bars) or during the second hour (stippled bar) following the single (Groups A and B) or the second (Group D) PGF$_{2\alpha}$ injection. (Redrawn from Stacey and Goetz, 1982, courtesy of Canadian Journal of Fisheries and Aquatic Science)

The case for a role of PGs in spawning behavior of female goldfish is strengthened considerably by studies of changes in the circulating concentration of PGs at ovulation (Goetz, 1983). Although these experiments were designed to examine the relationship between PG levels and ovulation, their results lend support to the hypothesis that PG levels increase at the time when the female is sexually active. Female goldfish can be induced to ovulate by injections of human chorionic gonadotropin (hCG). Bouffard (see Goetz, 1983) showed that in females that ovulated, circulating concentrations of PGF in the plasma begin to increase at the time of ovulation (10 hours after hCG injection), and by 14 hours after ovulation (24 hours after hCG injection) are more than 10 times the level seen in fish which failed to ovulate. Significantly, if fish that ovulate are stripped of their eggs at the time of ovulation, plasma PGF declines 14 hours later, suggesting that the high PGF levels in fish which are not stripped are due to the continued presence of ovulated eggs. Bouffard also found that PGF levels in the ovarian fluid are higher than those in the blood, suggesting that PG synthesis by the ovary or oviduct is responsible for the increase in plasma PGF levels at ovulation.

More recent work by Cetta and Goetz (Goetz, 1983) shows that plasma PGF levels also increase at ovulation in the brook trout (*Salvelinus fontinalis*). As with goldfish, the ovary is the most likely source of increased plasma PGF concentrations. At ovulation, PGF levels increase in the ovary, while concentrations of PGF in the coelomic fluid exceed those in the plasma. Unlike goldfish, which release the ovulated eggs into an oviduct continuous with the ovary, trout release ovulated eggs directly into the body cavity. As will be discussed below, there is only suggestive evidence at present that PGs play a role in sexual behavior of female trout.

The fact that spawning behavior in female goldfish can be induced either by intraovarian injection of ovulated eggs or by injection of PGs suggests three ways by which egg injection might increase PG levels. The most straightforward might seem to be that ovulated eggs normally produce PGs and continue to do so after being stripped from one female and injected into another. However, the fact that a physical substitute for ovulated eggs (petroleum jelly) can induce spawning behavior when injected into the ovarian cavity (Stacey, 1977) indicates that, although eggs might produce PGs, they probably are not the only source.

The second explanation for the ability of egg injection to induce spawning behavior is that, as ovarian fluid contains high levels of PGF, spawning is induced not through stimulated PG synthesis in the recipient (egg-injected) female, but simply by injection of PGF already synthesized in the donor female. The effectiveness of an egg substitute would already argue against such a mechanism. Further, if injection of eggs triggers spawning simply by introducing ovarian fluid containing PGF, then we would have to conclude that indomethacin blocks the spawning response to egg injection not by inhibiting PG synthesis, but by inhibiting behavioral responsiveness to PG. The data presented in Figure 2.5, however, clearly show that the spawning response to injected PGF is *not* affected by indomethacin treatment. Thus, it is unlikely that indomethacin blocks the spawning response to egg injection by rendering the female unable to respond to PG injected with the eggs.

From these considerations, we are left with the third explanation— namely that injection of ovulated eggs induces spawning behavior by stimulat-

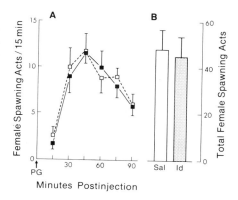

Figure 2.5. Indomethacin does not affect prostaglandin-induced spawning behavior in female goldfish (*Carassius auratus*). (A) Time course of spawning in females injected with indomethacin (ID, ■——■; 20 μg/g; n = 13) or saline (Sal, □——□; n = 10) 2 hours before testing and prostaglandin $F_{2\alpha}$ (0.1 μg/g) at start of test. (B) Total spawning acts performed during the 90-minute test. (Redrawn from Stacey and Goetz, 1982, courtesy of Canadian Journal of Fisheries and Aquatic Sciences)

ing PG synthesis in the recipient female. Unfortunately there is yet no direct experimental evidence which would either support or reject this hypothesis.

The PG proposed to be synthesized by the reproductive tract in response to the presence of ovulated eggs evidently stimulates spawning behavior by an action on the brain. The evidence for this comes from two types of experiment (Liley and Stacey, 1983). The first focuses on whether peripheral structures might mediate the effect of injected PG on spawning. In this instance, the ovipore, oviduct, and posterior portions of the ovaries are surgically removed from female goldfish. When these operated fish are injected with PG, their spawning responses are no different from those of intact fish. This demonstrates that if PGs do act peripherally to induce spawning, the site of action is not the posterior reproductive tract. Direct evidence for a central site of action comes from the second type of experiment in which PGs are injected directly into the brain. Injection of a "low" dose of $PGF_{2\alpha}$ (10 ng/g) into the third ventricle of the brain causes more fish to spawn, and with a shorter latency, than does the same dose injected into the body cavity or body musculature.

From the information so far presented, it seems reasonable to conclude that spawning behavior in female goldfish is stimulated by PGs synthesized in the reproductive tract in response to the presence of ovulated eggs, and carried in the bloodstream to the brain where they exert their effect. The temporal aspects of this proposed mechanism are presented in Figure 2.6. While there appear to be no inconsistencies among the various data supporting a role for PG in spawning behavior, it must be emphasized that much of the evidence is rather indirect. In particular, it remains to be demonstrated that blood concentrations of PGs increase after egg injection, and that these PGs actually reach the brain. Many questions regarding the regulation of spawning in the female goldfish are presently unanswered. For example, how do eggs stimulate PG synthesis, what PGs are produced, and where in the brain do they act? What also is not clear is whether ovarian steroid hormones, well known to regulate female sexual behaviors of internally fertilizing species by acting within the brain, may perform a similar function in the female goldfish.

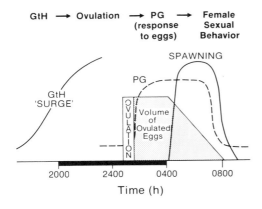

GtH → Ovulation → PG → Female
(response Sexual
to eggs) Behavior

Figure 2.6. Schematic diagram of mechanisms proposed to regulate spawning behavior in the female goldfish (*Carassius auratus*). Spawning is ultimately regulated by a photoperiodically synchronized surge of blood gonadotropin which induces ovulation before dawn. Ovulated eggs in the reproductive tract stimulate synthesis of prostaglandin (PG), which enters the bloodstream and acts within the brain to trigger spawning behavior when there is sufficient light. As spawning depletes the ovulated eggs, PG synthesis decreases, PG levels in the blood fall, and spawning behavior ceases.

An extremely intriguing aspect of PG-induced female spawning behavior in the goldfish is that it occurs in both sexes. That is, normal levels of female spawning behavior can be induced in male goldfish simply by injecting PGs (Stacey and Kyle, 1983). Male goldfish treated with PGs are not inhibited from performing male sexual behaviors; when placed with both male and receptive female partners, PG-injected males will repeatedly alternate between performance of male and female behaviors.

This full and operational behavioral bisexuality of the male goldfish might at first seem surprising, for the adults of many mammal and bird species only infrequently display reproductive behaviors characteristic of the opposite sex (see Chapter 4). However, as discussed in Chapter 4, many species of fish are hermaphrodites, and are capable of behaving and functioning both as male and female after reaching sexual maturity. In simultaneous hermaphrodites, for example, both sexes are functional at the same time. The effect of PG treatment on male goldfish—stimulation of female behavior without inhibition of male behavior—is strikingly similar to the normal sequence of events in the spawning of some simultaneous hermaphrodites, in which the ovulated individual switches between male and female roles a number of times during the course of one spawning encounter. Is it possible that the behavioral bisexuality of simultaneous hermaphrodites is not an evolutionary specialization for that mode of reproduction, but rather the expression of a physiological capability normally latent in gonochoristic species?

Other Externally Fertilizing Species

The mechanism proposed to synchronize sexual behavior with ovulation in the female goldfish may be widespread among fishes, for PGs have recently been shown to stimulate female-typical behaviors in a variety of externally fertilizing species (Table 2.1). Not all of these studies have yielded results as consistent as those obtained with the goldfish. For example, injection of PGs induces spawning of female paradise fish (*Macropodus opercularis*) and two-spot cichlids (*Cichlosoma bimaculatum*) which are not

TABLE 2.1 Evidence that prostaglandin (PG) stimulates female sexual behavior in vertebrate species exhibiting external fertilization.

Species	Effect of PG Injection	Effect of Injecting PG Synthesis Inhibitor	Source
Fish			
Goldfish	+	−	Stacey and Goetz, 1982
Lampan jawa	+	NT	Liley and Tan, 1985
(*Puntius gonionotus*)			
Paradise fish	+	0	Villars et al., 1985
Two-spot cichlid	+	0	Cole and Stacey, 1984
Three-spine stickleback	(+)	(−)	Lam, unpubl.[1]
(*Gasterosteus aculeatus*)			
Rainbow trout	0	−	Liley, unpubl.[1]
Amphibia			
Leopard frog	+	−	Diakow and Nemiroff, 1981
Xenopus laevis	+	−	Weintraub et al., 1985

+ = full response, (+) = partial response, − = complete inhibition, (−) = partial inhibition, 0 = no response, NT = not tested.
[1]See Liley and Stacey, 1983.

ovulated; however, injecting ovulated females with the PG synthesis inhibitor indomethacin does not inhibit spawning (Villars et al., 1985; Cole and Stacey, 1985). In rainbow trout (*Salmo gairdneri*), on the other hand, indomethacin blocks nest-digging and spawning of ovulated fish, but PG treatments to date have not induced these behaviors (N. R. Liley, unpublished results). Perhaps the most intriguing departure from what has been seen in goldfish comes from work on the paradise fish.

Spawning behavior of paradise fish is typical of Belontiids, a group which includes the Siamese fighting fish (*Betta splendens*) and gouramis popular among home aquarists. These fish occur naturally in the warm, shallow ponds and ditches of South-East Asia where levels of dissolved oxygen can be very low. Presumably as a means of increasing oxygen availability to the eggs, the territorial and parental males construct a floating nest by blowing many small bubbles which are stabilized by mucous from glands in the mouth. When the female ovulates, she approaches the male and initiates a sequence of behavioral interactions which culminate in oviposition.

If female paradise fish are permitted to spawn with a male, left with the male until the following day, and then injected with $PGF_{2\alpha}$, they will perform the full range of female reproductive behaviors, including the postoviposition retreats from the nest site, although they have no ovulated eggs in the reproductive tract (Villars et al., 1985). As with goldfish, female paradise fish begin to spawn within minutes of being injected with PG and reach peak spawning activity within an hour. In other respects, however, the action of PG on female paradise fish is quite different.

For example, if female paradise fish are injected with PG either before they have ovulated and spawned with a male (Villars et al., 1985) or 3 to 5 days after they have spawned (Villars and Burdick, 1982), the treatment fails to induce any spawning behavior. The reason for this unresponsiveness is not known. It does not seem to be due to gonadal immaturity, for the females which failed to respond to PG before they had spawned with a male all ovulated and spawned normally the following day. Neither is the unresponsiveness due to "unfamiliarity" with the male, for females held with a male for 5 days were uniformly unresponsive to PG treatment. The most likely explanation would seem to be that some event associated with ovulation—perhaps steroid changes induced by the ovulatory surge of GtH—briefly sensitizes the female to PG, although this remains to be investigated.

The behavioral effects of injecting PGs and inhibiting PG synthesis in the few species so far studied suggest variability in what appears to be a widespread mechanism utilized by externally fertilizing fish to synchronize sexual behavior with ovulation. Just how widespread this mechanism might be becomes clear when we consider that the rapid and dramatic effects of PG on female sex behaviors are not restricted to fish.

Prostaglandin has been implicated in the stimulation of female reproductive behavior of the leopard frog (*Rana pipiens*) and the South African clawed frog (*Xenopus laevis*), both of which are externally fertilizing species (see Chapter 3). Female *Rana* which are not ovulated will emit a "release call" which inhibits clasping attempts by the male. However, if the female is ovulated, or if water accumulation has been induced experimentally by ligating the cloaca or injecting arginine vasotocin (AVT), she does not emit the release call when clasped (Diakow and Raimondi, 1981). Although these various conditions could act through different mechanisms to inhibit the release call, it seems more likely that all act by stimulating PG synthesis. Indomethacin restores release calling (i.e., inhibits receptivity) in females which have been injected with AVT, whereas injection of PG inhibits the release call (i.e., stimulates receptivity) in females which are not ovulated and are otherwise untreated (Diakow and Nemiroff, 1981). Similar results have been obtained with *Xenopus*. Receptive females fail to emit a release call when approached or clasped by a male, and also exhibit a leg adduction movement which facilitates the male's clasping attempts. Both of these receptive responses are blocked by injecting a PG synthesis inhibitor, and can be induced in unreceptive females by injecting a very low dose of PG (Weintraub et al., 1985).

Role of Prostaglandins in Internally Fertilizing Vertebrates

Prostaglandins also have been shown to have rapid stimulatory or inhibitory effects on female sexual behavior in some internally fertilizing terrestrial vertebrate species. Although these studies have so far been conducted on only a few species, there is a good correlation between the effect of injected PG on behavior (that is, whether PG is stimulatory or inhibitory) and the behavioral effect resulting from physical stimulation of the peripheral reproductive tract during intromission.

For example, in the rat (*Rattus norvegicus*), where physical stimulation of the vagina and cervix can produce a rapid increase in the display of lordosis behavior—the female receptive posture which allows mounting and intromission by the male—injection of PG stimulates receptivity in the ovariectomized female. On the other hand, in the female guinea pig (*Cavia porcellus*), vaginocervical stimulation or mating rapidly terminate receptivity (Marrone et al., 1979). As discussed by Whittier and Crews (1986), similar inhibitory responses to mating have been reported in the green anole lizard (*Anolis carolinensis*) and the red-sided garter snake (*Thamnophis sirtalis parietalis*). In all three of these species administration of PGs has a pronounced inhibitory effect on receptivity (Marrone et al., 1979; Whittier and Crews, 1986). It should be emphasized that these actions of PGs in reptiles and mammals likely serve to modulate ongoing behavior. That is, a period of receptivity is first induced by ovarian steroid hormones and then either extended or abbreviated by coital stimuli via synthesis of PG.

Is it merely a coincidence that PG affects female sexual behaviors in species as distantly related as goldfish, leopard frogs, green anoles, garter snakes, and guinea pigs? Or are these widespread actions indicative of an ancestral mechanism utilized by the externally fertilizing early fishes and retained and modified during vertebrate evolution? Allowing that the limited information available can justify only speculation, the second alternative would seem to be favored by the number of apparent similarities in when and how PG is proposed to regulate sex behaviors of the species examined. These similarities, discussed in more detail by Liley and Stacey (1983), can be summarized as: increase of PG synthesis by physical stimulation of the reproductive tract; change in gender-typical behavior within minutes; direct action of PGs within the brain. More recent studies suggest that there also are similarities in how PGs act within the brain (see Chapters 3 and 4). For example, it has been suggested (Irving et al., 1981) that PG inhibits receptivity in female guinea pigs by interfering with an adrenergic brain mechanism, because the effect of PG is blocked by the adrenergic agonist, clonidine. Thus, it is interesting that in the female goldfish, where PGs stimulate rather than inhibit sex behavior, the effect of PGs also is blocked by clonidine (Stacey, 1984).

Perhaps the most compelling reason to suspect homology in the various sex-behavior functions of PG is that all appear to be activated by a common factor, physical stimulation of the reproductive tract. If true, we might then expect that the same mechanism also functions to stimulate nonsexual behaviors which normally are tied to genital-tract perturbations: i.e., behaviors associated with oviposition in reptiles and birds and parturition in mammals. This interesting possibility remains to be explored.

HORMONES AND MALE REPRODUCTIVE BEHAVIOR

In hormone-reproductive behavior studies of fish, the male has received more attention than the female, likely for reasons of experimental practicality. Male reproductive behaviors generally are more quantifiable than are those of the female, for they are more visually obvious and of longer duration. This is true of species with "simple" spawning behaviors such as the goldfish, but particularly evident in many species with more elaborate behaviors, where the male may prepare and defend a nest site and care for the eggs and young (e.g., Belontiids). These behavioral differences between the sexes result in part from differences in gonadal function. Sexual activity in males can occur over extended periods due to prolonged production and storage of viable sperm, whereas that in females tends to be restricted to a relatively brief period after ovulation.

Although it is difficult to summarize the diverse studies of hormones and reproductive behavior in male fish, it does seem clear that gonadal androgens can stimulate the full range of male reproductive behaviors, whether these simply entail a brief shedding of milt or also include a variety of prespawning and postspawning activities. This broad involvement of gonadal androgens is suggested by several kinds of evidence.

Probably the most straightforward evidence is provided by experiments involving castration and androgen replacement therapy. In many species, male-typical reproductive behaviors are eliminated or reduced by castration and can be restored in castrated males, or induced in females, by androgen treatment (Liley and Stacey, 1983). A Belontiid, the blue gourami (*Trichogaster trichopterus*), provides a good example. Castrated males do not build bubble nests or court females. However, if castrated males are injected with methyltestosterone, all reproductive behaviors are restored, including care of the unfertilized eggs. Although nest-building and parental activities are normally exhibited only by the male, these behaviors can be induced in female blue gouramis by methyltestosterone treatment. These results are consistent with other lines of evidence implicating testicular androgens in the control of sexual behavior in the male: that is, circulating concentrations of androgen in the blood increase prior to spawning (Fostier et al., 1983); sex-steroid hormones are concentrated in brain areas believed to regulate male reproductive behavior (Demski and Hornby, 1982); an androgen antagonist, cyproterone acetate, can reduce sexual behaviors in males (Liley and Stacey, 1983).

The results of some other studies, however, have been interpreted as indicating that male reproductive behaviors of some species are not regulated by testicular androgen. This apparent contradiction has been reviewed recently (Liley and Stacey, 1983) and will only be summarized here. There seem to be two major problems.

The first problem is that some studies have used hormones and pharmacological agents (antiandrogen, antigonadotropin) to alter the reproductive behaviors of intact male fish. The effect, or lack of effect, of these hormonal and pharmacological treatments often have been attributed to their *presumed* inhibitory and negative feedback effects on the endocrine system. However, these studies generally do not provide clear evidence that the treatments have acted in the purported way. Interpreting the results of such pharmacological approaches would be aided considerably if the studies included measurements of blood hormone levels in treated fish.

The second problem concerns the interpretation of castration experiments which fail to inhibit behavior. Such negative results are difficult to interpret and can lead to confusion, unless it can be ascertained that the castration was complete. Fish are notorious for their ability to regenerate gonadal tissue. Further, some of the behaviors under study are normally displayed in nonsexual contexts. Studies of the blue gourami illustrate both sources of confusion.

When Johns and Liley (1970; see Liley and Stacey, 1983) castrated adult male blue gouramis, eleven individuals failed to build bubble nests and court females until they were treated with methyltestosterone. In contrast, four other castrates spawned normally without steroid hormone treatment, even though autopsy failed to detect any testicular regeneration. The behavior of the four sexually active castrates would at first seem to imply that male spawning behavior in this species is not strictly dependent on androgen. However, the dorsal fins (an androgen-dependent male secondary sex character) of these fish remained long, indicating the presence of biologically significant levels of endogenous androgen.

When castration appears to be complete—i.e., when the dorsal fin shortens and there is no apparent testicular regeneration—male gouramis show none of the aggressive behavior normally associated with defense of their nest site. On the other hand, the *nonterritorial* agonistic behavior of these castrates does not differ from that of intact males. This latter finding in other species has led to the erroneous conclusion that *male-typical* behaviors are not regulated by androgen because it was not realized that nonsexual aggression often is displayed by females and juveniles (see Liley and Stacey, 1983).

Although it seems clear that androgens stimulate male reproductive behaviors in many fish species, important aspects of this behavioral control are almost completely unexplored. A good case in point concerns the question of which endogenous steroid hormone(s) stimulates male-typical behaviors. The fact that exogenous testosterone is effective in inducing courtship and spawning in the male does not necessarily mean that testosterone acts on the presumed target neurons within the brain. Numerous studies in other vertebrate groups indicate that testosterone often does not act directly, but only after it is converted within the brain to other steroids such as estradiol or dihydrotestosterone (Adkins-Regan, 1981; Callard, 1983; see Chapter 10). Indeed, blood levels of testosterone in a number of fish are higher in the female than in the male (Fostier et al., 1983); thus, it is difficult to account for the regulation of male-typical reproductive behaviors solely in terms of a direct action of testosterone. Unfortunately, it is not yet known whether reproductive behaviors in male fish can be stimulated by 11-ketotestosterone, a steroid hormone known to exceed blood levels of testosterone in a number of male fish. This hormone appears to be more potent than testosterone in stimulating the development of male secondary sex characters (Fostier et al., 1983).

Behavioral Effects on the Endocrine System

Measurements of hormone concentrations in the blood have done more than demonstrate how little is known of how steroid hormones regulate sexual behavior in male fish. They also have revealed that hormone levels in male fish are not static but can change rapidly and dramatically as a result of sexual activity. Although the reciprocal interactions between hormones and behavior in males has been well documented in other vertebrate groups (Crews and Silver, 1985), this exciting aspect of male reproductive function has so far been demonstrated in only two fish species, the white sucker (*Catostomus commersoni*) and the goldfish.

The white sucker is a common North American freshwater fish which spawns in spring when water temperature reaches about 10°C. Typically, mature fish leave lakes and rivers and ascend small streams to spawn on shallow, rocky riffles. Females ovulate all of their mature eggs at once, spawn for a day or two, and then return downstream. Males, on the other hand, remain on the spawning riffles for a week or more, during which time they may spawn with a number of females. The white sucker is an excellent species in which to study hormone levels present in the blood during natural spawning. Because the spawning stream often is very small—only several meters wide—blood samples can be obtained within several minutes of disturbing the fish.

If white suckers are captured on spawning riffles throughout a spawning season and their blood assayed for gonadotropin (GtH) and other hormones, clear differences are found between females and males (Scott et al., 1984). Females about to ovulate, or which have just ovulated, have elevated blood levels of GtH and a progesterone metabolite, 17α-hydroxy-20β-dihydroprogesterone (17,20P), the steroid generally accepted to be the endogenous promoter of oocyte final maturation in many fish (Goetz, 1983). Males show the same dramatic increases in GtH and 17,20P as seen in females. A striking difference between the sexes, however, is that hormonal increases in females are seen only around the time of ovulation, regardless of when in the spawning season this occurs, whereas hormonal increases in males appear to occur synchronously with the onset of spawning activity in the stream.

We have recently sought to determine whether this apparently synchronous increase of GtH levels in males might be due to some factor associated with the spawning riffles (N. Stacey, A. Kyle, and J. Dulka, unpublished results). This time, however, fish were sampled both from spawning riffles and from nonspawning sites—deep, mud-bottomed areas in the stream. Regardless of where females were captured, their GtH levels increased around the time of ovulation. In marked contrast, GtH levels in males captured at nonspawning sites remained low throughout the two-week spawning season, whereas levels in males captured at spawning sites increased significantly within the first few days of spawning and remained high thereafter (Figure 2.7).

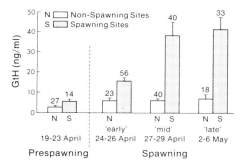

Figure 2.7. Blood gonadotropin levels in mature male white suckers (*Catostomus commersoni*) captured at spawning sites and nonspawning sites in a central Alberta stream.

The striking differences in GtH levels of males from spawning and nonspawning sites could be accounted for in two ways. Either males move from nonspawning to spawning areas when their GtH levels increase, or factors at the spawning sites stimulate GtH increase. Results of a simple laboratory experiment favor the latter alternative (Figure 2.8; N. Stacey and J. Dulka, unpublished results). Males were placed in two stream tanks which contained a pool and a spawning riffle. Ovulated females were placed in one of the stream tanks and they spawned actively with the males. Blood GtH levels in all males were undetectable (less than 1 ng/ml) at the time they were

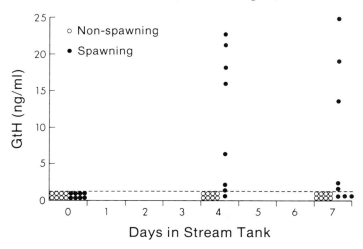

Figure 2.8. Spawning activity increases blood gonadotropin levels in laboratory-held male white suckers (*Catostomus commersoni*). Groups of 8 mature males were placed in two stream tanks, one of which contained ovulated females. Gonadotropin levels in all males not exposed to females remained undetectable throughout the experiment.

placed in the stream tanks and remained undetectable throughout the 7-day experiment in males which were not exposed to females. However, in many of the males which spawned with the females GtH levels increased dramatically.

Studies in goldfish also clearly demonstrate that sexual interaction increases blood GtH levels in the male. This effect can be seen within 20–40 minutes of the male's being placed with a receptive female (Kyle et al., 1985). Further, blood GtH levels can be shown to increase with the duration of spawning activity. For example, if male goldfish are allowed to spawn daily for up to one month, a "spawning season" which significantly depletes sperm stores, there is a steady and dramatic increase in blood GtH levels (Figure 2.9). This situation in male goldfish appears very comparable to what has been observed in the male white sucker under natural conditions (Figure 2.7).

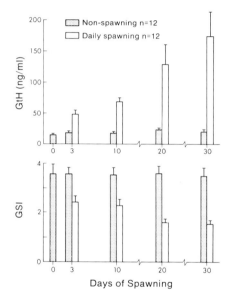

Figure 2.9. Changes in (A) blood gonadotropin levels and (B) gonadosomatic index (GSI: gonad weight/body weight $\times$ 100) during extended spawning in male goldfish (*Carassius auratus*). Males allowed to spawn every day exhibit progressive gonadotropin increase associated with sperm depletion; males under similar conditions but without access to females show no change in gonadotropin or GSI.

It is possible that a host of behavioral and physiological functions are influenced by the increase in blood GtH during spawning in male goldfish and white suckers. Although research in this area is only beginning, results to date suggest that one function of the increase in GtH is to replenish stores of releasable sperm which have been depleted by spawning.

Gonadotropin is well known to increase the volume of milt which can be stripped from a variety of fish species, although how GtH exerts this effect is not well understood (Billard et al., 1982). Thus it is significant that 17,20P and its precursor 17α-OH-progesterone (17P), both known to increase during spawning in male white suckers (Scott et al., 1984), dramatically increase the amount of milt which can be stripped from male goldfish, whereas injections of other steroid hormones are without effect (Stacey, unpublished results). It is easy to see the adaptive value of a mechanism whereby spawning activity triggers a neuroendocrine reflex stimulating rapid sperm production, for male reproductive success in group-spawning species such as the goldfish and white sucker must depend to a large extent on the ability to release large amounts of sperm.

REPRODUCTIVE PHEROMONES

External chemical signals or pheromones also play important roles in a wide range of reproductive and nonreproductive social interactions of fishes (Liley, 1982; Stacey et al., 1986). Here we will be concerned only with those situations where release of a chemical by one individual can be shown to alter the reproductive development or the likelihood of sexual behavior in another individual.

Undoubtedly, the best-known examples of vertebrate pheromone systems come from terrestrial species, where the sender of the chemical signal generally has glands developed for the secretion of one or more specialized products. In the case of fish, however, the situation is rather different, for the mechanisms generating the chemical signals appear to be much less sophisticated than those of many terrestrial species. Pheromone-producing structures, so obvious and widespread in terrestrial forms, have been identified in only a few fish species. In the few cases where the chemical identity of a fish reproductive pheromone has been proposed, the compound is simply a metabolite of a sex hormone, rather than a substance synthesized solely for its pheromonal function; however, whether this is the general case remains to be determined.

Why should the signalling aspects of pheromonal communication in the fishes appear to be so "simple" in comparison to many of their terrestrial vertebrate relatives? Certainly the incredible diversity of fishes indicates their adaptive potential is not the limiting factor. A more reasonable explanation would seem to be that there are very different constraints on the evolution of pheromone systems in aquatic and terrestrial habitats due to the obvious differences in the way water and air transport chemicals (Wilson, 1975).

To function as a pheromone in a terrestrial environment, chemicals generally must be volatile, a characteristic which restricts the size and chemical nature of airborne pheromones and generally requires the evolution of novel biochemical pathways and structures specialized for phero-mone synthesis and release. In the aquatic environment, however, the range of biochemicals which could potentially serve as pheromones is virtually limitless, for here the major prerequisite for pheromonal activity is solubil-ity. Thus, simply by evolving responsiveness to a preexisting metabolite, fish should have been able to readily incorporate latent chemical signals into their communication repertoires without obvious development and special-ization on the part of the signaller. However, while the aquatic environment does provide the advantage of increasing the opportunities for the origin of pheromone systems, it also presents disadvantages for their further evolution. Slow diffusion in water increases both the latency between sending and receiving the message and the time the receiver is exposed to the message. In view of these latter constraints, it perhaps is not surprising that fish reproductive pheromones appear to transmit simple tonic messages of arousal and orientation.

As with other types of pheromones, reproductive pheromones have been said to have either *primer* or *releaser* effects. A relatively slow response in the pheromone recipient would be considered a primer effect. An example of such an effect is the occurrence of ovulation in female zebra danios (*Brachydanio rerio*) exposed to water from males (Chen and Martinich, 1975; see Liley and Stacey, 1983). Releaser effects, on the other hand, are induced almost immediately after exposure to the pheromone. A good example is seen in the goldfish, where the male's locomotory behavior and investigation of tankmates are rapidly stimulated by adding water from ovulated females (Sorensen et al., 1986). The terms releaser and primer are useful in indicating the latency to a pheromone-induced response. However, it should be kept in mind that these terms refer to differences in the physiological response times of pheromone-induced effects and do not necessarily imply any differences in the pheromones per se.

Behavioral responses to fish reproductive pheromones are most commonly measured by two simple procedures which allow delivery of the pheromone and quantification of its effects under reasonably controlled conditions (Figure 2.10). In one approach, a fish's behavior is observed prior to and after addition of experimental or control water sources. Often, a sexually inactive conspecific of the opposite sex is placed in the testing container to determine whether the pheromone stimulates social or sexual

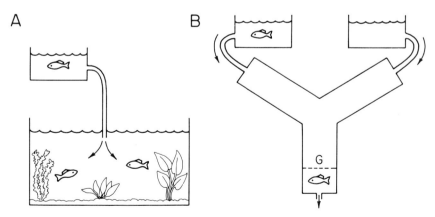

Figure 2.10. Two types of apparatus commonly used to investigate pheromone function in fish. (A) Water from container holding pheromone donor is added to aquarium containing one or more conspecifics. (B) Fish in stem of Y-maze must choose between stimulus and control water sources after gate (G) in stem of Y is removed.

interactions. The second approach is to use some form of Y-maze, which has a water inlet at the end of each arm and a drain in the stem of the Y. To carry out a test, a fish is placed in the stem and observed to determine whether it swims into the arm containing the pheromone. Between each test of a series, the arm which will receive pheromone should be altered on a random schedule to eliminate any inherent bias in the maze, and the maze should be washed to prevent contamination of the control arm.

Types of Pheromone Response

To appreciate how the roles of fish reproductive pheromones are related to reproductive strategy, it is helpful to consider that these chemical signals induce three basic categories of behavioral and physiological response: responses of males to pheromones released by females, responses of females to pheromones released by males, and responses induced in both sexes by the same pheromone.

Undoubtedly, the clearest and most numerous examples are those in which males respond to pheromones released by females. Studies in a number of oviparous species have shown that water from a female which has recently ovulated is more attractive to males, and more effective in stimulating male courtship, than is water from a female which has not ovulated. In the loach (*Misgurnus anguillicaudatus*), pheromone release begins at the time of ovulation and persists for only 3–4 hours (Honda, 1980). In the goldfish, where a number of males may compete for a single ovulated female, the female's postovulatory pheromone may be extremely important in enabling the male to locate the female during the frenzied courtship activities. Restricting pheromone production to the postovulatory period ensures that males are most attracted when the female is physiologically ready for oviposition. As sexual receptivity of the female also is dependent on the physiological changes at ovulation, the effect is coordination of the behaviors of male and female.

Pheromone production and female receptivity also are synchronized in the viviparous Poeciliids such as the guppy. Female guppies that have mated and produced a brood (nonvirgin females) are maximally receptive to male courtship for several days after parturition, the time when their odor is most stimulating to males (Meyer and Liley, 1982). Virgin females, on the other hand, appear to be constantly receptive until they have mated, after which their receptivity becomes cyclic. Thus it is interesting that in the related Poeciliid, *Poecilia chica*, samples of water from virgin and from early postpartum females are equally stimulating for males (Brett and Grosse, 1982). Studies in the guppy suggest that estrogen acts on the ovary to produce female sex pheromone in the postpartum period (Meyer and Liley, 1982).

There are fewer demonstrations of sex pheromone production in male fish than there are in female fish, although good examples of this category are seen in fish such as the Belontiids, in which the ovulated female is attracted to the bubble nest of the territorial male. Lee and Ingersoll (1979) have shown that females of several Belontiid species are attracted to water from conspecific males only if they are ovulated. The more recent findings (Villars et al., 1985) that injection of PGs can rapidly stimulate female spawning behavior in one of these Belontiids—the paradise fish—thus raises the interesting possibility that PGs synthesized at ovulation are responsible for rapidly increasing the female's behavioral responsiveness to chemical signals from the male. It seems likely that a similar mechanism may regulate female response to male pheromone in the marine goby, *Gobius jozo*. Normally, only ovulated females respond to the territorial male's pheromone by approaching his nest site; however, nonovulated females will show the same response after treatment with PG (Colombo et al., 1982 and unpublished results).

It perhaps is not surprising that the best evidence for male reproductive pheromones is found in species where males hold spatially fixed spawning territories, for in such conditions reproductive success will depend on the male's attracting, and the female's locating, a spawning partner. However, this consideration need not imply that in such species the only chemical communication between the sexes is from male to female. Male Belontiids are more attracted to water from ovulated females than from nonovulated females (Lee and Ingersoll, 1979), while in the frillfin goby (*Bathygobius soporator*), where the territorial males would be expected to release a sexual pheromone, the demonstration that a pheromone from ovulated females triggers courtship in males constitutes one of the classic examples of reproductive pheromones in fish (Tavolga, 1956).

The third "category" of behavioral response to reproductive pheromones—in which both sexes show a similar reaction—appears to contain only a single example, the Pacific herring (*Clupea harengus pallasi*). On the western coast of North America, herring spawn in intertidal and shallow subtidal areas with good vegetation cover. Although the spawning individuals are difficult to observe directly, the results of their activities are extremely impressive. So great is the number of synchronously spawning fish that the milky milt released can soon discolor the water for a considerable distance offshore and along kilometers of coastline. The milt discoloration, which can reduce visibility to only a few centimeters, often continues for several days, despite the actions of tide and current. This mass spawning activity evidently is triggered by a sex pheromone (Stacey and Hourston, 1982).

When mature (ovulated and spermiated) herring are captured on the spawning grounds and held in large aquaria, they rarely display any spontaneous spawning behavior. However, when a small amount of herring milt is added to the aquarium, the previously regular schooling behavior immediately disappears, both sexes begin to extend their genital papillae, and the males usually begin to release ribbons of milt as they swim. On encountering a clean, smooth substrate, males and females then orient their ventral surfaces toward the substrate and deposit a track of eggs or milt. Apart from the initial reaction of females to milt, spawning of herring does not seem to involve any communication or cooperation between the sexes, for the full range of behaviors can be induced by adding milt to unisexual schools of either sex.

The effectiveness of a milt pheromone in stimulating spawning of herring is clear. What is not known is how release of this potent chemical signal is initiated in a natural population, and what benefit is derived from using this *apparently* unusual pheromonal mechanism for synchronizing spawning. As milt release in captive mature males can be induced simply by handling, milt release under natural conditions could be initiated by such a stress as predation, the effect being amplified when additional males respond by releasing milt. The possible benefits are more difficult to assess. For the population, mass milt release must ensure a high rate of fertilization and help to reduce predation on spawners by increasing turbidity. For the individual male, however, it is not clear what selective pressures might have favored a mechanism for sperm release which is not dependent on interaction with a female.

Mode of Action

One consistent feature of sex-pheromone function throughout the fish species so far examined is that the olfactory system is required to mediate the response (Liley, 1982; Stacey et al., 1986); evidence for involvement of taste mechanisms is so far equivocal (Pollack et al., 1978). Thus, male or female fish made anosmic by plugging the nares, cauterizing the olfactory epithelium, or cutting the olfactory nerves or tracts lose the ability to discriminate sources of sex pheromones and generally show reduced sexual behaviors. In some cases, however, anosmic individuals may still be quite capable of successful spawning if other sensory channels can be employed. For example, while the female blue gourami evidently uses the olfactory system to locate the source of male sex pheromone (Lee and Ingersoll, 1979), anosmia has little effect on the spawning of females which already are in visual contact with males (Pollack et al., 1978).

Recent studies indicate that sex pheromones act on a subdivision of the fish olfactory system (see Chapter 1). Basically, olfactory information reaches the brain through a series of neural connections which begins in the olfactory epithelium (Figure 2.11). From here, axons of the primary receptors run in the olfactory nerve to the olfactory bulb, where they synapse with dendrites of the mitral cells. Mitral cell axons then leave the bulb by either the lateral (LOT) or medial (MOT) subdivisions of the olfactory tract and run to various terminal fields in the brain. Electrophysiological evidence indicates the medial-lateral subdivision of the olfactory system originates in the bulbs, for bile steroids applied to the olfactory organ evoke greater electrical activity in the medial part of the bulb, while amino acids evoke greater activity in the lateral portion (Stacey et al., 1986).

The medial portion of the system appears to be involved in transmitting sex-pheromone information. The clearest evidence for this is that sexual

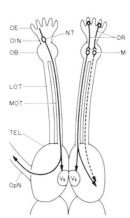

Figure 2.11. Highly simplified diagram of goldfish olfactory and *nervus terminalis* system (adapted from Demski and Northcutt, 1983, and von Bartheld et al., 1984). *Nervus terminalis* system shown on left and olfactory system on right; only centripetal and ipsilateral projections indicated. LOT, lateral olfactory tract; M, mitral cell; MOT, medial olfactory tract; NT, *nervus terminalis* neuron; OB, olfactory bulb; OE, olfactory epithelium; OlN, olfactory nerve; OpN, optic nerve; OR, olfactory receptor; TEL, telencephalon; V_s, supracommissural nucleus of area ventralis.

behavior in male goldfish is drastically reduced by cutting the MOT, but unaffected by cutting the LOT (Stacey and Kyle, 1983). Although many of the olfactory terminal fields in the goldfish brain are innervated by both the MOT and the LOT, only two terminal fields appear to be innervated by the MOT alone—the ventromedial telencephalon and the anterior preoptic area (von Bartheld et al., 1984). Significantly, if these brain areas are destroyed by lesioning, male sexual behavior is reduced (Koyama et al., 1984).

The evidence thus suggests that the medial portion of the olfactory system carries sex-pheromone information to specific brain areas to induce behavioral change. This may not be the entire story, however, for the MOT carries not only olfactory axons—those from the mitral cells in the medial portion of the olfactory bulb. The MOT also carries axons of the terminal nerve (*Nervus terminalis*—cranial nerve 0), whose ganglion is embedded in the olfactory system, and which projects to the forebrain and retina (Demski and Northcutt, 1983). Terminal nerve neurons are immunoreactive for mammalian luteinizing hormone-releasing hormone (LHRH), and some project to the ventromedial telencephalon, features which are tantalizingly suggestive of a reproductive function. As yet, however, there is no direct evidence that the terminal nerve is responsible for mediating responses to sex pheromones.

Sources and Chemical Nature

Certainly the gonads are the most commonly reported sources of sex pheromones in fish, although nongonadal sources such as the anal fin appendages of the blenny, *Blennius pavo*, also have been demonstrated (Stacey et al., 1986). The use of homogenates of testes dissected from mature donor fish (e.g., herring; Stacey and Hourston, 1982) has provided clear evidence that some gonadal constituent has pheromonal activity. Unfortunately, much of the evidence for gonadal pheromones in fish is not so clear, because it comes from experiments in which test preparations were obtained by stripping ovulated and spermiated donors. Such preparations will contain the gametes or genital cavity fluids suspected to contain the pheromone; however, they also are likely to contain urine, skin mucous, feces, and bile, all of which have been suggested as pheromone sources (Liley, 1982).

An interesting experiment with the goby, *Gobius jozo*, (Colombo et al., 1982) illustrates the need for caution in interpreting the effects of pheromone preparations obtained by stripping. Using both ovulated and nonovulated females as donors, Colombo and his colleagues compared the effectiveness of urine and ovarian fluid in stimulating courtship behavior of the male. To obtain urine, they ligated the external genital papilla and inserted a syringe into the swollen urinary bladder the following day. Ovarian fluid was obtained by rinsing dissected ovaries in a small amount of fish saline.

The potency of both urine and ovarian fluid was greater in preparations from ovulated females, while urine was consistently more effective than ovarian fluid. Although many interpretations of these results are possible, the simplest would be that a pheromone is produced in the ovary at the time of ovulation, released to the bloodstream and accumulated in the urine. Provided that she has some control over the timing of urine release, such a mechanism would enable the ovulated female to efficiently signal to the territorial male that she is ready to spawn.

Despite the considerable information on where and when sex phero-mones are produced in fish, surprisingly little is known of their chemical nature. This is unfortunate, for having access to a pure pheromone would greatly aid research by allowing quantification of the stimulus. Only in two species, the zebra danio (*Brachydanio rerio*) and *Gobius jozo*, is there good evidence for the molecular identity of a reproductive pheromone in fish. In both cases, the pheromones are steroid glucuronides, metabolites formed in the gonads by the addition of glucuronic acid to the steroid molecule. This conjugation increases solubility in water, an important feature for a waterborne pheromone.

In *Gobius*, the steroid glucuronide—etiocholanolone glucuronide—is produced by the territorial male (Colombo et al., 1982). The androgenic Leydig cells of the testes are gathered into large mesorchial glands evidently specialized for pheromone synthesis. This is one of the few examples in fish of structural modification associated with production of pheromone. When female *Gobius* ovulate, they are attracted to synthetic etiocholanolone glucuronide and in some cases will oviposit.

In female zebra danios, steroid glucuronides which attract males are produced in the ovary shortly after ovulation (van den Hurk and Lambert, 1983). However, there is no indication here of the structural specialization for pheromone production seen in the goby testis. In their studies of sex-pheromone production in female zebra danios, van den Hurk and Lambert first demonstrated that the pheromonal activity of a water-soluble ovarian extract was associated with a fraction containing glucuronides, and not with fractions containing steroid sulphates, steroid phosphates, or unconjugated steroids. They then attempted to identify the glucuronide(s) responsible for the activity of the ovarian extract by observing the behavior of males exposed to synthetic glucuronides. When each glucuronide was tested by itself, only estradiol glucuronide was effective in attracting males, and even then the response was minimal. However, when estradiol glucuronide was combined with testosterone glucuronide, which by itself was completely ineffective, the response of males was markedly increased. As the responses to combinations of these synthetic steroids were never as strong as those evoked by the total glucuronide complement extracted from ovulated ovaries, van den Hurk and Lambert suggested that the natural female pheromone in zebra danios is likely a complex glucuronide mixture.

The possibility of a multichemical sex pheromone in female zebra danios has several important implications for further attempts at pheromone identification. The first concerns the problem of identifying complex pheromones. The positive interaction between estradiol and testosterone glucuronides was uncovered only because both were suspected of being components of the active ovarian fraction known to contain glucuronides. However, as testosterone glucuronide is inactive when tested alone, it is entirely possible that other components of the proposed *glucuronide* mixture are not glucuronides and are contained in inactive ovarian fractions. In other words, if full activity of a fish sex pheromone depends on the interaction of unrelated chemicals, identification of these chemicals may prove extremely difficult.

The second issue raised by the possibility of complex sex pheromones is that the message transmitted could be changed not only by increasing the concentration, as would be expected in the case of a single chemical pheromone, but also by modifying the chemical mixture. In goldfish, for example, water from ovulated females is more attractive to males than is water from mature, nonovulated females, although males are attracted to both water sources (Colombo et al., 1982; Sorensen et al., 1986). Unfortunately, nothing is known of the chemical basis of these attractions. Males may prefer ovulated to nonovulated females simply because the ovaries of ovulated females produce more of the same chemical or mixture of chemicals. Alternatively, the pheromone from nonovulated females, presumably signalling "female goldfish" to the male, may receive an additional component at the time of ovulation, changing the message to "ovulated female goldfish."

Some very indirect evidence suggests this may be the case. Male goldfish can be stimulated to court hypophysectomized males which have been fed a diet containing estradiol (Yamazaki and Watanabe, 1979); the estradiol treatment presumably stimulates production of a "female" pheromone. On the other hand, male goldfish in an open-field maze exhibit minimal response to water from females which have not ovulated, but show strong and indistinguishable responses to water either from ovulated females or from nonovulated females injected with PGs (Sorensen et al., 1986). Presumably the PG treatment stimulates release of an "ovulatory" pheromone.

If female fish release distinct pheromones to indicate their gender and ovulatory condition, a problem arises when the protocol for characterizing the "ovulatory pheromone" simply involves measuring the attraction of males to various chemical fractions. Unless the behavioral assay can distinguish male responses to an ovulatory odor from simple attraction to females, it cannot be claimed that an active fraction contains the "ovulatory" pheromone.

SUMMARY

Considering that many important contributions to our understanding of hormonal and pheromonal function in fish reproductive behavior have been made quite recently, it seems entirely reasonable to expect that there soon will be greatly increased research activity in this important area of vertebrate reproductive psychobiology.

In the case of female reproductive behaviors, it will be important to determine whether prostaglandin regulation of female sexual activity is widespread among the externally fertilizing fishes, and how this mechanism for behavioral control varies among those species employing it. Perhaps of equal importance is the question of how the presumably ancestral prostaglandin regulation of female sexual behavior in externally fertilizing species might have given rise to sex-steroid control of female behavior in those species which have evolved internal fertilization. As discussed by Liley and Stacey (1983), some insight into this problem might be gained by examining those oviparous species which exhibit courtship or copulatory behaviors prior to ovulation. On a more practical level, certain kinds of research on the sexual behaviors of externally fertilizing species should be greatly facilitated by the use of prostaglandins to induce female sexual activity, for it no longer will be necessary to use only females which are ovulated.

Although reproductive behaviors in male fish have been shown to be stimulated by sex-steroid hormones, it is not yet known which steroids are involved, or whether different aspects of male reproductive behaviors (aggression, nest-building, spawning, parental care) might be regulated by different steroids. Rapid hormonal changes induced by sexual stimuli so far have been demonstrated in only the goldfish and white sucker, species which exhibit quite similar spawning strategies. It remains to be determined what functions these rapid hormonal changes might perform and whether sexual stimuli induce similar hormonal change in species with different spawning strategies.

Our understanding of sex-pheromone function in fish has been hampered to a considerable extent by a lack of information on the chemical identity of sex pheromones. Recent evidence that sex pheromones in two fish species are steroid glucuronides of gonadal origin should stimulate further research to determine how these pheromones are synthesized and released, and how they exert their behavioral effects.

ACKNOWLEDGMENTS

The author gratefully acknowledges both his financial support (Grant A2903) from the Natural Sciences and Engineering Research Council of Canada (NSERC) and the helpful comments of Dr. P.W. Sorensen on an earlier draft of the manuscript. I also thank Diane Hollingdale for preparing Figures 2.3, 2.10, and 2.11.

REFERENCES

ADKINS-REGAN, E. (1981) Hormone specificity, androgen metabolism, and social behavior. Amer. Zool. *21*:257–271.

BEHRMAN, H.R. (1979) Prostaglandins in hypothalamo-pituitary and ovarian function. Ann. Rev. Physiol. *41*:685–700.

BILLARD, R., A. FOSTIER, C. WEIL, and B. BRETON (1982) Endocrine control of spermatogenesis in fish. Can. J. Fish. Aquatic Sci. *39*:65–79.

BRETT, B.L.H., and D.J. GROSSE (1982) A reproductive pheromone in the Mexican poeciliid fish *Poecilia chica*. Copeia, pp. 219–223.

CALLARD, G.V. (1983) Androgen and estrogen actions in the vertebrate brain. Amer. Zool. *23*:607–620.

CHEN, L.C., and R.L. MARTINICH (1975) Pheromonal stimulation and metabolite inhibition of ovulation in the zebrafish, *Brachydanio rerio*. Fish. Bull. *73*:889–894.

COLE, K.S., and N.E. STACEY (1984) Prostaglandin induction of spawning behavior in *Cichlasoma bimaculatum* (Pisces Cichlidae). Horm. Behav. *18*:235–248.

COLOMBO, L., P.C. BELVEDERE, A. MARCONATO, and F. BENTIVEGNA (1982) Pheromones in teleost fish. In *Proc. Int'l. Symp. Reprod. Physiol. Fish*. C.J.J. Richter and H.J.Th. Goos, eds., pp. 84–94, Pudoc, Wageningen, Netherlands.

CREWS, D., and R. SILVER (1985) Reproductive physiology and behavior interactions in nonmammalian vertebrates. In *Handbook of Behavioral Neurobiology*, Vol. 7. N. Adler, D. Pfaff, and R.W. Goy, eds., pp. 101–182, Plenum Press, New York.

DEMSKI, L.S., and P.J. HORNBY (1982) Hormonal control of fish reproductive behavior: brain-gonadal steroid interactions. Can. J. Fish. Aquatic Sci. *39*:36–47.

DEMSKI, L.S., and R.G. NORTHCUTT (1983) The terminal nerve: a new chemosensory system in vertebrates? Science *220*:435–437.

DIAKOW, C., and A. NEMIROFF (1981) Vasotocin, prostaglandin, and female reproductive behavior in the frog, *Rana pipiens*. Horm. Behav. *15*:86–93.

DIAKOW, C., and D. RAIMONDI (1981) Physiology of *Rana pipiens* reproductive behavior: a proposed mechanism for inhibition of the release call. Amer. Zool. *21*:295–304.

FOSTIER, A., B. JALABERT, R. BILLARD, B. BRETON, and Y. ZOHAR (1983) The gonadal steroids. In *Fish Physiology*, Vol. IXA, *Endocrine Tissues and Hormones*.

W.S. Hoar, D.J. Randall, and E.M. Donaldson, eds., pp. 277–372, Academic Press, New York.

GOETZ, F.W. (1983) Hormonal control of oocyte final maturation and ovulation in fishes. In *Fish Physiology*, Vol. IXB, *Behavior and Fertility Control*. W.S. Hoar, D.J. Randall, and E.M. Donaldson, eds., pp. 117–170, Academic Press, New York.

HONDA, H. (1980) Female sex pheromone of the loach, *Misgurnus anguillicaudatus*, involved in courtship behavior. Bull. Jap. Soc. Sci. Fish. *46*:1109–1112.

IRVING, S.M., R.W. GOY, R.V. HANING, and G.A. DAVIS (1981) Prostaglandins, clonidine and sexual receptivity in the guinea pig. Brain Res. *204*:65–77.

KOYAMA, Y., M. SATOU, Y. OKA, and K. UEDA (1984) Involvement of the telencephalic hemispheres and the preoptic area in sexual behavior of the male goldfish, *Carassius auratus*: a brain-lesion study. Behav. Neural Biol. *40*:70–86.

KYLE, A.L., N.E. STACEY, R.E. PETER, and R. BILLARD (1985) Elevations in gonadotropin concentrations and milt volumes as a result of spawning behavior in the goldfish. Gen. Comp. Endocrinol. *57*:10–22.

LEE, C.T., and D.W. INGERSOLL (1979) Social chemosignals in five Belontiidae (Pisces) species. J. Comp. Physiol. Psychol. *93*:1171–1181.

LILEY, N.R. (1982) Chemical communication in fish. Can. J. Fish. Aquatic Sci. *39*:22–35.

LILEY, N.R., and W.P. WISHLOW (1974) The interaction of endocrine and experiential factors in the regulation of sexual behavior in the female guppy *Poecilia reticulata*. Behaviour *48*:185–214.

LILEY, N.R., and N.E. STACEY (1983) Hormones, pheromones, and reproductive behavior in fish. In *Fish Physiology*, Vol. IXB, *Behavior and Fertility Control*. W.S. Hoar, D.J. Randall, and E.M. Donaldson, eds., pp. 1–63, Academic Press, New York.

LILEY, N.R., and E.S.P. TAN (1985) The induction of spawning behavior in *Puntius gonionotus* (Bleeker) by treatment with prostaglandin $PGF_{2\alpha}$. J. Fish Biol. *26*:491–502.

MARRONE, B.L., J.F. RODRIGUEZ-SIERRA, and H.H. FEDER (1979) Differential effects of prostaglandins on lordosis behavior in female guinea pigs and rats. Biol. Reprod. *20*:853–861.

MEYER, J.H., and N.R. LILEY (1982) Hormonal control of pheromone production in the guppy (*Poecilia reticulata* Peters). Can. J. Zool. *60*:1505–1510.

POLLACK, E.I., L.R. BECKER, and K. HAYNES (1978) Sensory control of mating in the blue gourami, *Trichogaster trichopterus* (Pisces, Belontiidae). Behav. Biol. *22*:92–103.

SCOTT, A.P., D.S. MACKENZIE, and N.E. STACEY (1984) Endocrine changes during natural spawning in the white sucker, *Catostomus commersoni*. II. Steroid hormones. Gen. Comp. Endocrinol. *56*:349–359.

SORENSEN, P.W., N.E. STACEY, and P. NAIDU (1986) Release of spawning pheromone(s) by naturally ovulated and prostaglandin-injected, nonovulated female goldfish. In *Chemical Signals in Vertebrates, Vol. IV: Ecology, Evolution and Comparative Biology*. D. Duvall, D. Muller-Schwarze, and R.M. Silverstein, eds., pp. 149–154, Plenum Press, New York.

STACEY, N.E. (1977) The regulation of spawning behavior in the female goldfish, *Carassius auratus*. Ph.D. Thesis, University of British Columbia, Vancouver, B.C., Canada.

STACEY, N.E. (1984) Clonidine inhibits female spawning behavior in ovulated and prostaglandin-treated goldfish. Pharm. Biochem. Behav. *20*:887–891.

STACEY, N.E., and N.R. LILEY (1974) Regulation of spawning behavior in the female goldfish. Nature (*London*) *247*:71–72.

STACEY, N.E., A.F. COOK, and R.E. PETER (1979) Ovulatory surge of gonadotropin in the goldfish, *Carassius auratus*. Gen. Comp. Endocrinol. *37*:246–249.

STACEY, N.E., and F.W. GOETZ (1982) Role of prostaglandins in fish reproduction. Can. J. Fish. Aquatic Sci. *39*:92–98.

STACEY, N.E., and A.S. HOURSTON (1982) Spawning and feeding behavior of captive Pacific herring, *Clupea harengus pallasi*. Can. J. Fish. Aquatic Sci. *39*:489–498.

STACEY, N.E., and A.L. KYLE (1983) Effects of olfactory tract lesions on sexual and feeding behavior in the goldfish. Physiol. Behav. *30*:621–628.

STACEY, N.E., A.L. KYLE, and N.R. LILEY (1986) Fish reproductive pheromones. In *Chemical Signals in Vertebrates, Vol. IV: Ecology, Evolution and Comparative Biology*. D. Duvall, D. Muller-Schwarze, and R.M. Silverstein, eds., pp. 117–133, Plenum Press, New York..

TAVOLGA, W.N. (1956) Visual, chemical and sound stimuli as cues in the sex discriminatory behavior of the gobiid fish *Bathygobius soporator*. Zoologica *41*:49–64.

VAN DEN HURK, R., and J.G.D. LAMBERT (1983) Ovarian steroid glucuronides function as sex pheromones for female zebrafish, *Brachydanio rerio*. Can. J. Zool. *61*:2381–2387.

VILLARS, T.A., and M. BURDICK (1982) Rapid decline in the behavioral response of female paradise fish to prostaglandin treatment. Amer. Zool. *22*:4948.

VILLARS, T.A., N. HALE, and D. CHAPNICK (1985) Prostaglandin $F_{2\alpha}$ stimulates reproductive behavior of female paradise fish (*Macropodus opercularis*). Horm. Behav. *19*:21–35.

VON BARTHELD, C.S., D.L. MEYER, Z. FIEBIG, and S.O.E. EBBESSON (1984) Central connections of the olfactory bulb in the goldfish, *Carassius auratus*. Cell Tiss. Res. *238*:475–487.

WEINTRAUB, A.S., D.B. KELLEY, and R.S. BOCKMAN (1985) Prostaglandin E2 induces receptive behavior in female *Xenopus laevis*. Horm. Behav. *19*:386–399.

WHITTIER, J.M., and D. CREWS (1986) Effects of prostaglandin $F_{2\alpha}$ on sexual behavior and ovarian function in female garter snakes (*Thamnophis sirtalis parietalis*). Endocrinology (in press).

WILSON, E.O. (1975) *Sociobiology: The New Synthesis*. Harvard University Press, Cambridge, Mass.

YAMAZAKI, F., and K. WATANABE (1979) The role of sex hormones in sex recognition during spawning behavior of the goldfish, *Carassius auratus* L. Proc. Indian Natl. Sci. Acad. Part B *45*:505–511

THREE
Behavioral Actions
of Neurohypophysial Peptides

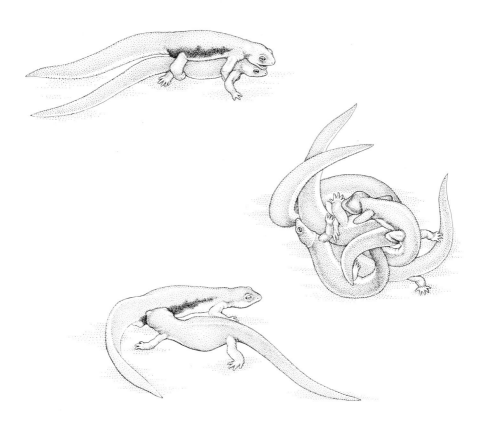

Frank L. Moore
Department of Zoology
Oregon State University
Corvallis, Oregon

Arginine vasotocin (AVT), arginine vasopressin (AVP), and oxytocin (OXY) are among the first hormones to be isolated and identified in vertebrates (Norris, 1985). These three hormones are often referred to as neurohypophysial hormones, because they are stored in and secreted from the neurohypophysis, a neurohemal organ that is sometimes called the pars nervosa or posterior pituitary gland.

There are striking structural similarities among the neurohypophysial hormones. The primary structure of AVT differs from AVP and OXY by only a single amino acid (Figure 3.1). Furthermore, AVT, AVP, and OXY each contain nine amino acids that are linked together by cysteine residues which form a six-amino-acid ring with a three-residue tail. Each of these peptides is synthesized from a larger precursor peptide that contains neurophysin, a presumed carrier molecule. These biochemical similarities among AVT, AVP, and OXY have stimulated many questions about the evolution of this family of peptides.

Studies of the evolutionary relationship among these neurohypophysial hormones take into account not only the primary structures of these peptides, but also their distribution among the vertebrate taxa. Of particular importance is the fact that AVT is found in all vertebrates, from primitive fishes to mammals, whereas AVP and OXY are restricted to mammals (Figure 3.2). Most scientists agree, as a result, that AVT is an ancestral neuropeptide and that AVT gave rise to AVP through divergent evolution (Acher, 1983; 1985).

By comparing the behavioral functions of AVT in the nonmammalian vertebrates with the behavioral functions of AVP and OXY in mammals, it is possible to gain insights into how hormones and their functions evolve. Although the traditional functions of these hormones (hydromineral balance, cardiovascular change, milk-ejection, uterine contraction, etc.) have been the focus of much research, there is increasing evidence for behavioral actions of AVT, AVP, and OXY in species from each major class of vertebrates.

The reports of behavioral effects of AVP and OXY in mammals are paralleled by reports of behavioral effects of AVT in nonmammalian vertebrates. These reports are reviewed in this chapter in order to address the following questions about the evolution of the role of neurohypophysial peptides in the control of behavior:

1. Are the behavioral actions of AVP and OXY in mammals newly acquired functions, or are there evolutionary precedents for behavioral actions by neurohypophysial peptides?
2. Do neurohypophysial peptides have neurotransmitterlike functions

SCHEMATIC OF ARGININE VASOPRESSIN

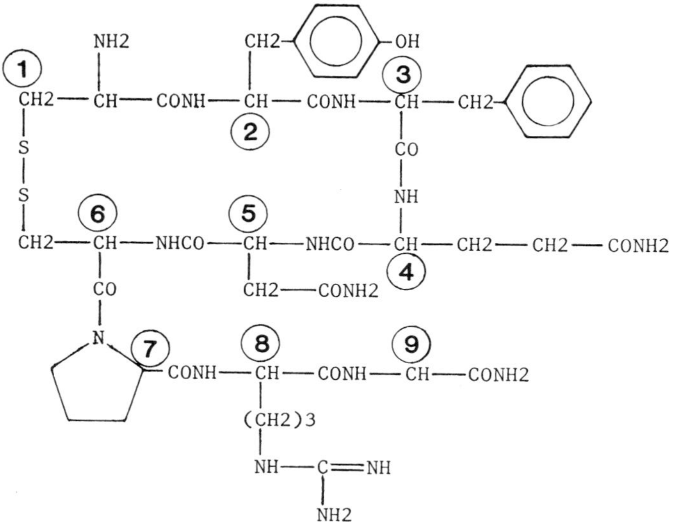

HORMONE	AMINO ACID SEQUENCE
	1 2 3 4 5 6 7 8 9
Arginine Vasotocin	Cys-Tyr-Ile-Gln-Asn-Cys-Pro-Arg-Gly-NH2
Arginine Vasopressin	Cys-Tyr-Phe-Gln-Asn-Cys-Pro-Arg-Gly-NH2
Oxytocin	Cys-Tyr-Ile-Gln-Asn-Cys-Pro-Leu-Gly-NH2

FIGURE 3.1. Schematic representation of the primary structure of arginine vasopressin, a nonapeptide that occurs in most mammals. The numbers in the schematic correspond with the numbers at the bottom of the figure, indicating the amino acid sequence for three related nonapeptides. Note that the primary structures for arginine vasotocin, arginine vasopressin, and oxytocin differ only at positions 3 and 8.

and mediate behavioral responses by acting directly on neurons in the brain?

3. What are the evolutionary selective pressures which favor multiple behavioral regulators of particular behaviors?

BEHAVIORAL EFFECTS OF AVT, AVP, AND OXY

Nonmammalian Vertebrates

Of the neurohypophysial hormones that are present in nonmammalian vertebrates, only AVT has been associated strongly with behavioral actions. The other nonmammalian neurohypophysial hormones, such as mesotocin

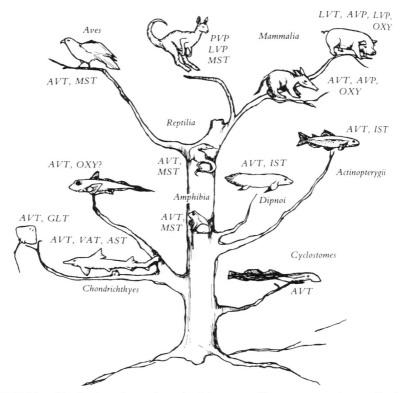

FIGURE 3.2. Distribution of neurohypophysial nonapeptides among vertebrates. Evolutionary relationships, as represented by the tree, indicate that an ancestral amphibian gave rise to extant amphibians, reptiles, birds, and mammals. AST, aspargtocin; AVP, arginine vasopressin; AVT, arginine vasotocin; GLT, glumitocin; IST, isotocin; LVP, lysine vasopressin; LVT, lysine vasotocin; MST, mesotocin; OXY, oxytocin; VAT, valitocin. (Reprinted with permission from Norris, 1985)

and isotocin, have not been linked to behavioral actions, most likely because these hormones are not readily available and have not been studied extensively. There is evidence that AVT can activate particular behaviors in certain species of fish, amphibians, reptiles, and birds. The studies of amphibians (frogs and salamanders) provide the best evidence for behavioral actions of AVT.

In amphibians, AVT regulates sexual behaviors. Evidence of a functional link between amphibian sexual behaviors and AVT comes from two species: leopard frogs (*Rana pipiens*; Diakow, 1978) and rough-skinned newts (*Taricha granulosa*; Moore, 1983). Laboratory experiments indicate that AVT stimulates sexual receptivity in female leopard frogs and male courtship behaviors in rough-skinned newts.

Diakow (1978) was the first to demonstrate an effect of AVT on an amphibian sexual behavior, the "release call" of female leopard frogs. The release call consists of a repetitive series of vibrations and vocalizations that apparently communicate to a sexually active male that he has clasped an unreceptive female or a conspecific male. Female frogs that are sexually receptive remain silent. When female leopard frogs are injected with synthetic AVT (or a suspension of whole pituitary gland), release calls are inhibited (Diakow and Raimondi, 1981). This inhibition of release calls by AVT is interpreted as evidence that AVT enhances sexual receptivity in female frogs.

In rough-skinned newts, the behavior that has been studied is the amplectic clasping behavior (Figure 3.3). This is the first overt component of the mating sequence and is used by sexually active males to "capture" prospective female partners. When male rough-skinned newts are injected with synthetic AVT, the incidence of amplectic clasping increases significantly (Moore and Zoeller, 1979; Moore and Miller, 1983; Zoeller and Moore, 1982). This increase has been observed in intact males and in castrated males that are treated with testosterone and dihydrotestosterone.

The minimally effective dose of AVT depends on the mode of administration. If AVT is administered systemically by an injection into the abdominal cavity, from 10 to 100 μg of AVT can activate newt clasping behaviors. In contrast, if AVT is administered intracranially by a microinjection into the third ventricle of male newts, as little as 1 ng of AVT can stimulate sexual behaviors (Moore and Miller, 1983). Thus, newts are at least 10,000 times more sensitive to AVT that is administered intracranially

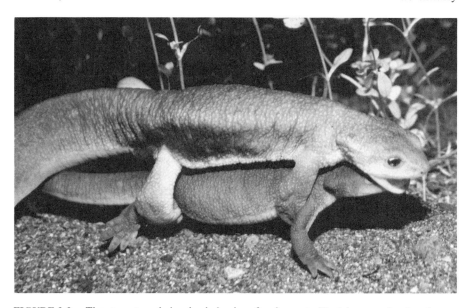

FIGURE 3.3. The stereotyped clasping behavior of male newts (*Taricha granulosa*) makes an excellent model for studying the neuroendocrine basis of reproductive behaviors. This photograph shows a male newt clasping a female in amplexus and rubbing his chin against the nares of the female. The up-lifted head of the female signals sexual receptivity and precedes spermatophore transfer. (Photo by author)

than systemically, an observation which suggests that AVT is acting on cells in the brain rather than at some peripheral site.

If AVT is indeed a necessary component in the activation of newt sexual behaviors, experimental suppression of endogenous AVT activity would be expected to inhibit sexual behaviors. This is what was found in male rough-skinned newts, using two separate approaches to suppress endogenous AVT activity. In one experiment an antiserum to AVT was injected into the ventricle of the brain (Moore and Miller, 1983). Sexual behavior was suppressed in male newts. Thus, antiserum administered into the brain is thought to bind to the endogenous AVT and thereby reduce the amount of AVT that is available to the receptors. In a second experiment, a synthetic antagonist to AVT [d(CH2)5Tyr(Me)AVP] was injected into the ventricle of the brain, and the incidence of amplectic clasping decreased significantly (Moore and Miller, 1983). This chemical is thought to compete with endogenous AVT for available receptor sites and thereby reduce the AVT responses.

Furthermore, one would expect that if AVT regulates sexual behaviors in male rough-skinned newts, the concentration of AVT in at least some regions of the brain will vary with changes in the occurrence of newt sexual behaviors. In two separate studies, that is what was found. One study investigated whether seasonal changes in AVT are correlated with seasonal changes in sexual behavior; the other investigated whether, on a particular date, males that exhibit sexual behaviors have higher levels of AVT in particular brain areas than males not exhibiting sexual behaviors. Both studies measured AVT in specific brain regions in male rough-skinned newts, using the microdissection procedures of Palkovits and Brownstein (1982; Figure 3.4) and a radio-immunoassay that is specific for AVT (Zoeller and Moore, 1986a).

For the seasonal study, AVT was measured in the optic tectum of male rough-skinned newts that were collected during each season of the year (Zoeller and Moore, 1986b). As can be seen in Figure 3.5, the concentration of AVT in the optic tectum begins to increase during February and reaches peak levels in April. Since male newts are most sexually active from February through April, the concentration of AVT in the optic tectum is seasonally correlated with the occurrence of sexual behaviors. Until comparable studies are performed with other animals, it will not be known whether a seasonal correlation between behavioral state and brain neuropeptide content is the exception among vertebrates—or the rule.

Further evidence of the causal relation between AVT and sexual behavior comes from measurements of AVT in particular brain areas of male newts that are either sexually active or inactive. Near the end of the breeding season, when some of the males have become sexually inactive, newly captured male newts were placed in pondside tanks containing sexually attractive females. The behaviors of the males were closely monitored, and males were classified as either sexually active (those that exhibited amplectic clasping) or sexually inactive (those that failed to exhibit any sexual behaviors during a one-hour behavior test). Brain AVT levels were measured in brain tissue from each group of males.

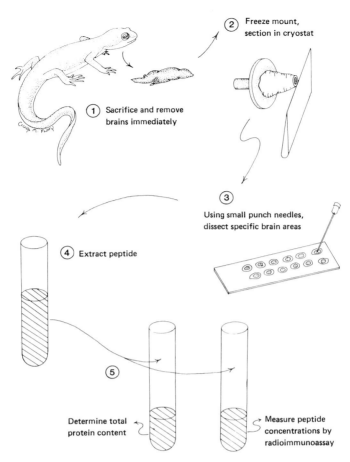

FIGURE 3.4. Microdissection procedure uses frozen sections of brain tissue mounted on glass slides. Concentrations of particular chemical messengers—for example, arginine vasotocin—are determined by radioimmunoassay.

As can be seen in Figure 3.6, AVT levels are significantly higher in sexually active than in inactive male newts, particularly in the dorsal preoptic area, optic tectum, cerebral spinal fluid (third ventricle), and ventral infundibulum. AVT levels in other areas, such as the interpeduncular nucleus and dorsal infundibulum, were no higher in the sexually active than in inactive males. These data support the conclusion that endogenous AVT is causally related to the male's propensity to exhibit sexual behaviors.

To summarize this research on amphibians, three different types of evidence indicate that AVT is involved in activating sexual behaviors. Nanogram injections of synthetic AVT stimulate the behavior; injections of an AVT antagonist or AVT antiserum inhibit the behavior; brain concentrations of AVT are higher in sexually active than inactive males on a seasonal or daily basis.

Evidence that AVT is involved in regulating fish behaviors comes from

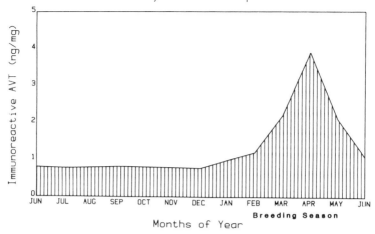

Seasonal Study: AVT in Optic Tectum

FIGURE 3.5. Seasonal changes in immunoreactive arginine vasotocin (AVT) were determined using microdissection/radioimmunoassay procedures on male rough-skinned newts (*Taricha granulosa*). Elevated concentrations of AVT occur in the optic tectum during the months when male newts have the highest propensity to exhibit courtship behaviors. (From data in Zoeller and Moore, 1986b)

studies with killifish, *Fundulus heteroclitus* (Wilhelmi et al., 1955; Pickford and Strecker, 1977). The S-shaped spawning reflex, exhibited by both male and female killifish, can be elicited by systemic injections of AVT and other neurohypophysial peptides. There are differences, however, between the AVT-induced behavior and the behavior pattern that occurs during spontaneous spawning. When these fish spawn, the S-shaped spawning reflex is oriented toward the sexual partner in order to facilitate external fertilization. When killifish are injected with AVT, however, the S-shaped reflex occurs independently of any sexual partner. Thus, AVT appears to mediate this behavioral response by activating the reflex, not by increasing the propensity to respond to sexual stimuli.

In reptiles, published reports on the behavioral effects of AVT are limited to behaviors associated with oviposition and parturition. In several lizard species—*Hemidactylus frenatus, Lepidodactylus lugubris, Sceloporus aeneus,* and *Sceloporus jarrovi*—the administration of synthetic AVT not only induces oviposition or parturition, but also elicits associated behaviors (Guillette and Jones, 1982; Jones and Guillette, 1982). For example, when gravid *H. frenatus* and *L. lugubris* are injected with AVT, they climb the cage walls and remain perched there until eggs are deposited. These geckoes normally deposit eggs in trees, so this climbing behavior probably represents the behaviors of nest-site selection.

In birds, AVT has been associated with two types of behaviors: sexual behaviors and imprinting. Kihlstrom and Danninge (1972) reported that in domestic fowl (*Gallus domesticus*) and pigeons (*Columba livia*) the fre-

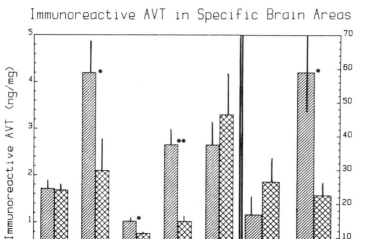

FIGURE 3.6. Immunoreactive arginine vasotocin (AVT) concentrations were determined using microdissection/radioimmunoassay procedures on male rough-skinned newts (*Taricha granulosa*). In specific brain regions, AVT concentrations are significantly higher in sexually active than inactive males, particularly in the dorsal preoptic area (dPOA), optic tectum (OpTect), third ventricle (CSF), and ventral infundibulum (vInf). Other brain regions—such as the ventral preoptic area (vPOA), interpeduncular nucleus (InPN), and dorsal infundibulum (dInf)—apparently have AVT concentrations that are independent of the behavioral state of the male, indicating regional specificity in functions for this neuropeptide. (Data from Zoeller and Moore, unpublished)

quency and duration of copulatory behaviors are significantly increased by injections of AVT or OXY. Evidence that AVT may be involved in imprinting in birds comes from a few studies with ducklings (Martin and van Wimersma Greidanus, 1979). Imprinting is the phenomenon whereby precocial birds learn to recognize their mother by approaching and following a moving object during a critical period after hatching. In newly hatched Pekin ducks, injections of an AVT analog altered the imprinting phenomenon in such a way to support the interpretation that this neuropeptide stimulated information retrieval (Martin and van Wimersma Greidanus, 1979). Thus, although much yet remains to be learned about the behavioral effects of AVT in birds, these two studies provide evidence that AVT may enhance male sexual behaviors and memory processes in birds.

Mammals

There is increasing evidence that in mammals both AVP and OXY have behavioral actions, in addition to having traditional actions such as antidiuresis and milk ejection. Research on these behavioral actions is abundant and varied—from the recent studies of sexual and maternal behaviors to the large volume of research on memory and learning processes.

Sexual and maternal behaviors. Although the phenomenon has received relatively little research attention, recent evidence indicates that OXY and AVP may modulate copulatory behaviors in mammals. Arletti et al. (1985) report that the administration of synthetic OXY to sexually active male rats improves copulatory performance; it significantly shortens both the ejaculation latency and postejaculatory interval during controlled tests for copulatory performance. Because rats are more sensitive to intracranial than systemic administration, OXY appears to mediate this behavioral response by acting on the central nervous system and not by acting on peripheral targets such as the vas deferens.

In contrast to OXY, AVP appears to interfere with sexual performance. When male rabbits are injected with AVP, ejaculatory latency increases (Kihlstrom and Agmo, 1974). Likewise, in a study measuring lordosis quotients in female rats—a standard method to quantify female sexual receptivity—AVP administration significantly inhibited sexual receptivity (Sodersten et al., 1983). These authors also report that the behavioral response to AVP (1) does not occur in female rats that are pretreated with an antiserum to AVP; (2) is not observed when closely related peptides such as lysine vasopressin are used instead of AVP; (3) occurs in response to intracranial administration of nanogram quantities of AVP. These observations support the conclusion that AVP acts specifically on the brain to inhibit sexual receptivity in female rats.

Recent studies indicate that OXY may be involved in the regulation of maternal behaviors in mammals. Intracerebroventricular infusion OXY into virgin female rats that have been ovariectomized and estrogen-primed can elicit maternal behaviors toward foster pups (Pedersen et al., 1982). Furthermore, brain injections of a synthetic OXY antagonist or an antiserum to OXY significantly suppress maternal behavior in female rats (Fahrbach et al., 1985). The role of OXY in eliciting maternal behaviors in rats is still controversial, because several laboratories have failed to observe any effects of OXY injections on rat maternal behaviors (Rubin et al., 1983; Bolwerk and Swanson, 1984).

In addition to these investigations on sexual behaviors and maternal behaviors, other studies have demonstrated that AVP and OXY can influence a variety of adaptive behaviors. For example, in mice, the administration of AVP or OXY can elicit hyperactivity, foraging, grooming, scratching, and squeaking (Delanoy et al., 1978). In rats, AVP injections enhance exploratory behaviors and other components of open-field test measurements (e.g., King et al., 1982). When hamsters are injected with AVP into the medial preoptic area, they exhibit a stereotyped flank-marking behavior (Ferris et al., 1984). These studies provide evidence that AVP and OXY may be involved in a variety of adaptive behaviors, but firm conclusions must be reserved until these behavioral responses have been more thoroughly researched.

Memory and learning. Studies on the effects of AVP and OXY on memory and learning are varied in experimental approaches, utilizing a wide range of learning paradigms and numerous analogs of naturally occurring peptides (see reviews by deWied and Jolles, 1982; Bloom, 1982). Although these studies are not without controversy, there is growing agreement that substances structurally related to AVP and OXY can influence measurements of learning and memory. In general, AVP appears to enhance the storage and retrieval of information, whereas OXY appears to impair these processes.

Most studies of the effects of AVP-like peptides on memory and learning measure the latencies to extinction of either a conditioned avoidance response or a passive avoidance situation. For example, an experiment with a conditioned avoidance response would involve training rats to jump onto a pole in response to a flash of light (the conditioned stimulus) in order to avoid an electrical shock (the unconditioned stimulus). Following a training period, the rate of extinction is determined by recording the persistence of the pole-jump response to the conditioned stimulus in the absence of the unconditioned stimulus.

The evidence that AVP enhances learning comes from studies in which this peptide is administered at the time of the training sessions. For example, deWied (1976) demonstrated that a single subcutaneous injection of AVP during the last training session for the pole-jump response increases the resistance to extinction of this conditioned avoidance response. His interpretation is that AVP enhances the learning of the avoidance response by acting on information-consolidation processes.

On the other hand, the evidence that AVP enhances memory (the retrieval of information) comes from studies in which AVP is injected during the testing period. For example, the administration of AVP during the extinction trials results in increased resistance to extinction of the conditioned avoidance response. There are studies which demonstrate that the administration of AVP to rats reduces the rate of extinction of conditioned avoidance responses. Because some authors have suggested that the effects of AVP on conditioned avoidance situations might reflect some component of a fear or stress response, instead of learning and memory, a few studies have tested the effects of AVP on training with a positive reinforcer. For example, Bohus (1977) trained rats by reinforcing correct choices in a T-maze with access to sexually receptive female rats and found that injections of an AVP analog enhanced the learning of this positively reinforced behavior.

Several types of evidence suggest that the effects of AVP on measurements of learning and memory are mediated by central rather than peripheral actions. One type of evidence comes from studies which demonstrate that AVP is more effective when administered centrally than peripherally. For example, in deWied's (1976) investigation of the pole-jump avoidance response, rats showed a greater resistance to extinction of the response if injected intracranially, rather than systemically.

A second type of evidence comes from studies in which antiserum to AVP is administered in the brain in order to interfere with endogenous AVP activities. Passive avoidance behaviors can be retarded by intracranial, but not systemic, administration of antiserum to AVP (van Wimersma Greidanus, 1984). A third type of evidence comes from studies which compare the relative effectiveness of different synthetic analogs of AVP on behavioral responses and peripheral functions, such as memory effects compared to antidiuretic and vasopressor effects. Using synthetic analogs to AVP, deWied et al. (1984) demonstrated that certain analogs which were devoid of any apparent peripheral actions, significantly enhanced passive avoidance behaviors. All of these studies support the interpretation that AVP (and structurally related peptides) can enhance measurements of memory and learning by acting at the level of the brain.

There is also evidence that the levels of AVP in the brain are associated with the acquisition and retention of passive avoidance behaviors. The concentrations of immunoreactive AVP decrease in the hippocampus and increase in the cerebrospinal fluid immediately after the learning trial for passive avoidance (Laczi et al., 1983). These results indicate that the learning of passive avoidance behaviors is associated with central release of AVP.

In summary, the evidence that AVP is involved in the performance and retention of particular learned behaviors is fairly strong. The administration of AVP and related peptides improves performance, whereas the administration of antagonists or antiserum impairs it. Likewise, the acquisition of the avoidance behaviors is associated with changes in AVP content in specific brain areas. It seems reasonable to conclude that there are peptides in the brain—either AVP or peptides that are structurally related to AVP—that enhance the performance of certain learned behaviors.

A word of caution is in order, however. Clearly, many behaviors can be activated by the administration of AVT, AVP, or OXY under controlled experimental conditions. However, injection experiments alone do not prove that the peptide in question is actually involved in regulating the behavior. That is, the scientist may be seeing instead a pharmacological effect. This is analogous to the behavioral changes that are associated with the intake of alcohol. Behavioral changes may result, after alcohol intake, but alcohol is not the natural regulator of these behaviors. Similarly, pharmacological effects of administering neurohypophysial peptides may account for the observed behavioral changes yet not be involved in their normal regulation. For this reason, injection experiments should be followed by experiments in which the endogenous peptide activity is specifically suppressed and in which endogenous peptide levels are measured.

In experiments in which endogenous peptide levels have been measured—the regulation of newt sexual behavior by AVT and the modification of rat avoidance behaviors by AVP—the evidence demonstrates quite convincingly that these behaviors must be regulated, at least in part, by endogenous molecules which are structurally identical to, or similar to, AVT and AVP. Therefore, because neurohypophysial hormones can function as behaviorally active neuropeptides in newts and rats, the other behavioral responses to injections of AVT, AVP, or OXY warrant further investigations.

Evolution of the Behavioral Actions

Are there any evolutionary precedents for the behavioral actions of AVP and OXY in mammals? Yes, there is evidence that AVT functions as a behaviorally active neuropeptide in representative species of fish, amphibians, reptiles, and birds. There is even evidence from invertebrates; an AVT-like peptide appears to activate behaviors in *Aplysia*, a gastropod mollusc (Thornhill et al., 1981). If this proves to be true and if this molluscan AVT-like peptide is evolutionarily related to vertebrate AVT, then it would appear that the behavioral functions of these neuropeptides may have preceded the hormonal functions. In any case, there are definitely evolutionary precedents for behavioral actions of neurohypophysial hormones.

Certain types of behaviors are more often regulated by these neurohypophysial peptides than other types. In nonmammalian vertebrates, for example, AVT appears to be almost exclusively associated with sexual behaviors or the nest-site-selecting behaviors of reptiles. There are fundamental similarities, in terms of parental care, between the selection of a nest site in reptiles and maternal behaviors of mammals. Thus, there does appear to be some type of evolutionary conservation in the sense that neurohypophysial peptides are associated with sexual or maternal behaviors in species from each class of vertebrates.

This example of evolutionary conservation is not unique. Nature provides other cases wherein a particular peptide appears to control a particular type of behavior in diverse vertebrate taxa. For example, sexual behaviors of amphibians, reptiles, birds, and mammals have been shown to be enhanced by the administration of gonadotropin-releasing hormone (GnRH), another hypothalamic neuropeptide (Moore, 1983). This conservation of behavioral function across vertebrate taxa is similar to the well-documented conservation of the peripheral functions of vertebrate hormones (e.g., testosterone and male sexual behaviors in most vertebrates). As discussed later, the selective pressures that are associated with the acquisition of new behavioral functions and new homeostatic functions are interrelated.

What about the other behavioral responses to AVP and OXY that are unique to mammals, such as the miscellaneous adaptive behaviors? Does this mean that AVP and OXY have acquired new behavioral functions since the appearance of the first primitive mammals? Unfortunately, there are too few studies to answer these questions with any degree of confidence. For example, at this time, no studies have investigated the effects of AVT or any other neurohypophysial peptide on the performance of learned behaviors in any species of fish, amphibian, or reptile.

BRAIN ACTIONS OF NEUROHYPOPHYSIAL PEPTIDES

Given the above evidence that neurohypophysial hormones are involved in controlling particular behaviors, it is appropriate to question where and how these peptides modulate behaviors. While it may be decades before the answers to these questions are complete, some recent experimental results provide insights into where and how behaviors are controlled by AVT, AVP, and OXY.

Neuroanatomical Distribution

Although neurohypophysial peptides have been known for nearly half a century to be synthesized in brain neurons, recent studies indicate that their distribution in the brain is more widespread than previously suspected. Similarly, other peptide hormones—such as the pituitary and gastrointestinal peptides—have been found in neurons of the central nervous system (Krieger, 1983).

Two powerful techniques have identified the neuroanatomical distribution of neurohypophysial peptides, immunocytochemistry and microdissection with radioimmunoassay. The immunocytochemical technique employs antigen-antibody binding phenomena in order to visualize the location of AVT, AVP, or OXY on carefully prepared microscope slides of sectioned brain tissue. Immunocytochemistry provides good resolution and accurate detail about the anatomical sites, but it is limited by the specificity of the antisera. Antisera with low specificity will react with other peptides or with fragments of the peptide, misleading investigators. Immunocytochemistry also is not adequate for quantification of the peptides in the tissue.

The microdissection/radioimmunoassay procedure, as described in Figure 3.3, can quantify the amount of peptide in a particular anatomical location. This procedure also is limited by the specificity of the antisera, but the problems of specificity can be resolved by employing special extraction and purification procedures, such as reverse-phase high-pressure liquid chromatography. The microdissection/radioimmunoassay procedure, however, does not have the resolution of immunocytochemistry. Thus both techniques are useful.

Immunocytochemical studies confirm that neurohypophysial peptides are synthesized in cell bodies in the magnocellular neurosecretory system, which in mammals includes the supraoptic nucleus (SON), paraventricular nucleus (PVN), and parvocellular suprachiasmatic nucleus (SCN). These peptides are transported to the posterior pituitary gland, where they are stored until secreted into the blood (Silverman and Zimmerman, 1983). This pathway, of course, is critical to the traditional hormonal functions of the neurohypophysial hormones.

In addition to the neurohypophysial secretory system, AVP and OXY have been identified in a variety of other locations, some of which relate to the behavioral actions of these peptides (Doris, 1984). In mammals, AVP-

and OXY-containing cell bodies have been found in magnocellular nuclei (SON, PVN, and SCN) and in the medial amygdaloid nucleus and locus coeruleus. From the SON and PVN, AVP-containing fibers project to the substantia nigra, solitary tract nucleus, dorsal vagal nucleus, and substantia gelantinosa of the spinal cord (Doris, 1984). From the SCN, AVP-containing fibers enter the lateral septum, amygdala, thalamus, habenula, and brain stem. Microdissection procedures confirm the above observations and provide evidence that AVP and OXY are present in the thalamus, hippocampus, septum, amygdala, striatum, substantia nigra, cerebellum, medulla oblongata, globus pallidus, periaqueductal grey, locus coeruleus, and cerebral spinal fluid (Hawthorn et al., 1984).

Although there are fewer studies of the neuroanatomical distribution of neurohypophysial peptides in nonmammalian vertebrates compared to mammals, the evidence is still quite good that AVT is widely distributed in the brain. Immunocytochemical studies of fish, amphibians, and reptiles confirm that AVT-containing cell bodies are present in the magnocellular preoptic nucleus (PON) and that neuronal fibers project to the neurohypophysis (Schreibman and Halpern, 1980; Jokura and Urano, 1985). Microdissection/radioimmunoassay studies of rough-skinned newts provide evidence that AVT immunoreactivity occurs in many brain areas that are homologous to those listed above for mammals (Zoeller and Moore, 1986a).

Thus all vertebrates appear to have neurohypophysial peptides located in diverse structures in the brain, spinal cord, and cerebral spinal fluid. This neuroanatomical distribution is consistent with the notion that these peptides regulate behaviors by actions in the central nervous system which are independent of the systemic hormonal actions.

Independent Neurohypophysial Systems

A current hypothesis states that the secretion of AVP (or any other neurohypophysial peptide) into the blood is controlled independently of the secretion of AVP within the central nervous system. In support of this hypothesis, several recent studies in mammals showed that the concentrations of AVP and OXY in the cerebral spinal fluid fluctuate independently of the AVP and OXY concentrations in the plasma (Reppert et al., 1982). However, other studies fail to support the hypothesis; AVP concentrations in cerebral spinal fluid and plasma exhibited parallel changes following osmotic stress or hypoxia to rats and sheep (Stark et al., 1984).

In nonmammalian vertebrates, separate AVT systems appear to control hydromineral balance and sexual behaviors. A microdissection/radioimmunoassay study of rough-skinned newts (Zoeller and Moore, unpublished) showed changes in AVT content in response to osmotic stress in the ventral preoptic area, an area in which AVT content is not correlated with sexual behaviors. This suggests that newts have separate AVT systems in the brain—one associated with hydromineral balance (peripheral hormone function) and the other with sexual behavior (central behavioral function).

In summary, recent data with several species of mammals and one amphibian indicate that the neurohypophysial peptides which are secreted into the blood can be controlled separately from those which are secreted centrally. Such independence of peripheral and central neurohypophysial systems makes it theoretically possible for these peptides to have both traditional hormonal functions and central behavioral functions.

Direct Effects of Neuropeptides on Neurons

Given that neurohypophysial peptides are behaviorally active and are widely distributed in the brain, it is possible that they may have neurotransmitterlike functions in the brain. Neurotransmitters are usually defined as chemical messengers which act quickly and over short distances transiently to alter cell excitability. Neurotransmitters are distinguished from neuromodulators, which modify the response of a neuron to a distinct chemical input, and from neurohormones, which act on target cells that are at a distance from the site of release. Because these three categories of chemical messengers are defined by the mode of action, any given chemical messenger can theoretically function as neurotransmitter, neuromodulator, and neurohormone.

There is anatomical and electrophysiological evidence that, indeed, neurohypophysial peptides have neurotransmitterlike functions (Muhlethaler et al., 1984). Anatomical evidence comes from ultrastructural studies of the cellular and synaptic interactions between neurohypophysial-containing neurons and adjacent somata. For example, AVT-containing axon terminals in the goldfish brain possess ultrastructural arrangements and membrane specializations which are indicative of synaptic interactions (Cumming et al., 1982). Furthermore, specific neurons in the central nervous system possess receptors for neurohypophysial peptides (Brinton et al., 1984; Cornett and Dorsa, 1985).

Electrophysiological changes have been observed in neurons that are exposed to neurohypophysial peptides. Specific neurons in the hippocampus, locus coeruleus, and spinal cord are sensitive to iontophoretic application of AVP. For example, neurons in the rat hippocampus respond to AVP with a slow and prolonged enhancement in electrical activity; both spike discharge rate and excitatory postsynaptic potential increase (Mizuno et al., 1984). Likewise, the administration of AVP alters hippocampus neurons physiologically by modulating catecholamine turnover and synthesis (Kovacs et al., 1977). Studies of other neurons showed that dopamine secretion from the nucleus caudatus is enhanced by AVP (van Heuven-Nolsen and Versteeg, 1985). Therefore, it appears that neurohypophysial peptides can have neurotransmitterlike functions acting directly on neurons in the central nervous system.

However, important differences between neuropeptides and classic neurotransmitters exist. With classic neurotransmitters, like serotonin or dopamine, the electrophysiological state of target neurons is modulated rapidly and briefly; postsynaptic responses to classic neurotransmitters usually last for only fractions of a second. In contrast, certain neuropeptides have the capacity to alter excitability in target neurons for many minutes, even hours, after initial exposure (Mayeri et al., 1979).

The duration and type of response to a particular neuropeptide seems to depend upon target neuron. Studies with *Aplysia* indicate that one neuropeptide can cause several types of long-lasting responses, depending on the identity of the target neuron. In the abdominal ganglion of *Aplysia*, for example, the administration of egg-laying hormone causes target neuron R15 to have augmented bursts of action potentials and target neuron L3 to have prolonged inhibition of spontaneous activity (Mayeri et al., 1979).

Long-lasting neuronal responses to neuropeptides could be critical to the regulation of behaviors. Perhaps neuropeptides control particular behaviors by activating specific neurons in the central nervous system, sensory afferent pathways, and/or motor efferent pathways.

Studies show that the administration of neurohypophysial peptides can elicit certain behaviors in the absence of the normal releasing stimuli. For example, the spawning reflex of *F. heteroclitus* can be evoked in sexually isolated individuals by AVT injections (Pickford and Strecker, 1977). Even when appropriate sexual partners are present in the aquaria, AVT-injected fish do not orient the spawning behaviors toward a partner. This example and others are interpreted as evidence that neuropeptides can sometimes activate neuronal motor units directly, such as by activating central neurons which control motor efferent pathways.

Other studies, in contrast, indicate that neuropeptides can activate stereotyped behaviors by increasing or decreasing sensitivities to releasing stimuli. For example, AVT injections into male newts increases their responsiveness to female sexual stimuli. This example and others are interpreted as evidence that neuropeptides can sometimes influence the propensity to respond to external stimuli, perhaps by acting on neurons in the sensory afferent pathway or on central neurons which integrate sensory input. Additional research may support these interpretations, substantiating that neuropeptides can control behaviors by acting on neurons in the sensory, motor, and central pathways in the nervous system.

It will be interesting when researchers discover whether a particular neuropeptide acts on all levels of the nervous system or whether specific neuropeptides function predominantly as either transducers of sensory inputs or activators of motor outputs. Kelley (1980) provided evidence that testosterone, a steroid hormone, may influence sexual behaviors in amphibians by acting on sensory, motor, and central neuronal units.

In summary, there is evidence that neurohypophysial peptides occur in extrahypothalamic neurons in the brain and spinal cord and that these peptides can act directly on neurons with neurotransmitterlike functions. Neuropeptides may act on sensory, motor, and/or central neuronal units. Characteristics of neuropeptides, including prolonged neuronal responses, make them candidates for the neurophysiological regulation of behavioral states.

EVOLUTION OF BEHAVIORAL REGULATORS

Although there is good evidence that neurohypophysial peptides regulate a variety of behaviors, none of these behaviors is thought to be regulated by just one neuropeptide. It is probably more typical that a suite of chemical messengers (steroid hormones, neuropeptides, classic neurotransmitters, and prostaglandins) participate in the regulation of particular behaviors. From an evolutionary perspective, why are certain chemical messengers functionally linked to particular behaviors?

The claim that each type of behavior is controlled by a suite of chemical messengers is inferred from the observation that, when particular behaviors are studied extensively, multiple regulators usually are discovered. This, of course, does not mean that all behaviors have multiple regulators, but it does indicate that multiplicity in behavioral regulators is the norm rather than the exception. The lordosis behaviors of female rats and the courtship behaviors of male rough-skinned newts are two examples among many.

Lordosis behaviors, which include arching the back and raising the hindquarters, are exhibited by sexually receptive female rats during mating (Figure 3.7). This sexual behavior appears to be influenced by several steroid hormones, neuropeptides, prostaglandins (Morali and Beyer, 1979). The ovarian steroids that are important include estradiol, which activates lordosis, and progesterone, which either stimulates or inhibits lordosis, depending on concentration and previous exposure to estrogen. Under certain conditions, androgenic steroids, which are secreted by ovarian and adrenal tissue, also may activate lordosis in female rats.

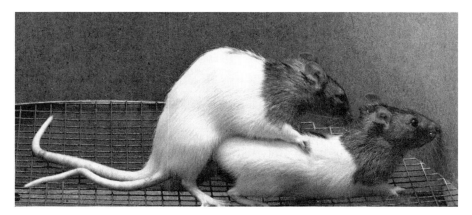

FIGURE 3.7. Lordosis in female rats has been used extensively as a research model for determining the neuroendocrine basis of reproductive behaviors. (Photo by Michael J. Baum)

Besides these steroid hormones, several neuropeptides also influence lordosis in female rats. Gonadotropin-releasing hormone (GnRH) has been shown to activate lordosis in estrogen-primed rats by acting directly on neurons in the brain and independently of the pituitary-ovarian axis (Mauk et al., 1980). There is also evidence that prolactin (PRL) enhances lordosis in estrogen-primed female rats by acting on neurons in the dorsal midbrain (Harlan et al., 1983). Other investigators have found that injections of prostaglandins or ACTHlike peptides, including αMSH, can either stimulate or inhibit rat lordosis, depending on dosage and mode of administration (Beckwith and Sandman, 1982). Several hormones appear to inhibit lordosis: AVP, corticotropin-releasing factor (CRF), β-endorphin, met-enkephalin, and corticosteroids (deCatanzaro and Gorzalka, 1980; Sirinathsinghji, 1984; Sirinathsinghji et al., 1983; Sodersten et al., 1983). These studies provide evidence that more than one chemical messenger regulates rat lordosis behaviors.

Sexual behaviors of male rough-skinned newts (*T. granulosa*) appear to be controlled by many of the same steroid hormones and neuropeptides as rats (Moore, 1983). Specifically, male courtship behaviors (amplectic clasping) can be activated by testicular steroid hormones, including testosterone, dihydrotestosterone, estradiol (Moore, 1978; Moore and Miller, 1983), and the following neuropeptides: AVT, LHRH, ACTH, and αMSH (Moore and Miller, 1983; Moore et al., 1982; Miller and Moore, 1983). Several hormones appear to inhibit male courtship behaviors during periods of stress: CRF, corticosterone, and opioid peptides (Moore and Miller, 1984).

These comparative data from female rats and male newts suggest three points. First, particular behaviors typically are controlled by more than one chemical messenger. Second, certain hormones are more likely to be associated with the control of a particular type of behavior than are other hormones. Third, there are differences among species in the control of a particular type of behavior.

Multiple Regulators of Behaviors

Why are there multiple regulators of a particular behavior? Considering that some chemical messengers mediate the actions of others, such as cAMP functioning as a "second messenger" for certain hormones, it is likely that some multiple regulators simply reflect different levels of the control mechanism. For example, there is evidence that β-endorphin inhibits lordosis behavior in female rats by suppressing GnRH activity in the mesencephalic central gray (Sirinathsinghji, 1984). Other such functional links between the behavioral regulators of sexual behaviors probably exist, but they do not explain all of the multiplicity.

Multiplicity in behavioral regulators can confer finer control of behavioral responses, particularly if different chemical messengers respond to different types of external and internal stimuli. The seasonal breeding cycle of rough-skinned newts is an example where finer behavioral control would be important. Males undergo seasonal changes in reproductive condition in response to changes in temperature and photoperiod, which in turn control the secretion of testicular steroids. Breeding activity peaks during periods of heavy, vernal rains, when newts migrate into the breeding ponds. Harsh environmental conditions suppress reproductive activities in this species.

Thus in newts under natural conditions, sexual behaviors are regulated so that mating occurs at the appropriate time and in the appropriate place. To accomplish this successfully, animals must initiate some developmental events prior to the breeding season. In newts and many other vertebrates, this phase of the control of sexual behaviors appears to be mediated by the gonadal steroid hormones. After these steroid-dependent changes, sexual behaviors are activated (or inactivated) by a variety of social and environmental stimuli, behavioral responses which could be mediated by neuropeptides.

Similar points can be made for female rats, except that, instead of seasonal cycles of reproduction, the estrous and pregnancy cycles are critically important. It appears that, in general, steroid hormones can mediate long-term changes and neuropeptides can regulate short-term changes in sexual behaviors. Multiple behavioral regulators can provide finer control of the behaviors, particularly when the regulators respond to different stimuli.

Evolution of Behavioral Regulators

Certain hormones are more likely to be associated with the regulation of particular behaviors than are other hormones. Gonadal steroid hormones, for example, are more likely to be associated with regulating sexual behaviors than are pancreatic hormones (insulin or glucagon). Likewise, certain neuropeptides have been found to regulate sexual behaviors, others have not. This observed conservatism in behavioral regulators has been explained in several ways.

One explanation is that the observed conservatism is an artifact due to research bias. There is a "bandwagon effect" in scientific research such that, for example, when behavioral endocrinologists discover a new phenomenon, others enthusiastically look for the phenomenon in their own research animal. Although the bandwagon effect tends to distort the amount of research effort on a given topic, it is counteracted by the fact that researchers are rewarded more by investigating new problems. It is unlikely that the observed conservatism in behavioral regulators is entirely the result of researchers' confirming findings in new species.

A second explanation is that the observed conservatism in behavioral regulators is a product of evolution. It follows that, for a particular behavior, evolutionary selective pressures favor certain hormones over others. Take for example the prevalence of testosterone as one of the regulators of male sexual behaviors; according to this explanation, selective pressures favor testosterone over other less common regulators such as progesterone or corticosterone.

Although the conservation in behavioral regulators has been emphasized, there are obvious differences among species. Even our most-used example, the activation of male sexual behaviors by testosterone, does not seem to fit for some species. Sexual behaviors of male garter snakes and white-crowned sparrows appear to be independent of plasma testosterone (Crews et al., 1984; Moore and Kranz, 1983). Another example of species differences is that GnRH can enhance female sexual behaviors in rats and mice but, apparently, not in voles or hamsters (Mauk et al., 1980; S. Peterson, unpublished data). Two species of newts from the same taxonomic family, Salamandridae, appear to differ in the control of male courtship behaviors; in the crested newt (*Triturus cristatus*), PRL, but not AVT, is a potent activator of courtship behaviors (Malacarne et al., 1982), whereas in the rough-skinned newt (*T. granulosa*), AVT activates courtship behaviors (Moore, 1983). Considering these examples, there are both species differences and similarities in behavioral regulators, all of which provide insights into how these systems have evolved.

Discussions of the evolution of behavioral control mechanisms in extant species should consider two interrelated phenomena, the evolutionary history of the species and selective pressures on the species. Evolutionary history encompasses all ancestral changes, from molecular to behavioral, and represents the evolutionary sequence leading to existing species. Each ancestral change can influence subsequent evolutionary changes; the acquisition or degeneration of particular structures, for example, can alter changes in future generations to subsequent selective pressures. It therefore follows that, in order to understand the evolution of behavioral regulators in extant species, we must understand the evolutionary history of that species. Ancestral forms of extant species are not available today for study, so it is not possible to directly study evolutionary history. The comparative approach to behavioral endocrinology is a viable option, however. Much can be learned about the evolutionary history of behavioral regulators by comparing systems in species with known phylogenetic relationships.

But what are the selective pressures which favor one hormone over another as a behavioral regulator? Since it is adaptive for individuals to exhibit particular behaviors at appropriate times and places, it follows that there are selective pressures to incorporate those hormones into the control mechanism which have peaks in activity that are temporally associated with the optimal times and places for expressing the particular behavior. It also follows that there are selective pressures against incorporating those hormones into the control system which have physiological constraints that restrict them from acquiring particular behavioral functions.

Testosterone, for example, typically increases prior to the onset of the breeding season and controls the development of many reproductive functions. Thus, testosterone can function as an adequate chemical messenger for activating male sexual behaviors in those species which mate at the time when (or shortly after) plasma testosterone levels are elevated. The converse may also be true, since Crews (1984) observed that, in species with dissociated reproductive patterns, testosterone is not elevated at the time of mating and is not a dominant regulator of male sexual behaviors.

As mentioned, certain hormones would be selected against because of physiological constraints. Imagine the problems an animal would have, for example, if male sexual arousal were activated by high plasma insulin levels; he would become aroused after every meal. The point is that, if the hormone already has vital functions and if these functions are incompatible with acquiring the new behavioral functions, then that hormone as a trigger (or signal) will be selected against. There are alternative solutions to this negative selection pressure, however, such as the one described below.

There are examples of neuropeptides which apparently have incompatible functions. In newts, AVT controls water balance and sexual behaviors, which means that, when males are in the pond mating, AVT levels should be low in order to avoid hydration and should be high in order to activate sexual behaviors. The solution to this apparent paradox is that, as presented earlier, AVT activity is controlled independently for behavior versus water balance. Furthermore, AVT functions in the brain are isolated anatomically from peripheral target tissues.

Neuropeptides and other chemical messengers with localized, short-distance actions are subject to different selective pressures. These localized chemical messengers can acquire regionally localized functions as well as regionally localized control mechanisms, functioning independently of plasma hormone patterns. Localization of function can be accomplished in several ways: by confining the chemical messenger to specific anatomical locations, such as in classic neurotransmitters, or by converting within a specific area a widely distributed chemical messenger into another biologically active form. Examples of the latter include the aromatization of testosterone to estrogen in specific brain areas and the enzymatic cleaving of AVP into a biologically active fragment (Burbach et al., 1983).

With regionally localized functions, there are more opportunities for diversification. This point has largely been overlooked by many scientists, which is unfortunate, because it provides insight into the multiple functions which have been attributed to localized chemical messengers, from prostaglandins to neuropeptides. Furthermore, this regional localization in the control of and activity of neuropeptides should be considered in discussions of the evolution of behavioral control mechanisms.

ACKNOWLEDGMENTS

Many thanks to the following people associated with my laboratory and the research on newt behaviors: S. Boyd, P. Deviche, L. Miller, C. Propper, J. Specker, S. Petersen, A. Weaver, and R.T. Zoeller. I also thank K. Moore for editorial advice. The recent research on newts was supported by the

Behavioral Actions of Neurohypophysial Peptides   Chap. 3

National Science Foundation (PCM 83-16006) and National Institutes of Health (1 K04 HD00407 and 2 R01 HD13508).

REFERENCES

ACHER, R. (1983) Principles of evolution: The neural hierarchy model. In *Brain Peptides*. Krieger, Brownstein, and Martin, eds., pp. 135–164, Wiley, New York.

ACHER, R. (1985) Biosynthesis, processing, and evolution of neurohypophysial hormone precursors. In *Neurosecretion and the Biology of Neuropeptides*. Kobayashi, Bern, and Urano, eds., pp. 11–25, Springer-Verlag, Berlin.

ARLETTI, R., C. BAZZANI, M. CASTELLI, and A. BERTOLINI (1985) Oxytocin improves male copulatory performance in rats. Horm. Behav. *19*:14–20.

BECKWITH, B., and C.A. SANDMAN (1982) Central nervous system and peripheral effects of ACTH, MSH, and related neuropeptides. Peptides *3*:411–420.

BLOOM, F.E. (1982) Strategies to investigate the behavioral effects of vasopressin. Proc. Ann. Meet. Soc. Neurosci. 1982: 227–236.

BOHUS, B. (1977) Effect of desglycinamide-lysine vasopressin (DG-LVP) on sexually motivated T-maze behavior of the male rat. Horm. Behav. *8*:52–61.

BOLWERK, E.L.M., and H.H. SWANSON (1984) Does oxytocin play a role in the onset of maternal behaviour in the rat? J. Endocr. *101*:353–357.

BRINTON, R.E., K.W. GEE, J.K. WAMSLEY, T.P. DAVIS, and H.I. YAMAMURA (1984) Regional distribution of putative vasopressin receptors in rat brain and pituitary by quantitative autoradiography. Proc. Nat. Acad. Sci. USA *81*:7248–7252.

BURBACH, J.P.H., G.L. KOVACS, D. DE WIED, J.W. VAN NISPEN, and H.M. GREVEN (1983) A major metabolite of arginine vasopressin in the brain is a highly potent neuropeptide. Science *221*:1310–1312.

CORNETT, L.E., and D.M. DORSA (1985) Vasopressin receptor subtypes in dorsal hindbrain and renal medulla. Peptides *6*:85–89.

CREWS, D. (1984) Gamete production, sex hormone secretion, and mating behavior uncoupled. Horm. Behav. *18*:22–28.

CREWS, D., B. CAMAZINE, M. DIAMOND, M. MASON, R. TOKARZ, and W.R. GARSTKA (1984) Hormonal-independence of courtship behavior in the male garter snake. Horm. Behav. *18*:29–41.

CUMMING, R., T.A. REAVES, JR., and J.N. HAYWARD (1982) Ultrastructural immunocytochemical characterization of isotocin, vasotocin and neurophysin neurons in the magnocellular preoptic nucleus of the goldfish. Cell Tissue Res. *223*:685–694.

DE CATANZARO, D., and B.B. GORZALKA (1979) Effects of dexamethason, corticosterone, and ACTH on lordosis in ovariectomized and adrenalectomized-ovariectomized rats. Pharm. Biochem. Behav. *12*:201–206.

DELANOY, R.L., A.J. DUNN, and R. WALTER (1979) Neurohypophysial hormones and behavior: Effects of intracerebroventricularly injected hormone analogs in mice. Life Sci. *24*:651–658.

DE WIED, D. (1976) Behavioral effects of intraventricularly administered vasopressin and vasopressin fragments. Life Sci. *19*:685–690.

DE WIED, D., and J. JOLLES (1982) Neuropeptides derived from pro-opiocortin: Behavioral, physiological and neurochemical effects. Physiological Rev. *62*:976–10l53.

DE WIED, D., O. GAFFORI, J.M. VAN REE, and W. DE JONG (1984) Central target for the behavioural effects of vasopressin neuropeptides. Nature *308*:276–278.

DIAKOW, C. (1978) Hormonal basis for breeding behavior in female frogs: Vasotocin inhibits the release call of *Rana pipiens*. Science *199*:1456–1457.

DIAKOW, C., and D. RAIMONDI (1981) Physiology of *Rana pipiens* reproductive behavior: A proposed mechanism for inhibition of the release call. Amer. Zool. *21*:296–304.

DORIS, P.A. (1984) Vasopressin and central integrative processes. Neuroendocrinology *38*:75–85.

FAHRBACH, S.E., J.I. MORRELL, and D.W. PFAFF (1985) Possible role for endogenous oxytocin in estrogen-facilitated maternal behavior in rats. Neuroendocrinology *40*:526–532.

FERRIS, C.F., H.E. ALBERS, S.M. WESLOWSKI, B.D. GOLDMAN, and S.E. LUMAN (1984) Vasopressin injected into the hypothalamus triggers a stereotypic behavior in golden hamsters. Science *224*:521–523.

GUILLETTE, L.J., and R.E. JONES (1982) Further observations on arginine vasotocin-induced oviposition and parturition in lizards. J. Herpetology *16*:140–144.

HARLAN, R.E., B.D. SHIVERS, and D.W. PFAFF (1983) Midbrain microinfusions of prolactin increase the estrogen-dependent behavior, lordosis. Science *219*:1451–1453.

HAWTHORN, J., V.T.Y. ANG, and J.S. JENKINS (1984) Comparison of the distribution of oxytocin and vasopressin in the rat brain. Brain Res. *307*:289–294.

JOKURA, Y., and A. URANO (1985) An immunohistochemical study of seasonal changes in luteinizing hormone-releasing hormone and vasotocin in the forebrain and the neurohypophysis of the toad, *Bufo japonicus*. Gen. Comp. Endocrinol. *59*:238–245.

JONES, R.E., and L.J. GUILLETTE, JR. (1982) Hormonal control of oviposition and parturition in lizards. Herpetologica *38*:80–93.

KELLEY, D.B. (1980) Auditory and vocal nuclei in the frog brain concentrate sex hormones. Science *207*:553–555.

KIHLSTROM, J.E., and A. AGMO (1974) Some effects of vasopressin on sexual behaviour and seminal characteristics in intact and castrated rabbits. J. Endocr. *60*:445–453.

KIHLSTROM, J.E., and I. DANNINGE (1972) Neurohypophysial hormones and sexual behavior in males of the domestic fowl (*Gallus domesticus* L.) and the pigeon (*Columba livia* Gmel.). Gen. Comp. Endocrinol. *18*:115–120.

KING, M.G., L. STINUS, M. LEMOAL, and M. GEFFARD (1982) Central administration of arginine vasopressin: Effects on exploratory behavior in the rat. Psychopharmacology *76*:40–43.

KOVACS, G.L., L. VECSEI, G. SZABO, and G. TELEGDY (1977) The involvement of catecholaminergic mechanisms in the behavioural action of vasopressin. Neuroscience Letters *5*:337–344.

KRIEGER, D.T. (1983) Brain peptides: What, where, and why? Science *222*:975–985.

LACZI, F., O. GAFFORI, E.R. DE KLOET, and D. DE WIED (1983) Arginine-vasopressin content of hippocampus and amygdala during passive avoidance behavior in rats. Brain Res. *280*:309–315.

MALACARNE, G., C. GIACOMA, C. VELLANO, and V. MAZZI (1982) Prolactin and sexual behaviour in the crested newt (*Triturus cristatus carnifex* Laur.) Gen. Comp. Endocrinol. *47*:139–147.

MARTIN, J.T., and T.B. VAN WIMERSMA GREIDANUS (1979) Imprinting behavior: Influence of vasopressin and ACTH analogues. Psychoneuroendocrinology *3*:261–269.

MAUK, M.D., G.A. OLSON, A.J. KASTIN, and R.D. OLSON (1980) Behavioral effects of LHR-RH. Neurosci. Biobehav. Rev. *4*:1–8.

MAYERI, E., P. BROWNELL, W.D. BRANTON, and S.B. SIMON (1979) Multiple, prolonged actions of neuroendocrine bag cells on neurons in *Aplysia*. I. Effects of bursting pacemaker neurons. J. Neurophysiology *42*:1165–1185.

MILLER, L.J., and F.L. MOORE (1983) Intracranial administration of corticotropin-like peptides increases incidence of amphibian reproductive behavior. Peptides *4*:729–733.

MIZUNO, Y., Y. OOMURA, N. HORI, and D.O. CARPENTER (1984) Action of vasopressin in CA1 pyramidal neurons in rat hippocampal slices. Brain Res. *309*:241–246.

MOORE, F.L. (1978) Differential effects of testosterone plus dihydrotestosterone on male courtship of castrated newts, *Taricha granulosa*. Horm. Behav. *11*:202–208.

MOORE, F.L. (1983) Behavioral endocrinology of amphibian reproduction. BioScience *33*:557–561.

MOORE, F.L., and L.J. MILLER (1983) Arginine vasotocin induces sexual behavior of newts by acting on cells in the brain. Peptides *4*:97–102.

MOORE, F.L., and L.J. MILLER (1984) Stress-induced inhibition of sexual behavior: Corticosterone inhibits courtship behaviors of a male amphibian (*Taricha granulosa*). Horm. Behav. *18*:400–410.

MOORE, F.L., L.J. MILLER, S.P. SPIELVOGEL, T. KUBIAK, and K. FOLKERS (1982) Luteinizing hormone-releasing hormone involvement in the reproductive behavior of a male amphibian. Neuroendocrinology *35*:212–216.

MOORE, F.L., and R.T. ZOELLER (1979) Endocrine control of amphibian sexual behavior: Evidence for a neurohormone-androgen interaction. Horm. Behav. *13*:207–213.

MOORE, M.C., and R. KRANZ (1983) Evidence of androgen independence of male mounting behavior in white-crowned sparrows (*Zonotrichia leucophrys gambelii*). Horm. Behav. *17*:414–423.

MORALI, G., and C. BEYER (1979) Neuroendocrine control of mammalian estrous behavior. In *Endocrine Control of Sexual Behavior*. C. Beyer, ed., pp. 33–75, Raven Press, New York.

MUHLETHALER, M., R. RAGGENBASS, and J.J. DREIFUSS (1984) Is oxytocin a neurotransmitter in the vertebrate hippocampus? In *Endocrinology, Excerpta Medica*. F. Labrie and L.L. Proulx, eds., pp. 899–902, Elsevier Science Publishers B.V., Amsterdam, New York.

NORRIS, D.O. (1985) *Vertebrate Endocrinology*. Lea and Febiger, Philadelphia.

PALKOVITS, M., and M.J. BROWNSTEIN (1982) Microdissection of brain areas by the punch technique. Proc. Ann. Meet. Soc. Neurosci.: 60–71.

PEDERSEN, C.A., J.A. ASCHER, Y.L. MONROE, and A. J. PRANGE, JR. (1982) Oxytocin induces maternal behavior in virgin female rats. Science 216:648–650.

PICKFORD, G.E., and E.L. STRECKER (1977) The spawning reflex response of the killifish, *Fundulus heteroclitus*: Isotocin is relatively inactive in comparison to arginine vasotocin. Gen. Comp. Endocrinol. 32:132–137.

REPPERT, S.M., H.G. ARTMAN, S. SWAMINATHAN, and D.A. FISHER (1981) Vasopressin exhibits a rhythmic daily pattern in cerebrospinal fluid but not in blood. Science 213:1256–1257.

RUBIN, B.S., F.S. MENNITI, and R.S. BRIDGES (1983) Intracerebroventricular administration of oxytocin and maternal behavior in rats after prolonged and acute steroid pretreatment. Horm. Behav. 17:45–53.

SCHREIBMAN, M.P., and L.R. HALPERN (1980) The demonstration of neurophysin and arginine vasotocin by immunocytochemical methods in the brain and pituitary gland of the platyfish, *Xiphophorus maculatus*. Gen. Comp. Endocrinol. 40:1–7.

SILVERMAN, A.J., and E.A. ZIMMERMAN (1983) Magnocellular neurosecretory system. Ann. Rev. Neurosci. 6:357–380.

SIRINATHSINGHJI, D.J.S. (1984) Modulation of lordosis behavior of female rats by naloxone, β-endorphin and its antiserum in the mesencephalic central gray: Possible mediation via GnRH. Neuroendocrinology 39:222–230.

SIRINATHSINGHJI, D.J.S., L.H. REES, J. RIVIER, and W. VALE (1983) Corticotropin-releasing factor is a potent inhibitor of sexual receptivity in the female rat. Nature 305:232–235.

SODERSTEN, P., M. HENNING, P. MELIN, and S. LUDIN (1983) Vasopressin alters female sexual behaviour by acting on the brain independently of alterations in blood pressure. Nature 301:608–610.

STARK, R.I., S.S. DANIEL, M.K. HUSAIN, A.B. ZUBROW, and L.S. JAMES (1984) Effects of hypoxia on vasopressin concentrations in cerebrospinal fluid and plasma of sheep. Neuroendocrinology 38:453–460.

THORNHILL, J.A., K. LUKOWIAK, K.E. COOPER, W.L. VEALE, and J.P. EDSTROM (1981) Arginine vasotocin, an endogenous neuropeptide of *Aplysia*, suppresses the gill withdrawal reflex and induces the evoked synaptic input to central gill motor neurons. J. Neurobiol. 12:533–544.

VAN HEUVEN-NOLSEN, D., and D.H.G. VERSTEEG (1985) Interaction of vasopressin with the nigro-striatal dopamine system: Site and mechanism of action. Brain Res. 337:269–276.

VAN WIMERSMA GREIDANUS, TJ.B., and J.P.H. BURBACH (1984) Behavioral effects of neurohypophysial hormones. In *Endocrinology, Excerpta Medica*. F. Labrie and L. Proulx, eds., pp. 129–132, Elsevier Science Publishers B.V., Amsterdam, New York.

WILHELMI, A.E., G.E. PICKFORD, and W. H. SAWYER (1955) Initiation of the spawning reflex response in *Fundulus* by the administration of fish and mammalian neurohypophysial preparations and synthetic oxytocin. Endocrinology 57:243–252.

ZOELLER, R.T., and F.L. MOORE (1982) Duration of androgen treatment modifies behavioral response to arginine vasotocin in *Taricha granulosa*. Horm. Behav. *16*:23–30.

Zoeller, R.T., and F.L. Moore (1986a) Arginine vasotocin immunoreactivity in hypothalamic and extrahypothalamic areas of an amphibian brain. Neuroendocrinology *42*:120–123.

Zoeller, R.T., and F.L. Moore (1986b) Correlation between immunoreactive vasotocin in optic tectum and seasonal changes in reproductive behaviors of male rough-skinned newts. Horm. Behav. *20*:148–154.

FOUR
Diversity and Evolution of Behavioral Controlling Mechanisms

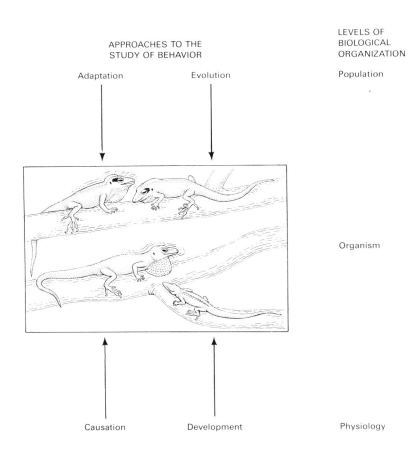

David Crews
Institute of Reproductive Biology
Department of Zoology
University of Texas at Austin

The study of behavior has traditionally been approached from two directions. One has emphasized proximate physiological mechanisms while the other has stressed ultimate evolutionary factors. Because these two approaches have asked different kinds of questions and concentrated on different kinds of animals, they have developed independently. This is unfortunate, since the advances in each address the problems of the other. For example, the issue of variation between species, individuals, or the sexes has proven to be a difficult problem to the behavioral physiologist. Evolutionary biologists, however, have developed a powerful set of theories and testable hypotheses that provide a context within which to consider the question of variance. On the other hand, evolutionary biologists know little, and appreciate less, the physiological mechanisms underlying the very behaviors they recognize to be on the leading edge of evolutionary change.

Why has there been a tendency for behavioral physiology and evolutionary biology to be mutually exclusive, almost opposite, endeavors? One reason may be that much of the theory in behavioral physiology is based on data obtained from highly inbred and domesticated species, whereas in evolutionary biology and behavioral ecology theory has focused on naturally occurring species. Another reason is that most behavioral physiologists eschew individual variation while the behavioral biologists emphasize individual variation.

The aims of this chapter will be twofold. The first is to show how the evolutionary perspective can increase our understanding of the proximate causes and development of behavioral controlling mechanisms. The second is the complement of the first—that is, to illustrate how knowledge of the mechanisms underlying behavior can supplement our understanding of the adaptation and evolution of these processes. Because these perspectives are complementary, they can, when considered together, provide insight into the constraints as well as the ultimate plasticity of fundamental behavioral controlling mechanisms.

This chapter will demonstrate that (1) there are multiple proximate mechanisms triggering sexual behavior and, further, these mechanisms have evolved to meet specific environmental challenges; (2) there are trends within this diversity of behavioral controlling mechanisms that point to new avenues of investigation; (3) the development of these mechanisms is in accord with the individual's life history; and (4) this diversity presents natural experiments, the study of which can reveal how brain-behavior relationships evolve.

Two thematic threads run throughout this chapter. While each has been open to controversy, it is not my intention to debate their validity.

Rather, they will provide the context in which to view the points to be made. The first is that evolution selects for individuals, with evolutionary fitness being measured by reproductive success, or survival of the young until they themselves reproduce. The second is that the brain, the organ of behavior, is like any other morphological structure and subject to selective pressures that have shaped both its structures and functions.

The central questions we will focus on in this chapter are (1) what is the meaning of variation for our understanding of the fundamental nature of behavioral controlling mechanisms, and (2) how has the brain come to exploit specific external and internal stimuli so that they come to serve as triggers for adaptive responses? Before addressing these questions, we must first consider the constraints on reproduction, and hence on the mechanisms underlying reproduction.

CONSTRAINTS ON THE TIMING OF REPRODUCTION

Reproduction is the single most important event in the life of any organism, for failure here means in most instances that the individual will not contribute its genes to subsequent generations. Since the brain receives and integrates stimuli from both the internal and external environments, it follows that the neural mechanisms regulating reproduction are as much adaptational responses to the environment as are any morphological or behavioral characters. Recent studies of wild, naturally occurring species have revealed that multiple mechanisms have evolved, even within the same species, to maximize reproductive success over the life history of the individual (Austad and Howard, 1984; Clutton-Brock et al., 1982; Crews and Moore, 1986a).

There is abundant evidence that the neural mechanisms subserving reproduction have been shaped by environmental and physiological constraints on the reproductive process (Crews and Moore, 1986a). These constraints have given rise to a great variety of reproductive strategies in vertebrates. Some of the evolutionary pressures leading to what has been termed r and K selection (Pianka, 1970) are: (1) the stability and predictability of the environment both historically and presently; (2) the differential cost of reproduction for males and females; (3) the availability of mating opportunities; (4) the number and survival of young and the attendant costs to the parent; and (5) the time required for maturation of the gametes, zygotes, and juveniles. Studies taking these and other variables into account hold particular promise for future research.

I will illustrate some of these issues by considering the problem of seasonal reproduction. Most animals are seasonal breeders, reproducing during those periods most propitious for the survival of both parent and young. It was recognized more than 50 years ago that the evolution of reproductive seasons is determined by "ultimate" factors which select against those individuals bearing young during times of food scarcity or other adverse environmental conditions (Immelmann, 1972; Whittier and

Crews, 1986a). Thus, the quality and quantity of food, the availability of appropriate nesting materials, and predation act as long-range factors determining the optimal time of breeding for a particular population or individual.

These ultimate factors must be distinguished from the variety of "proximate" factors that precede the optimal periods for reproduction (Immelmann, 1972; Whittier and Crews, 1986a). Because of their predictability, these proximate factors have come to trigger or cue the actual onset, maintenance, and termination of reproductive processes, thereby coordinating the individual's internal state with changing environmental conditions. The complexity of reproductive regulators is further increased by the fact that, in many species, responsiveness to external stimuli varies seasonally, presumably reflecting endogenous circannual rhythms in sensitivity to these proximate cues.

Photoperiod and temperature are well-known proximate cues utilized by animals. However, any physical, biotic, or social stimulus in the environment can potentially serve as a reproductive trigger and thereby help to fine-tune reproduction. The sole requirement is that the stimulus accurately predict the optimal period for breeding. Rainfall, humidity, soil moisture, trace elements, and secondary plant compounds are just a few examples. Behavior can also serve as a proximate stimulus initiating reproduction. For example, male copulatory and pheromonal stimuli are known to modulate female reproductive physiology and behavior in the Asian musk shrew (*Suncus murinus*) and in several species of microtine rodents (Dryden and Anderson, 1977; Crews and Moore, 1986a).

There are also physiological constraints inherent in the reproductive process that influence the evolution of neural mechanisms subserving reproduction. I will consider just one of those enumerated above. A significant limiting force is the time necessary to grow a gamete. In the case of mammals and birds, there appears to be an incompressible period of approximately six weeks necessary for spermatogenesis (Clermont, 1972). A similar time constraint applies to the female, although some small rodents are capable of generating ova in as little as three weeks (Greenwald, 1978). In other nonhomeothermic vertebrates it is common for gamete maturation to take many months or even years (Jones, 1978; Licht, 1984).

While this constraint does not pose problems for many species living in environments in which favorable conditions are predictable and/or prolonged, it does present serious difficulties for species living in (1) harsh environments that are predictable but with an abbreviated favorable period or (2) harsh environments having completely unpredictable favorable periods. In both situations the available time for the animals to mate, the female to reproduce, and the young to grow sufficiently so they might survive is extremely brief. This places great selective advantage on phenotypes in which the gametes are available and growth is maximized when propitious environmental conditions do occur.

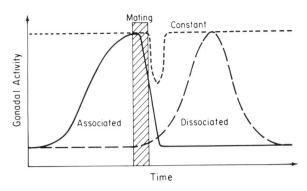

Figure 4.1. Three reproductive patterns exhibited in vertebrates. Gonadal activity is defined in terms of the maturation and shedding of gametes and/or the secretion of sex steroid hormones. In individuals exhibiting the *associated* reproductive pattern, gonadal activity increases immediately prior to mating. In species exhibiting the *dissociated* reproductive pattern, gonadal activity is minimal at mating. In species exhibiting the *constant* reproductive pattern, the gonads are maintained at or near maximum activity.

There is no question that these environmental and physiological constraints affect all aspects of reproduction. I will consider only three major reproductive patterns exhibited in vertebrates (Figure 4.1). The first, and most common, reproductive pattern is characterized by the gametes' attaining maturity coincident with breeding. A second reproductive pattern is characterized by gonadal recrudescence occurring only after all breeding activity has ceased; with the subsequent collapse of the gonad, the mature gametes are stored until the next breeding season. A third reproductive pattern is for the gonads to develop and maintain gametes in an advanced stage of development for prolonged periods. These reproductive patterns are discussed in greater detail below.

DIVERSITY OF NEUROENDOCRINE MECHANISMS CONTROLLING MATING BEHAVIOR

The diversity in reproductive patterns must reflect an equal diversity in neuroendocrine controlling mechanisms. To understand the relationship between the animal's environment, its reproductive pattern, and the underlying neuroendocrine mechanisms controlling reproduction, it is useful to first consider the reproductive process as having three major components: the production of gametes, the secretion of sex steroid hormones by the gonad, and the timing of mating behavior. Depending upon the environmental and physiological constraints operating on the individual, the relationship among these three components can differ profoundly.

It should be kept in mind that the three reproductive patterns to be discussed each are points on a continuum and thus are only representative of the great variety of reproductive patterns found in nature. For the purposes of this chapter, however, I will focus on these three reproductive patterns to show the coevolution of different cues and neuroendocrine mechanisms controlling mating behavior.

The Associated Reproductive Pattern

It is common to find that many vertebrates living in temperate regions are seasonal breeders in which maturation of the gametes and maximum sex steroid hormone secretion immediately precede or coincide with mating (Figure 4.1). In vertebrates exhibiting a close temporal relationship between gonadal activity and mating, the increase in circulating levels of sex steroid hormones accompanying gonadal growth activates mating behavior both in the male and in the female as adults (see Chapters, 2, 5, 6, 10-12). This activational role of sex steroid hormones in regulating mating behavior is clearly seen in the green anole lizard (*Anolis carolinensis*) (Crews, 1980).

The green anole is found throughout the southeastern United States, where it breeds in the late spring and summer months (Figure 4.2). Temperature is the major environmental cue stimulating the transition from reproductive inactivity to reproductive activity in this lizard. In addition to inducing the male's emergence from winter dormancy, rising ambient temperatures in the spring also stimulate testicular recrudescence. As the testes mature and androgen concentrations in the systemic circulation peak, the males establish territories. The frequency of male agonistic displays begin to wane as the females arrive on the breeding grounds. Although males court females vigorously, the first copulations are not seen for several weeks after the females have emerged.

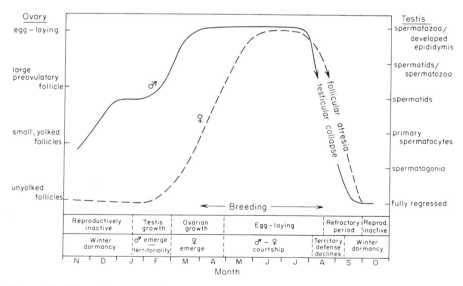

Figure 4.2. The major physiological and behavioral events in the annual reproductive cycle of the green anole lizard, *Anolis carolinensis*. (From Crews, 1975)

In both the male and the female green anole there is a close temporal association between the peak phase in gonadal activity (gamete maturation and maximal sex-steroid hormone secretion) and breeding (mating behavior). As in other animals exhibiting an associated reproductive pattern (Crews, 1984), including laboratory and domesticated mammals and birds (Leshner, 1978), courtship and copulatory behavior in the male green anole depends upon the functional integrity of the hypothalamic-pituitary-gonadal axis. Experiments have shown that the basal hypothalamus and preoptic area in the brain are major integrative areas for the internal and external stimuli that regulate reproduction; these areas also secrete hormones important in modulating sexual behavior (Crews, 1979a). Removal of the pituitary results in gonadal atrophy, whereas administration of pituitary gonadotropins to hypophysectomized or intact, winter-dormant animals will stimulate gametogenesis and steroidogenesis (Crews, 1979a). Finally, removal of the gonads abolishes sexual behavior, whereas sex hormone replacement therapy reinstates the complete repertoire of sexual behaviors (Crews, 1979a) (Figure 4.3).

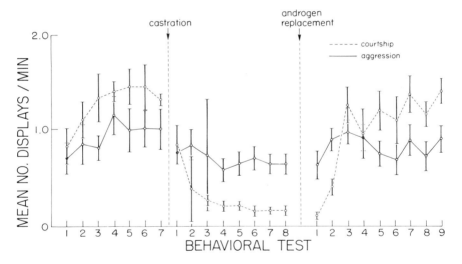

Figure 4.3. Effect of castration and testosterone replacement therapy on sexual and aggressive behavior in male green anole lizards, *Anolis carolinensis*. (From Crews, 1979a, The hormonal control of behavior in a lizard. Copyright © 1979 by Scientific American, Inc. All rights reserved)

The sites of action of testicular hormones in the green anole are known to resemble those found in other vertebrates studied. In addition to being selectively bound in the accessory sex structures, both testosterone (T) and dihydrotestosterone (DHT) are concentrated in specific areas of the brain. For example, a major site of androgen-concentrating cells is the anterior hypothalamus and preoptic area (AH-POA) (Morrell et al., 1979). Both areas are involved in the regulation of aggressive and sexual behavior in males as well as in hormone feedback regulation of pituitary gonadotropin secretion.

Destruction of the AH-POA results in an immediate and rapid decline in both sexual and aggressive behavior. Sexual behavior can be restored in long-term castrated, sexually inactive green anoles by implantation of minute amounts of T directly into the AH-POA (Crews, 1979a).

A similar reciprocal interaction between the external and internal milieu exists in the female green anole. Warm temperatures are necessary, but not sufficient, for stimulating ovarian activity. The rate and completion of ovarian growth is determined by the behavior of the male. Male courtship displays stimulate pituitary gonadotropin secretion, whereas aggressive displays inhibit environmentally-induced ovarian growth (Crews, 1980) (Figure 4.4).

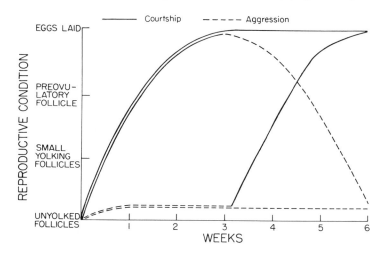

Figure 4.4. Interaction of male behavior and female reproductive status in the green anole lizard, *Anolis carolinensis*. Four groups of females are depicted. One of them (bottom curve) was exposed only to male aggressive behavior (hatched lines). Another group (top curve) was exposed only to male courtship displays (solid lines). The curve that ascends after three weeks of aggression represents a group that was exposed to three weeks of aggression and then three weeks of courtship. The curve that descends after three weeks represents a group that received the opposite treatment. (From Crews, 1979b)

In *Anolis* lizards, as in many higher primates, the ovaries alternate in the production of a single ovum during the breeding season (Figure 4.5). With these regular progressive changes in ovarian morphology are correlated fluctuations in the nature and pattern of sex steroid hormone secretion. Estrogen (E) concentrations in the blood increase as the largest ovarian follicle matures. At the time of ovulation E levels drop precipitously and progesterone (P) concentrations rise abruptly. This pattern of a preovulatory elevation of E in the plasma followed by high concentrations of P after ovulation appears to be common in all egg-laying vertebrates (Licht, 1984).

These cycles of ovarian growth and transitions in hormone secretion are correlated with regular periods of sexual receptivity in the female green anole (Figure 4.5). Sexual receptivity, identified by the neck-bending response of the female to male courtship, is seen only during the latter third of

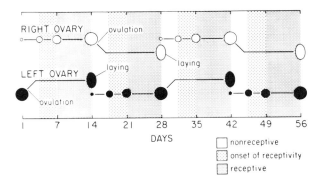

Figure 4.5. Relationship between maturation and ovulation of the largest ovarian follicle and sexual receptivity in female green anole lizards, *Anolis carolinensis*. During the breeding season, female green anoles undergo cycles of sexual receptivity which are correlated with the maturation and ovulation of a single follicle; the ovaries alternate in the production of the ovum. The exact onset of estrus varies among females. Females are no longer receptive to the courtship behavior of males shortly after ovulation or following mating.

the follicular cycle. During this period an unmated female will approach and solicit copulation from the male.

The Dissociated Reproductive Pattern

Many species inhabiting harsh environments in which there is a regular but narrow window of opportunity for breeding exhibit a pattern of reproduction in which there is a complete uncoupling of mating behavior from gamete maturation and sex steroid hormone secretion (Figure 4.1). In such species gonadal recrudescence occurs only after all breeding activity for the current season has ceased; that is, gametes are produced and stored many months before the next breeding season. In species exhibiting this *dissociated* reproductive pattern (Crews, 1984), a specific physical or behavioral cue usually serves as the trigger for sexual behavior, and gonadal sex steroid hormones may not be involved. A good example of this reproductive pattern is the Canadian red-sided garter snake (*Thamnophis sirtalis parietalis*).

In Manitoba, the red-sided garter snake spends much of its time underneath the ground in limestone caverns that serve as subterranean hibernacula (Figure 4.6). The snakes emerge in the spring, and the majority of matings occur during the next three weeks (Crews and Garstka, 1982). Courtship behavior in the adult male red-sided garter snake is not activated by testicular or pituitary hormones, but rather by the increase in ambient temperature following winter dormancy (Crews, 1983). Immediately after mating, snakes disperse to feeding grounds and return in the fall to the hibernaculum from which they had emerged the previous spring.

Testicular activity in emerging, mating male red-sided garter snakes is minimal. It is only 5–10 weeks later, after the males have left the den sites and will no longer court an attractive female, that the testes grow and

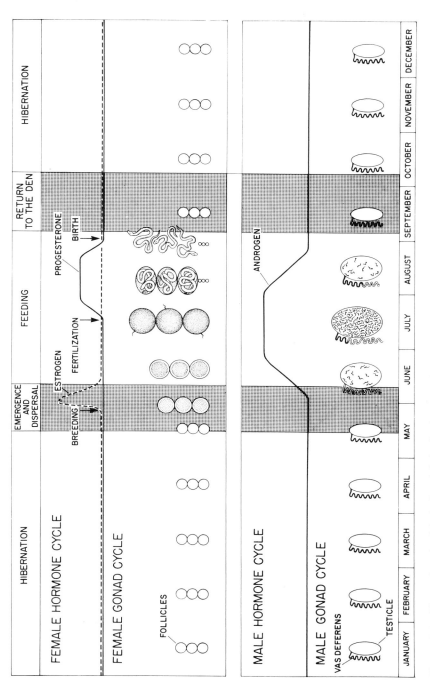

Figure 4.6. The major physiological and behavioral events in the annual reproductive cycle of the Canadian red-sided garter snake, *Thamnophis sirtalis parietalis*. (Redrawn from Crews and Garstka, 1982, The ecological physiology of a garter snake. Copyright 1982 by Scientific American Inc. All rights reserved.)

TABLE 4.1. Experimental manipulations and their effects on the courtship behavior of the male Canadian red-sided garter snake (*Thamnophis sirtalis parietalis*)

Manipulation	Response	Authority
Hibernation	+	Aleksuik and Gregory, 1974; Hawley and Aleksuik, 1975, 1976; Garstka et al., 1982
Castration:		
On emergence	−	Camazine et al., 1980
Before hibernation	−	Garstka et al., 1982; Crews et al., 1984
Breeding	−	Crews et al., 1984
Adrenalectomy + castration	−	Crews et al., 1984
Hypophysectomy:		
On emergence	−	Crews et al., 1984
Before hibernation	−	Crews et al., 1984
Systemic hormone treatment:		
Sex steroid hormones	−	Camazine et al., 1980; Garstka et al., 1982; Crews et al., 1984
Hypothalamic hormones	−	Garstka et al., 1982
Neurotransmitters	−	Garstka et al., 1982
Cyproterone acetate	−	Crews et al., 1984
Hypothalamic implants	−	Friedman and Crews, 1985a
Hypothalamic lesions:		
On emergence	+	Friedman and Crews, 1985b
Before hibernation	+	Krohmer and Crews, 1986

+ signifies an effect on courtship behavior; − signifies no effect on courtship behavior.

androgen levels increase. The sperm produced during this testicular growth period are then stored in the epididymides and vasa deferentia, where they remain until the next spring. Experiments have established that so long as male red-sided garter snakes have gone through a period of low-temperature dormancy, the display of sexual behavior will neither be inhibited nor prolonged by castration, removal of the pituitary gland, and/or androgen replacement therapy (Table 4.1). Further, administration of a variety of hypothalamic hormones and neurotransmitters (Crews, 1983) and even implantation of T directly into the AH-POA (Friedman and Crews, 1985a) will not activate courtship behavior in adult males maintained under summerlike conditions.

Courtship behavior in recently emerged red-sided garter snakes has been abolished only by electrolytic lesions in the AH-POA (Friedman and

Crews, 1985b) (Table 4.1). Similarly, males that have sustained lesions in this area prior to entering hibernation also fail to court on emergence (Krohmer and Crews, 1986). In addition to containing sex steroid hormone-concentrating neurons (Halpern et al., 1982), the AH-POA also contains temperature-sensitive neurons (Satinoff, 1978). In view of the lack of effect of sex steroid hormones on mating behavior in adult male snakes, it is likely this decline or absence in courtship behavior following lesions in the AH-POA is not due to destruction of hormone-sensitive neurons subserving courtship behavior, but rather is due to the destruction of temperature-sensing neurons. Indeed, experiments indicate that male red-sided garter snakes with lesions in the AH-POA are unable to integrate information derived from the seasonal shift in temperature (Krohmer and Crews, 1986). Thus, it appears that in the red-sided garter snake the neural mechanisms activating sexual behavior are triggered by a specific environmental cue—a shift in temperature—rather than by surges in sex steroid hormone levels.

It is important here to emphasize that while all available evidence indicates that gonadal sex steroid hormones *do not* play a role in activating the neural substrates underlying courtship behavior in adult male red-sided garter snakes, this is not the same thing as saying that sexual behavior is independent of all hormonal control. Indeed, it is probable that at some level neurohormones and neurotransmitters are involved in the control of courtship behavior (see Chapter 3). Nor does this mean, as will be pointed out below, that sex steroid hormones play *no* role in the development of sexual behavior in males.

Like the male, the female red-sided garter snake mates when her ovaries are small and contain only previtellogenic follicles (Crews and Garstka, 1982). Circulating concentrations of E are low at this time, but if the female mates, there is a marked but transient surge in E levels. Mating can actually initiate ovarian growth, with this increase in E both facilitating transport of recently deposited sperm as well as mobilizing stored phospholipids so that yolking can occur (Bona-Gallo, 1983; Garstka et al., 1985). Ovulation occurs about 6–8 weeks later and pregnancy lasts for approximately 6 weeks. However, mating is not essential for reproduction if the female is sexually experienced. Sperm can be stored throughout winter dormancy in specialized furrows located in the anterior portion of the oviducts, enabling a female to still become pregnant the following year even if she does not mate that spring (Halpert et al., 1982; Whittier and Crews, 1986b).

Females are attractive to males on emergence from the hibernaculum, and most matings occur at this time (Crews and Garstka, 1982). Although the female is courted by a number of males, who form a "mating ball" about the female, she usually will mate with only one of the males. Immediately following mating the female is unreceptive to the copulatory attempts of other males, and within 24 hours she is no longer attractive to males. These changes in the sexual receptivity and attractivity of the female are mediated by physiological changes that occur as a consequence of the mating (Whittier and Crews, 1986b). Prostaglandins from the copulatory plug deposited by the mating male and/or from the female herself may play a major role in regulating these changes (Whittier and Crews, 1986c) (see Chapter 2).

The Constant Reproductive Pattern

In other harsh environments, such as some deserts, the onset of suitable conditions for breeding is very sudden and unpredictable. In species living under these conditions, the entire breeding season is over very quickly, hence the term *opportunistic* or *explosive* breeders. These species often exhibit a reproductive pattern in which large gonads with mature gametes or zygotes are maintained for prolonged periods in a constant state of readiness (Figure 4.1). Unfortunately, there have been few studies of the mechanisms controlling sexual behavior among species exhibiting this *constant* reproductive pattern. Perhaps the best studied is the desert-dwelling zebra finch (*Taeniopygia guttata castanotis*). Zebra finches are found in the deserts of mid-western Australia, where rainfall is very rare and unpredictable. Despite droughts that can last for years, males will maintain spermatogenically active testes and high circulating levels of androgens, and females will maintain ovaries containing follicles in an advanced resting state until appropriate conditions are encountered (Serventy, 1971). Rainfall is the proximate cue initiating reproductive behavior (Immelmann, 1972). Indeed, zebra finches have been observed to copulate within 10 minutes, to nest-build within 4 hours, and to lay eggs within a week of the onset of rains. While the dependence of sexual behavior in adult male zebra finches on gonadal androgens is well established, the permissive role of water for this response is as yet untested, since in all of the previous studies water has been available *ad libitum*. Recent experiments in which natural conditions are simulated by maintaining animals under water deprivation reveal that the neuroendocrine mechanisms of animals maintained under these conditions are profoundly different from those of animals with free access to water (Priedkalns et al., 1984; Vleck and Priedkalns, 1985).

TRENDS IN THE DIVERSITY OF REPRODUCTION

Study of this diversity in reproductive patterns has revealed that the concept of sexual behavior being dependent upon sex steroid hormones, a concept central to vertebrate behavioral physiology, is overly simplistic. The abundant evidence that gonadal hormones activate mating behavior in species representing each vertebrate class was taken as evidence for an intrinsic functional association among gamete production, sex hormone secretion, and mating behavior—in effect reflecting an evolutionary conservatism of hormone-brain-behavior regulating mechanisms. However, it is important to keep in mind that all evidence supporting the hypothesis of a causal relationship between gonadal hormones and mating behavior has been gathered on species exhibiting the associated reproductive pattern. There is now experimental data obtained on species exhibiting other reproductive patterns to suggest an alternative explanation. That is, similarities in dependence of mating behavior on sex steroid hormones observed in different vertebrates could be due to repeated convergent evolution rather than to descent from a common ancestor. Thus, it now appears that the paradigm that gonadal sex hormones activate sexual behavior in all vertebrates reflects an unintentional bias in the species most studied rather than a general rule.

Not only do studies of species exhibiting alternative reproductive patterns reveal profound differences in the neuroendocrine mechanisms subserving sexual behavior, they can also provide a framework within which to regard the great diversity in reproduction found among sexually reproducing vertebrates. To take just one example, we can deliberately polarize what is obviously a complex continuum, namely the associated versus dissociated reproductive patterns, and represent them as extremes. If we next assume that most individuals can exhibit only one reproductive pattern at a time, at least four distinct reproductive strategies might be predicted among vertebrates. Indeed, representatives of each category have been found to exist (Crews, 1984) (Table 4.2). That is, in many species both the male and the female exhibit mating behavior in close association with maximum gonadal activity. There also are a number of species in which both the male and female show a dissociation between gonadal activity and mating behavior. Finally, there are species having "mixed" reproductive strategies in which one sex exhibits one pattern and the other sex exhibits the opposite pattern.

TABLE 4.2. Relationship between gonadal activity and mating behavior in vertebrates

		Male	
		Associated	Dissociated
Female	Associated	Many laboratory and domesticated mammals; most birds; many temperate and tropical lizards, crocodilians	Most temperate turtles (e.g., *Chrysemys picta; Gopherus polyphemus*), *Crotalus h. horridus, Virginia; Ambystoma tigrinum; Esox lucius*
	Dissociated	*Suncus murinus; Fulmarus glacialis; Hemiergis peronii, Eumesces egregius, Phyllodactylus marmoratus, Sceloporus a. bicanthalis, Sceloporus g. microlepidotus, Vipera aspis, Micrurus fulvius; Cymatogaster aggregata, Trachycorystes striatulus*	Vespertilionid and rhinolophid (hibernating) bats; several crotalid, elapid, and colubrid snakes; *Carphophis vermis; Desmognathus* spp; *Pleuronectes platessa; Cyprinus carpio*

The research with the garter snake shows that the mechanisms underlying reproductive behavior in animals exhibiting the dissociated reproductive pattern can be fundamentally different from those found in animals exhibiting an associated reproductive tactic. However, it is the species exhibiting a mixed strategy that are of particular interest. While there are few studies of these species, there is evidence that the sexes can depend upon different environmental cues in timing seasonal gonadal activity. For example, the painted turtle (*Chrysemys picta*) breeds in early spring, shortly after emergence from hibernation. The male exhibits a dissociated reproductive pattern, mating when the testes are small. High body temperatures are required for testicular growth, which occurs later in the summer (Licht, 1984). The female, on the other hand, exhibits an associated reproductive pattern, mating when the ovaries have large follicles. Low body temperatures experienced the preceding fall stimulate ovarian recrudescence. While it is obvious that males and females must have different mechanisms regulating gonadal activity, how and why the mechanisms differ is a subject for further study. Neuroendocrine mechanisms subserving mating behavior can also show such fundamental differences between the sexes. The Asian musk shrew also exhibits a mixed reproductive strategy. Mating behavior in the male coincides with testicular growth and is dependent on testicular androgens, yet in the female, sexual receptivity is independent of gonadal hormone control (Dryden and Anderson, 1977; Hasler et al., 1975). Why such differences exist between the sexes awaits further study.

DIVERSITY AND THE DEVELOPMENT OF BEHAVIORAL CONTROLLING MECHANISMS

Species exhibiting different reproductive patterns may also exhibit differences in the development of neuroendocrine mechanisms subserving reproductive behavior. Studies of these species may yield insight into when and where sex steroid hormones are likely to act on the CNS. For example, extensive research has established that in species in which both sexes exhibit an associated reproductive pattern, the gonadal hormones produced during embryogenesis organize neural areas that later regulate mating behavior and reproductive physiology in the adult (Goy and McEwen, 1980). This action may be expressed at the structural level in the growth and destruction of CNS neurons. Hormonal mediation of CNS organization may also be expressed at the functional level. That is, sex steroid hormones in the adult may act on these areas to activate sexual behavior. Finally, just as sex steroid hormones alter the sensitivity of neural substrates involved in the regulation of reproductive physiology, they may also play an important role in perception, causing the organism to respond adaptively to appropriate internal and external cues (Beach, 1983).

We have seen how in species exhibiting alternative reproductive patterns, mating behavior can be independent of direct sex steroid hormone control in the adult. This does not mean that in these species sex steroid hormones are unimportant. Indeed, the evidence indicates that in such species, sex steroid hormones do play an important role, but only early in life. In these species sex steroid hormones appear to prepare or imprint specific sensory and motor systems so as to insure that the animal responds appropriately as an adult. The exact neural substrates affected by early hormone influences can be predicted by considering those substrates involved in the adult in the detection of biologically important stimuli and the performance of mating behavior. An example of such a system is found in the red-sided garter snake.

Although sex steroid hormones are not necessary for the display of courtship behavior in the adult male red-sided garter snakes, these hormones are involved in the development of the ability to express reproductive behavior in adulthood. Unlike adult red-sided garter snakes, treatment of males castrated as neonates with T will cause them to court attractive females (Crews, 1985). Only those males that have experienced high levels of androgens early in life will exhibit courtship behavior when they are adults; males castrated as neonates never show courtship behavior (Crews, 1985). Such a system in which sex steroid hormones are necessary for the organization of the neural substrates underlying courtship behavior, but not for their activation in adulthood, would explain the seeming paradox of the temporal organization of the dissociated reproductive pattern. This stems from the question of how, if the gametes are reproduced only after mating, is the first breeding season not a wasted effort? It is believed that male red-sided garter snakes undergo their first testicular growth cycle (puberty) in the summer of their second year. The androgens produced during the first testicular development therefore would program the brain such that the warm temperatures experienced on emergence the following spring elicit courtship behavior.

In the same way as hormones, behavioral experiences can also have a permanent organizing effect on behavioral controlling mechanisms. For example, it is well established that in many domesticated birds and rodents the longer the isolated castrated adult is deprived of hormones, the higher the threshold for eliciting mating behavior with exogenous hormone treatment (Crews, 1986). Further, gonadal hormones can potentiate neuronal activity, particularly in those areas of the brain that concentrate sex steroid hormones. It is also well known that in adult vertebrates specific environmental and social stimuli can activate these neural systems. Thus, the behavioral interaction of the individual during development with its internal and external environment is a major directive force in the maturation, and ultimately in the evolution of neural systems. In one sense, then, sex steroid hormones can be viewed as allowing for the growth of neural connections during development, whereas the participation of these neural circuits in particular behaviors establishes and maintains their functional integrity.

The above observation, and the discovery that gamete production, sex steroid hormone secretion, and mating behavior may be uncoupled, could account for why in some species the effect of gonadectomy on mating behavior is less pronounced if the individual is sexually experienced. There is no question that mating behavior, and hence reproductive success, improve with experience. It has also been noted that in species in which sexual experience plays a major role in the control of mating behavior, individuals frequently mate when the gonads are not producing gametes. Mating when the gonads are regressed may indicate that the causal mechanisms underlying mating behavior are different at different times of the year or, alternatively, that in these species the mating behavior of one or both of the sexes is less dependent on hormones and more dependent on social context. The potential interdependence of experiential and physiological factors is illustrated by the finding that castrated, sexually experienced rodents and primates no longer exhibit a preference for the opposite sex although they retain the ability to discriminate the opposite sex (Crews, 1986). Finally, it is likely that certain functional associations allow for learning of the behavioral as well as the physiological responses attendant to mating. These in turn may form the bases for motivated behaviors.

Another area totally unexplored is the possibility that organisms displaying alternative life-history strategies have fundamentally different behavioral controlling mechanisms. Evolutionary biologists have discovered recently that individuals within a given population may adopt distinctly different physiologies, morphologies, and/or behaviors. For example, there are three types of male bluegill sunfish (*Lepomis macrochirus*): a large colorful male that defends territories and solicits females, a small male that sneaks matings when the territorial male is otherwise occupied, and a large but drab male that mimics females in appearance (Gross, 1984). These female mimics effectively insert themselves between a courting territorial male and the female he is courting; in this manner the female mimic fertilizes the female.

Recent studies of the red-sided garter snake have revealed that female mimicry by males can also be expressed as a physiological feminization (Mason and Crews, 1985). Some adult male red-sided garter snakes produce what had been believed to be a female-specific attractant pheromone. In more than 200 mating balls in which the individuals have been censused, a male was the object of courtship in 16% of the mating aggregations. These individuals, termed "she-males," release a pheromone that has similar, if not identical, properties to the estrogen-dependent attractiveness pheromone released by adult females. In competitive mating trials in which normal males and a she-male were placed in an arena with an unmated female, the she-male mated with the female significantly more often than did the normal males. This mating advantage was accomplished by the she-male confusing the other males in the mating ball, causing them to ignore the female and court the she-male.

Behavioral, morphological, and physiological studies have revealed that she-males are genetic males that do not differ significantly from other males in length and weight. Further, the she-males have fully functional testes and accessory sex structures identical to other males and will court and mate with females. Radioimmunoassay of circulating levels of sex steroid hormones indicate that she-males have very high concentrations of T. Although circulating levels of E are similar to those found in normal males, it is possible that aromatase enzymes that convert T into E in the liver and skin, the target organs involved in the production and release of the attractiveness pheromone, produce high local concentrations of E which effectively feminize the male.

These female mimics may develop as a result of hormones experienced early in life (Mason and Crews, 1986). That is, this trait could be developmentally transmitted rather than genetically fixed. It is now known that in mice and rats, fetal position in the uterus has an influence on both the morphology and behavior of the adult. That is, males that develop between two females are feminized as compared to males that develop between two males (Vom Saal, 1983). We have recorded the intrauterine position of garter snake embryos and find that 16% of the males develop between two females. Although identical to the percentage of she-males found in the population, this is not evidence of a causal relationship. However, experiments indicate that early hormone environment may indeed be important. Administration of exogenous E to adult males will cause the production of the female attractiveness pheromone by its action on the liver (Garstka and Crews, 1981). This pheromone is carried in the blood but, unlike females, does not percolate through the skin and so is not released. This indicates that the skin of adult males and females is fundamentally different in its ability to transfer the pheromone from the blood to the skin surface. Like females, the skin of she-males does transport the attractiveness pheromone. Similarly, E administered to neonatal males will cause these baby males to be courted by adult males (Crews, 1985), indicating that administration of E early in life can feminize both the physiology and morphology of the male red-sided garter snake.

EVOLUTION OF HORMONE-BRAIN-BEHAVIOR CONTROLLING MECHANISMS

A basic tenet of neuroethology is that the structure and function of the central nervous system are adaptational responses to the environment of the organism (Ingle and Crews, 1985). While we know that neural mechanisms underlying behavior can be modified by artificial selection or by hybridization of closely related species, there is little direct evidence demonstrating how brain-behavior relationships evolve in naturally occurring species. Recent studies with two closely related species, one the direct evolutionary ancestor of the other, provide further proof that the brain will exploit any available stimulus to serve as a trigger for behaviors important for reproductive success.

The whiptail lizards (*Cnemidophorus*) are unusual in that some species are gonochoristic, having both male and female individuals that reproduce sexually, whereas other species are unisexual, consisting only of females that reproduce by true parthenogenesis. The parthenogenetic species are secondarily evolved from sexual species, and in many instances the ancestry of the parthenogen is known. For example, *C. uniparens* is believed to have resulted from the hybrid union of two sexual species, *C. inornatus* and *C. gularis* (Lowe and Wright, 1966) (Figure 4.7). Both of these ancestral species exist today, making it possible to study the evolution of behavioral control-

Evolution of the Triploid *Cnemidophorus uniparens*

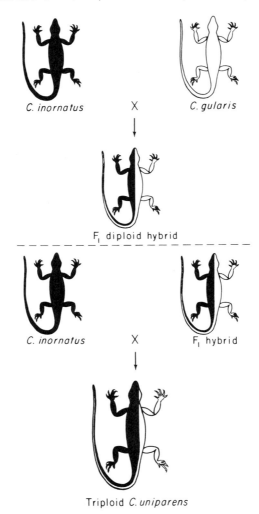

Figure 4.7. The hypothetical evolution of the parthenogenetic, all-female whiptail lizard *Cnemidophorus uniparens*. Two closely related sexual species, *C. inornatus* and *C. gularis*, are believed to have hybridized and the resulting F_1 backcrossed with *C. inornatus* to form the triploid (XXX) parthenogenetic *C. uniparens*.

ling mechanisms by examining the physiological control of species-typical behaviors in both the parthenogenetic species and its direct evolutionary ancestors.

The behavior of concern here is male courtship and copulatory behavior. *Cnemidophorus* lizards exhibit a highly stereotyped behavioral sequence during mating. In gonochoristic species, the male will approach and investigate the female with his bifed tongue, presumably indicating involvement of chemical senses via the vomeronasal organ as occurs in snakes (Figure 4.8). If the female is sexually receptive, she will stand still for the male, allowing him to mount her back. Usually just before the male mounts the female, he will grip with his jaws either a portion of the skin on the female's neck or her foreleg. As the male rides the female he will scratch her sides and press the female's body against the substrate. The male will then begin to maneuver his tail beneath the female's tail, attempting to appose the cloacal regions. During mating one of two hemipenes is everted through the male's cloacal opening and is intromitted into the female's cloacal. Simultaneous with intromission, the male will shift his jawgrip from the female's neck to her pelvic region, thereby assuming a contorted copulatory posture I have termed the doughnut posture (Crews and Fitzgerald, 1980). This posture will be maintained for 5–10 minutes, after which the male rapidly dismounts and leaves the female.

A similar sequence of events has been observed in at least five species of unisexual whiptail lizards (Figure 4.9). That is, one female will approach and mount another female and, after riding for a few minutes, the mounting female will swing her tail beneath that of the mounted female, apposing the cloacal regions. At the same time the mounting female will shift her jawgrip from the neck of to the pelvic region of the mounted female, forming the doughnut posture. Since parthenogenetic lizards are morphologically female, there are no hemipenes and intromission does not occur. Thus, while male individuals are absent in parthenogenetic lizards, this loss has been compensated for by the display of behaviors identical to the courtship and copulatory behavior of their ancestral species. Although we have yet to observe female-female mounting in our captive colony of intact *C. inornatus*, this behavior has been reported to occur, albeit rarely, between females of other gonochoristic whiptail species.

I have mentioned above that in addition to insuring fertilization of female ova by male sperm, the courtship and copulatory behavior of the male facilitates ovarian growth in conspecific females. This results in the synchronization and coordination of the reproductive physiologies of the male and the female; in many instances the female will not undergo normal ovarian development in the absence of sexually active males. This represents a powerful selective force in maintaining the display of male-typical behaviors.

Behavioral facilitation of reproduction is crucial even in species that do not reproduce sexually (Crews, 1982; Crews and Moore, 1986b). While isolated *C. uniparens* will lay viable eggs, the presence and behavior of

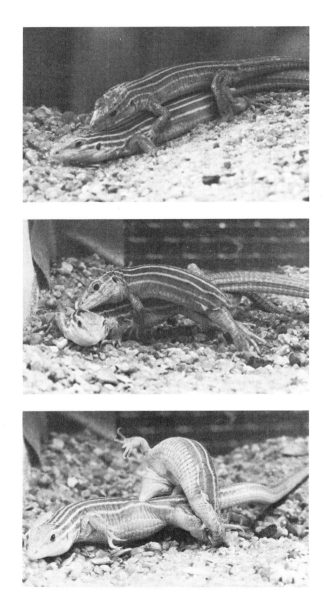

Figure 4.8. Mating sequence in the sexually reproducing whiptail lizard, *Cnemidophorus inornatus*, a direct evolutionary ancestor to the parthenogenetic whiptail, *C. uniparens*. See text for further details.

conspecifics has a marked facilitatory effect on an individual's reproductive effort. Females housed with other females, particularly if those females are hormonally treated so that they display male-like behavior, will lay significantly more eggs than will females housed alone (Gustafson and Crews, 1981; Crews et al., 1986; Crews and Moore, 1986b). This suggests that the

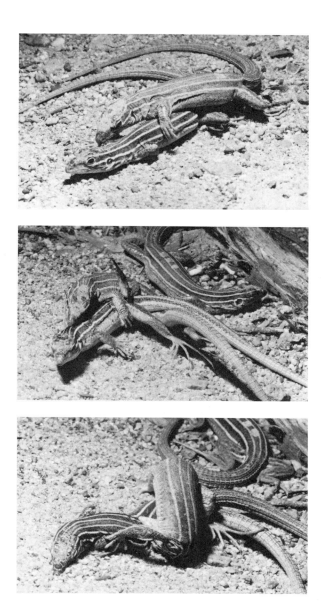

Figure 4.9. Pseudosexual behavior in the all-female parthenogenetic whiptail lizard *Cnemidophorus uniparens*. Note the similarity in the behavioral sequence to that of the gonochoristic whiptail species shown in Figure 4.8. (From Crews and Fitzgerald, 1980)

function of this pseudosexual behavior in parthenogenetic whiptails is similar to the male courtship facilitation of female ovarian growth in gonochoristic species.

Does this similarity in form and function of "sexual" behaviors between *C. inornatus* and *C. uniparens* also reflect similarity in physiological controlling mechanisms? It is in the answer to this question that we find clear evidence for the concept that the brain will exploit any stimulus that maximizes reproductive success.

Male *C. inornatus* are seasonal breeders, exhibiting courtship and copulatory behavior only during the late spring and early summer months. At this time the circulating levels of DHT and T are elevated, with plasma levels of DHT 2–3 times higher than plasma levels of T. The circulating concentrations of P during this period are low and unchanging, whereas the levels of E are undetectable (Moore and Crews, 1986).

The courtship and copulatory behavior of male *C. inornatus* is dependent upon testicular androgens (Lindzey and Crews, 1986). Castrated males court females significantly less often than do intact, sexually active males. Further, implantation of Silastic capsules containing DHT or T will reinstate sexual behavior in long-term castrated males (Figure 4.10). Significantly, a few castrated males receiving P also exhibited intense courtship behavior and even copulated.

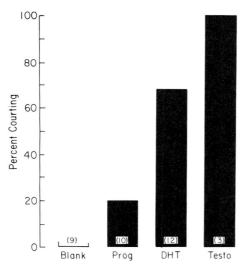

Figure 4.10. The level of courtship behavior exhibited by castrated male *Cnemidophorus inornatus* treated with hormones. Blank indicates those castrated males that received empty Silastic capsules. (From Lindzey and Crews, 1986)

In *C. uniparens* only reproductively active individuals exhibit pseudosexual behavior (Moore et al., 1985a). Female-like behavior is limited to the preovulatory stage of the follicular cycle, whereas the expression of male-like behavior occurs most frequently during the postovulatory stages of the cycle (Crews and Fitzgerald, 1980; Moore et al., 1985a) (Figure 4.11). Further, intact individuals when housed together will establish and maintain a complementarity in their reproductive conditions and alternate in their roles in pseudosexual encounters as they progress through their respective reproductive cycles (Moore et al., 1985a) (Figure 4.12). These changes in behavioral roles during pseudocopulations in *C. uniparens* are paralleled by transitions in the circulating levels of sex steroid hormones produced by the ovary (Figure 4.13).

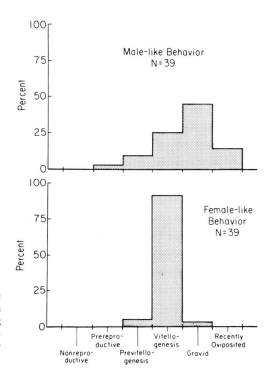

Figure 4.11. Exhibition of male-like (top panel) and female-like (bottom panel) pseudosexual behavior during different stages of the reproductive cycle of parthenogenetic *Cnemidophorus uniparens*. (From Moore et al., 1985a)

While it might be expected that *C. uniparens* would show elevated circulating levels of DHT and T that would coincide with the occurrence of male-like behavior, this is not the case (Moore et al., 1985b). Radio-immunoassay of these androgens reveals uniformly undetectable levels of these hormones at all stages of the reproductive cycle. The pattern and nature of sex steroid hormone secretion in *C. uniparens* is similar to that observed in female *C. inornatus*.

The circulating levels of sex steroid hormones in *C. uniparens* engaged in pseudocopulatory behavior are similar to those found in individuals in comparable stages of the reproductive cycle (Moore et al., 1985b). Preovulatory animals expressing female-like behavior are characterized by elevated levels of E and moderate levels of P. Postovulatory animals exhibiting male-like behavior have a twofold lower level of E and a threefold greater level of P.

It is clear that the neural substrates of male-typical courtship and copulatory behavior have been retained in the parthenogen *C. uniparens* and, further, that these substrates have retained their sensitivity to androgens. Male-like behaviors can be induced readily in either intact or ovariectomized *C. uniparens* by administration of exogenous DHT or T (Gustafson and Crews, 1982; Crews and Moore, 1986b). However, there is no evidence of even a transient elevation of either androgen during any phase of the ovarian cycle. Therefore, a cue other than DHT or T must

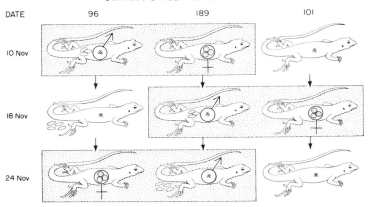

Figure 4.12. Schematic representation of the alternation of behavioral roles of captive parthenogenetic *Cnemidophorus uniparens*. In this experiment three animals were caged together and their reproductive states and behavioral interactions monitored. Stippled areas connect animals that pseudocopulated together, the generic emblem indicates the behavioral role assumed, and the structure within the body illustrates the stage of the reproductive cycle of each female at the time of the observation. In every instance, the female performing the female role was preovulatory, having large yolking follicles, whereas the female performing the male role was gravid with eggs in the oviduct or had recently ovulated.

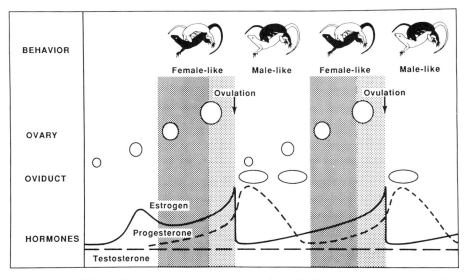

Figure 4.13. Relationship between the alternation in behavioral role during a pseudocopulation, changes in ovarian state, and the circulating levels of sex-steroid hormones in the parthenogenetic whiptail lizard, *Cnemidophorus uniparens*.

trigger male-like behavior in this parthenogen. If androgens are not involved in the activation of male-like pseudosexual behavior in *C. uniparens*, which hormone(s), if any, are?

The correlation between the transition from female-like to male-like behavior and the decrease in circulating levels of E and rise in P that accompanies ovulation suggest that the surge in P may be the trigger. To determine this, ovariectomized *C. uniparens* were given a Silastic implant of either P or E or a blank capsule (Grassman and Crews, 1986). Only when P-treated females were paired with E-treated females was pseudocopulation observed. Further, in every instance the P-treated female consistently performed male-like behavior (Table 4.3). When P-treated females were paired with females having blank implants, or when E-treated females were paired with females having blank implants, no pseudocopulations were observed. This indicates two things.

TABLE 4.3. Activation of pseudocopulatory behavior in unisexual *Cnemidophorus uniparens* by administration of progesterone and 17β-estradiol. The data are based on observations of pair-housed females. Lizards were ovariectomized and implanted with a Silastic capsule containing either progesterone (P), 17β-estradiol (E2), or a blank (B) Silastic capsule.

Experimental group	Number of pairs observed	Number of pairs in which pseudocopulations were observed	Number of pseudocopulations in which mounting individual was P-treated
Ovex + P			
Ovex + E2	21	15	15/15
Ovex + P			
Ovex + B	10	0	0/0
Ovex + B			
Ovex + E2	10	0	0/0

First, pseudosexual behavior is under ovarian hormone control in both participants. That is, high circulating levels of P stimulate male-like pseudosexual behavior in ovariectomized female *C. uniparens*. This is in contrast to results obtained in domesticated rats, quail, and ring doves, in which administration of exogenous P suppresses androgen-dependent sexual behaviors in males (Crews and Moore, 1986a). Female-like behavior, on the other hand, is induced in ovariectomized females with exogenous estradiol, which renders them both attractive and receptive to other females exhibiting male-like pseudosexual behavior. Thus, the hormonal basis of female-like behavior in *C. uniparens* is similar to that controlling sexual receptivity in females of many tetrapod vertebrates exhibiting an associated reproductive pattern.

Second, these results indicate that a complementarity in hormonal conditions is necessary if a pair of *C. uniparens* are to exhibit pseudosexual behavior.

In view of the facts that (1) DHT, T, and P are potent activators of male-like pseudosexual behavior in *C. uniparens* and (2) various progestigens can bind to androgen receptors and translocate to the nucleus, we are presently seeking to determine whether P is acting directly by binding to androgen receptors or is serving as a precursor and being converted to androgen at the site of action in the brain.

CONCLUDING REMARKS

For historical reasons the associated reproductive pattern, as the first discovered and the most investigated, has been viewed as the sole possible reproductive pattern. Further, all of the data supporting the popular belief of a deterministic relationship between sex steroid hormone secretion and sexual behavior in vertebrates have been obtained from species in which both the male and the female exhibit an associated reproductive pattern. However, it is obvious that in order to reproduce, all animals have evolved a sensitivity to the environment in which they live. Thus, given the abovementioned constraints, it is reasonable to assume that species have evolved a variety of mechanisms controlling mating behavior. For example, research on species exhibiting alternative reproductive patterns or strategies indicates that (1) gonadal activity and mating behavior are not necessarily temporally associated, (2) mating behavior need not depend upon increasing concentrations of sex steroid hormones, and (3) the stimuli regulating breeding, and hence the causal mechanisms underlying mating behavior, can be fundamentally different both within and between individuals of the same species, population, and sex.

With the exception of behavioral genetics and animal husbandry, the issue of species and individual variation has not been a focus of research by laboratory-oriented behavioral physiologists. However, variation is the fabric of evolution. Thus, the evolutionary perspective can provide a context in which to regard species and individual differences, while, at the same time, the physiological perspective uncovers the true nature of the mechanisms by which these differences arise. For example, the discovery of alternative life-history strategies within the same species (Austad and Howard, 1984) presents important challenges to current concepts. Similarly, the finding that in some species of microtine rodents, individuals within the same population may respond to different stimuli to initiate reproduction (Bronson, 1985; see Chapter 8) raises important questions regarding the meaning of variation in neuroendocrine mechanisms controlling reproduction. Finally, comparative study of closely related species can lead to insights into the evolution of behavioral controlling mechanisms. Thus, consideration of evolutionary theory can illuminate aspects that are not intuitively obvious yet are fundamental to the question of evolution of behavioral controlling mechanisms.

I have pointed out that any stimulus from the internal or external environments may evolve a signal function and serve as a trigger for mating behavior (Crews and Moore, 1986a) (Figure 4.14). For example, among

Figure 4.14. Because the expression of mating behavior must be synchronized with the occurrence of optimum environmental conditions, differences in the mechanisms controlling mating behavior can be viewed as alternative informational pathways between the physical environment and the central nervous system. Solid lines indicate possible direct effects of the physical environment on the organism; dashed lines indicate possible secondary pathways influencing the expression of sexual behavior. For example, in the most thoroughly studied vertebrates with associated reproductive patterns, the pathway consists of environmental stimulation of gonadal recrudescence and hence gonadal sex-steroid hormone action on the brain. In species exhibiting dissociated or constant reproductive patterns, the pathway is more direct, with environmental stimuli activating mating behavior without the mediating influence of sex-steroid hormones. (From Crews and Moore, 1986a)

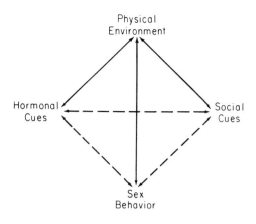

species exhibiting an associated reproductive pattern, sex steroid hormones are particularly well suited as internal signals, for they reliably predict gamete maturation. In certain environments, however, sex steroid hormones would be inappropriate as a proximate cue for reproductive behavior. In these instances specific physical, biotic, or social factors may serve as the proximate trigger for mating behavior and reproduction.

The purpose of this chapter has not been to provide answers so much as to point to new directions in research—namely, the need for more investigations of diverse organisms. As the evolutionary and physiological perspectives are integrated, another view of the relation of the different levels of organization necessary for reproduction will emerge. Evolutionary biology and behavioral ecology can provide new directions for investigations of behavioral controlling mechanisms, just as laboratory studies of the causes and functions of similar behaviors in different species can contribute to a better understanding of behavioral evolution. Such integrated studies will reveal the constraints and ultimate plasticity of proximate mechanisms controlling mating behavior.

ACKNOWLEDGMENTS

I thank the following individuals for reading earlier drafts of this manuscript: J. Blank, F. Bronson, J. Bull, N. Greenberg, J. Lindzey, H. Miller, G. Myers, R. Nelson, E. Rissman, J. Rosenblatt, M. Ryan, C. Sisk,

H. Snell, J. Whittier, W. Wilcyznki, I. Zucker. The research reported in this paper was supported by grants from NICHHD, NSF, and a NIMH Research Scientist Development Award.

REFERENCES

AUSTAD, S.N., and R.D. HOWARD (1984) Alternative reproductive tactics. Amer. Zool. *24*:305–418.

BEACH, F.A. (1983) Hormones and psychological processes. Can. J. Psychol. *37*:193–210.

BONA-GALLO, A., and P. LICHT (1983) Effects of temperature on sexual receptivity and ovarian recrudescence in the garter snake, *Thamnophis sirtalis parietalis*. Herpetol. *39*:173–182.

BRONSON, F.H. (1985) Mammalian reproduction: An ecological perspective. Biol. Reprod. *32*:1–26.

CLERMONT, Y. (1972) Kinetics of spermatogenesis: Seminiferous epithelium cycle and spermatogonial renewal. Physio. Rvw. *52*:198–231.

CLUTTON-BROCK, T.H., F.E. GUINNES, and S.D. ALBON (1982) *Red Deer: Behavior and Ecology of Two Sexes*. The University of Chicago Press, Chicago.

CREWS, D. (1975) Psychobiology of reptilian reproduction. Science *189*:1059–1065.

CREWS, D. (1979a) The neuroendocrinology of reproduction in reptiles. Biol. Reprod. *20*:51–73.

CREWS, D. (1979b) The hormonal control of behavior in a lizard. Sci. Amer. *241*: 180–187.

CREWS, D. (1980) Interrelationships among ecological, behavioral and neuroendocrine processes in the reproductive cycle of *Anolis carolinensis* and other reptiles. In *Advances in the Study of Behavior*, Vol. 11. J.S. Rosenblatt, R.A. Hinde, C.G. Beer, and M.C. Busnel, eds., pp. 1–74, Academic Press, New York.

CREWS, D. (1982) On the origin of sexual behavior. Psychoneuroendocrinol. *7*:259–270.

CREWS, D. (1983) Control of male sexual behavior in the Canadian red-sided garter snake. In *Hormones and Behavior in Higher Vertebrates*. J. Balthazart, E. Prove, and R. Gilles, eds., pp. 398–406, Plenum Press, London.

CREWS, D. (1984) Gamete production, sex hormone secretion, and mating behavior uncoupled. Horm. Beh. *18*:22–28.

CREWS, D. (1985) Effects of early sex hormone treatment on courtship behavior and sexual attractivity in the red-sided garter snake, *Thamnophis sirtalis parietalis*. Physiol. Behav. *35*:569–575.

CREWS, D. (1986) Functional associations in behavioral endocrinology. In *Masculinity/Feminity: Concepts and Definitions*. J.M. Reinisch, L.A. Rosenblum, and S.A. Sanders, eds. (in press), Oxford University Press, Oxford, England.

CREWS, D., and K. FITZGERALD (1980) "Sexual" behavior in parthenogenetic lizards (*Cnemidophorus*). Proc. Natl. Acad. Sci. *77*:499–502.

CREWS, D., and W. GARSTKA (1982) The ecological physiology of a garter snake. Sci. Amer. *247*:158–168.

CREWS, D., and M.C. MOORE (1986a) Evolution of mechanisms controlling mating behavior. Science *231*:121–125.

CREWS, D., and M.C. MOORE (1986b) Psychobiology of reproduction of unisexual whiptail lizards. In *Biology of Cnemidophorus Lizards*. J.W. Wright, ed. (in press), University of Washington Press, Seattle.

CREWS, D., M. GRASSMAN, and J. LINDZEY (1986) Behavioral facilitation of reproduction in sexual and parthenogenetic whiptail (*Cnemidophorus*) lizards. Proc. Natl. Acad. Sci. (in press).

DRYDEN, G.L., and J.N. ANDERSON (1977) Ovarian hormone: Lack of effect on reproductive structure of female Asian musk shrews. Science *197*:782–784.

FRIEDMAN, D.W., and D. CREWS (1985a) Role of the anterior hypothalamus-preoptic area in the regulation of courtship behavior in the male Canadian red-sided garter snake (*Thamnophis sirtalis parietalis*): Intracranial implantation experiments. Horm. Behav. *19*:122–136.

FRIEDMAN, D., and D. CREWS (1985b) Role of anterior hypothalamus–preoptic area in the regulation of courtship behavior in the male Canadian red-sided garter snake (*Thamnophis sirtalis parietalis*): Lesion experiments. Behav. Neurosci. *99*:942–949.

GARSTKA, W.R., and D. CREWS (1981) Female sex pheromone in the skin and circulation of a garter snake. Science *214*:681–683.

GARSTKA, W.R., R.R. TOKARZ, M. DIAMOND, A. HALPERT, and D. CREWS (1985) Behavioral and physiological control of yolk synthesis and deposition in the red-sided garter snake (*Thamnophis sirtalis parietalis*). Horm. Behav. *19*:137–153.

GHISELIN, M. (1974) *The Economy of Nature and the Evolution of Sex*. The University of California Press, Berkeley.

GOY, R.W., and B.S. MCEWEN (1980) *Sexual Differentiation of the Brain*. The MIT Press, Cambridge.

GRASSMAN, M., and D. CREWS (1986) Hormonal mediation of male- and female-like behaviors in an all-female lizard species. Horm. Behav. (in press).

GREENWALD, G.S. (1978) Follicular activity in the mammalian ovary. In *The Vertebrate Ovary*. R.E. Jones, ed., pp. 639–690, Plenum Press, New York.

GROSS, M.R. (1984) Sunfish, salmon, and the evolution of alternative reproductive strategies and tactics in fishes. In *Fish Reproduction: Strategies and Tactics*. G.W. Potts and R.J. Wooton, eds., pp. 55–76, Academic Press, London.

GUSTAFSON, J.E., and D. CREWS (1981) Effect of group size and physiological state of a cagemate on reproductive effort in the parthenogenetic lizard *Cnemidophorus uniparens* (Teiidae). Behav. Ecol. Sociobiol. *8*:267–272.

HALPERN, M., J. MORRELL, and D.W. PFAFF (1982) Cellular 3H-estradiol and 3H-testosterone localization in the brains of garter snakes: An autoradiographic study. Gen. Comp. Endocr. *46*:211–224.

HALPERT, A., W. GARSTKA, and D. CREWS (1982) Sperm transport and storage and its relation to the annual sexual cycle of the female red-sided garter snake, *Thamnophis sirtalis parietalis*. J. Morphol. *174*:149–159.

HASLER, M.J., R.E. FAVO, and A.V. NALBANDOV (1975) Testicular development and testosterone concentrations in the testis and plasma of young male shrews (*Suncus murinus*). Gen. Comp. Endocr. *25*:36–41.

IMMELMANN, K. (1972) Roles of the environment in reproduction as a source of "predictive" information. In *Breeding Biology of Birds*. D.S. Farner, ed., pp. 121–146, National Academy of Sciences, Washington, D.C.

INGLE, D., and D. CREWS (1985) Vertebrate neuroethology: Definitions and paradigms. Ann. Rvw. Neurosci. *8*:457–494.

JONES, R.E. (1978) Ovarian cycles in nonmammalian vertebrates. In *The Vertebrate Ovary*. R.E. Jones, ed., pp. 731–762, Plenum Press, New York.

KROHMER, R.W., and D. CREWS (1986) Neural control of courtship behavior in male garter snakes. Behav. Neurosci. (in press).

LESHNER, A.I. (1978) *An Introduction to Behavioral Endocrinology*. Oxford University Press, New York.

LICHT, P. (1984) Reptiles. In *Marshall's Physiology of Reproduction*: Vol. 1. *Reproductive Cycles of Vertebrates*. G.E. Lamming, ed., pp. 206–282, Churchill Livingstone, Edinburgh.

LINDZEY, J., and D. CREWS (1986) Control of sexual behavior in male *Cnemidophorus inornatus*. Gen. Comp. Endocr. (in press).

LOWE, C.H., and J.W. WRIGHT (1966) Evolution of parthenogenetic species of *Cnemidophorus* (whiptail) lizards in western North America. J. Ariz. Acad. Sci. *4*:81–87.

MASON, R.T., and D. CREWS (1985) Female mimicry in garter snakes. Nature *316*:59–60.

MASON, R.T., and D. CREWS (1986) Pheromonal mimicry in garter snakes. In *Chemical Signals in Vertebrates*. D. Duval and D. Muller-Schwartz, eds. (in press), Plenum Press, New York.

MOORE, M.C., J.M. WHITTIER, A.J. BILLY, and D. CREWS (1985a) Male-like behavior in an all-female lizard: Relationship to ovarian cycle. Anim. Behav. *33*:284–289.

MOORE, M.C., J.M. WHITTIER, and D. CREWS (1985b) Sex steroid hormones during the ovarian cycle of an all-female, parthenogenetic lizard and their correlation with pseudosexual behavior. Gen. Comp. Endocr. *60*:144–153.

MOORE, M.C., and D. CREWS (1986) Sex steroid hormone levels in male and female *Cnemidophorus inornatus*, a direct sexual ancestor of a unisexual, parthenogenetic lizard. Gen. Comp. Endocr. (in press).

MORRELL, J.I., D. CREWS, A. BALLIN, A. MORGENTALER, and D.W. PFAFF (1979) 3H-estradiol, 3H-testosterone, and 3H-dihydrotestosterone localization in the brain of the lizard, *Anolis carolinensis*: An autoradiographic study. J. Comp. Neurol. *188*:201–224.

PIANKA, E. (1970) On *r* and *K* selection. Amer. Natl. *100*:592–597.

PRIEDKALNS, J., A. OKSCHE, C. VLECK, and R.K. BENNETT (1984) The response of the hypothalamo-gonadal system to environmental factors in the zebra finch, *Poephila guttata castanotis*. Cell Tiss. Res. *238*:23–35.

SATINOFF, E. (1978) Neural organization and the evolution of thermoregulation in mammals. Science *201*:16–22.

SERVENTY, D.L. (1971) Biology of desert birds. In *Avian Biology*. D.S. Farner and J.R. King, eds., pp. 287–339, Academic Press, New York.

VLECK, C.M., and J. PRIEDKALNS (1985) Reproduction in zebra finches: Hormone levels and effect of dehydration. Condor *87*:37–46.

Vom Saal, F. (1983) The interaction of circulating oestrogens and androgens in regulating mammalian sexual differentiation. In *Hormones and Behaviour in Higher Vertebrates*. J. Balthazart, E. Prove, and R. Gilles, eds., pp. 159–177, Springer-Verlag, Berlin.

Whittier, J.M., R.T. Mason, and D. Crews (1985) Mating in the red-sided garter snake, *Thamnophis sirtalis parietalis*: Differential effects on male and female sexual behavior. Behav. Ecol. Sociobiol. *16*:257–261.

Whittier, J. M., and D. Crews (1986a) Seasonal reproduction: Patterns and control. In *Regulation of Reproductive Cycles in Nonmammalian Vertebrates*. K. Norris and R.E. Jones, eds. (in press), Plenum Press, New York.

Whittier, J., and D. Crews (1986b) Ovarian development in red-sided garter snakes, *Thamnophis sirtalis parietalis*: Relationship to mating. Gen. Comp. Endocrin. *61*:5–12.

Whittier, J.M., and D. Crews (1986c) Effects of prostaglandin F-2alpha on sexual behavior and ovarian function in female garter snakes, *Thamnophis sirtalis parietalis*. Endocr. *119*:787–792.

FIVE
Circadian Rhythms in Avian Reproduction

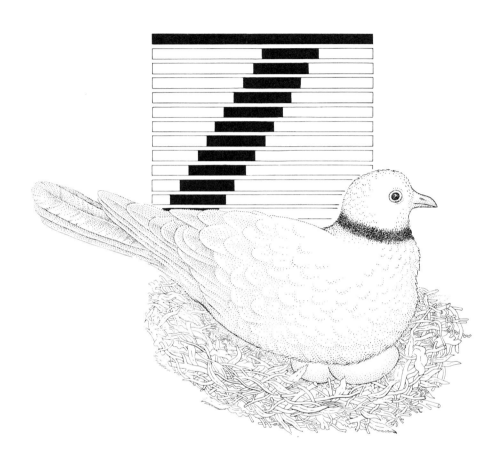

Rae Silver and Robert B. Norgren, Jr.
Barnard College of Columbia University
New York, NY

In order to breed successfully, animals must perform a series of behavioral responses in correct temporal order and in synchrony with specific physiological and morphological changes. In birds, for example, establishment of a territory and nest site is followed, over a period of days or weeks, by courtship and nest building, incubation, and care of the young. Activities such as feeding and caring for the young, as well as physiological responses such as ovulation, tend to occur at a particular time of day. Thus, reproduction in birds, as in other forms, can be viewed as a set of nested activities which must fit together appropriately if reproduction is to be successful. The way in which we understand these nested processes is in part determined by the "time-window" we use for the analysis.

In a broad temporal context, it is clear that the optimal time for initiating breeding activities for most species is ultimately determined by the availability of food necessary for the survival of young. Many seasonally breeding animals, especially those birds living in temperate zones, anticipate the optimal time for breeding by using daylength to predict the arrival of the annual breeding season. That is, birds use information present in daylength to anticipate the long days of summer and the appropriate time for seasonal growth of the gonads. Nonphotic factors also influence the onset of breeding, with differences among species, populations, and even among individuals in the relative importance of environmental effects (see Chapter 6) (Wingfield, 1983; Desjardins and Lopez, 1983). In some species, the measurement of time using daylength as an environmental cue depends on endogenous neural rhythms with circadian periodicity. In this chapter, we explore daily rhythms of behavioral and physiological changes in the reproduction of birds, and the relationship of these daily events to longer-duration breeding cycles (see Farner, 1985, for review of annual rhythms).

ANALYSIS OF DAILY ACTIVITY PATTERNS

In nature, organisms exhibit daily rhythms in many responses. Rats are active at night and sleep in the daytime, while most birds, like people, are active in the daytime and sleep at night. Intuitively we might expect that these activity rhythms are the direct result of exposure to daily rhythms which result from the earth's rotation about the sun. This is not the case. In fact, evidence from different kinds of organisms and for several responses within a single organism indicate that many circadian rhythms persist in the absence of periodic environmental input (see Aschoff, 1979, for review).

In laboratory conditions, where temporal cues from the environment can be eliminated, many activities continue to be expressed rhythmically, with a period very close to, but not precisely, 24 hours. Hence the term *circadian*. This suggests that some pacemaker system within the animal is capable of supporting continued, self-sustained oscillations which can serve to synchronize internal processes within the animal. The daily rhythms seen in nature result from the action of periodic environmental cues (such as the day-night cycle) acting to synchronize or entrain the animals' internal oscillator(s). In this way, physiological and behavioral rhythms expressed by the animal are synchronized with the environment.

Circadian rhythms were viewed as an interesting biological curiosity until it was recognized that they function to measure time. This conception stimulated modern scientific inquiry in the analysis of circadian rhythms. An example of the use of the circadian timer as a true clock that can be consulted at any time is seen in the sun-compass orientation of bees and birds (Hoffman, 1960). Here, animals respond to where the sun "should" be at a given time of day and modify their flight direction relative to the sun's position, as if they had an internal "time sense." To the extent that the internal clock can be used to measure daylength, it can also provide organisms with predictive information about season, thereby serving as an internal calendar.

Research on the analysis of circadian rhythms has proceeded in two directions. The first involves the development of mathematical models based on analogies between the endogenous circadian system (the circadian "clock") and physical oscillators. The second involves identification of the anatomical location and physiological and biochemical properties of the circadian clock. We will discuss each of these lines of research in turn.

Oscillator Model of Circadian System

In the first approach, the internal clock that regulates the expression of responses with a circadian period is considered to be a "black box." The properties of the clock itself are inferred from the response of any of a number of overt rhythms expressed by organisms. This method of studying the clock rests on the assumption that the period of the rhythm expressed in the response under study represents the period of the pacemaker or clock. Of necessity, the circadian response reflects not only the functioning of the clock itself, but also the properties of the input system that carries information from the external and internal milieu to the clock, as well as the output system from the clock to the physiological processes that control behavioral and physiological rhythms. Thus, it is important to separate experimental effects on the clock itself from those which affect the input and output pathways.

To an impressive degree, the control of the endogenous circadian oscillator by an exogenous driving oscillator obeys the laws of oscillation theory of physics. This has led to the development of mathematical models based on the analogy between biological clocks and physical oscillators and to the widespread adoption of an often complex terminology and methods of data analysis. A few concepts are necessary to an understanding of the literature. Definitions of terms are provided in Table 5.1.

TABLE 5.1.   Glossary of Terms Used to Describe Biological Rhythms

Circadian rhythm. An endogenous oscillation with a free-running period that is close to the period (24 hr) of the solar day.

Circadian system. The sum of all the circadian oscillations, including the pacemakers (driving oscillators), slave (driven) oscillators, and overt circadian rhythms of an organism.

Entrainment. The process by which an endogenous rhythm becomes coupled to and assumes the period of an environmental cycle (Zeitgeber).

Free-running period. The period of an endogenous rhythm when it is not entrained by an external cycle.

Period. The length of time between recurring phase reference points (see Figure 5.1) in a continuing oscillation—i.e., the time required for a rhythm to complete one full cycle.

Phase. An instantaneous state in an oscillation or some larger fraction of its period.

Phase angle. The time (e.g., in hours or degrees) between phase reference points in a rhythm and a Zeitgeber or between phases of two rhythms.

Phase shift. A single displacement of an oscillation along its time axis involving a temporary change in the rhythm's period.

Photoinducible phase. That phase or portion of the circadian cycle in which light can trigger a long-day photoperiodic response.

Photoperiod. Daylength; the length (in hours) of the light phase in a light-dark (LD) cycle.

Zeitgeber. An environmental cycle or perturbation that is capable of entraining a biological rhythm.

The basic principle of the analogy is that rhythmic behavioral and physiological functions can be analyzed in terms of known properties of physical oscillators (like pendulums or capacitors). This can be visualized by analogy with the rolling tire of a car. Consider the movement of a point marked on the tire, as the car moves forward. If you plot the distance of the mark above ground as a function of time, the result is a sinusoidal wave, as seen in Figure 5.1. The distance from d to d' is the *time* taken to complete one revolution or oscillation of the tire and is the *period* of the oscillation. The *period* stays constant as long as the tire moves forward at the same speed. Another measure of the speed of the rolling tire is the *frequency* of its rotation per unit time. This is the reciprocal of period, so that if the rolling tire slows down, the period increases and the frequency decreases. Any particular point in the cycle of oscillation is called a *phase*. If the tire were to strike a large stone as it moved forward, it would spin for a fraction of a revolution, and a given point on the tire would then be *phase-advanced* relative to comparable points on the other tires. The word *rhythm* is used to

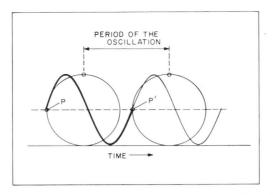

Figure 5.1. The principles of oscillations and cycles. The thick line plots the sine-wave displacement over time of point *p* on a wheel. The period of a biological rhythm is the time it takes for one complete rotation of the tire (represented by the circle) and is represented in the distance from *d* to *d'*. Biologists often use the term *amplitude* to describe the maximum peak-to-trough deviation of the rhythm.

describe the overt, observable response, while the word *oscillator* refers to the unseen but presumed underlying clock that drives the overt rhythms.

When an endogenous oscillation is modified by an outside force so that it assumes the period of the driver, it is said to be entrained or synchronized to the driving oscillator. If both oscillators are self-sustained, the term *entrainment* can be applied; in biological parlance the driving oscillator is called a *Zeitgeber* or "time-giver." In the absence of a driving oscillator, such as is seen in constant darkness (DD), the endogenous clock oscillates at its natural period (usually slightly different from the 24-hour period of the driving oscillator) and it is said to *free-run*.

Reproductive Behavior of Parent Ring Doves

Our interest in timing mechanisms stems from studies of the reproductive behavior of the ring dove, *Streptopelia roseogrisea*. The breeding cycle of ring doves has three major functional components: courtship and nest building, incubation of eggs, and brooding of the young. In the laboratory, when a pair of doves is placed in a breeding cage, courtship and nest building is observed for a 7–9-day period. The courtship and sexual behaviors displayed by the mates are known to be dependent on secretions of gonadal steroids—androgens in the male, and estrogen and progesterone in the female (Silver, 1978; Cheng, 1979). Also in this period, two ovarian follicles grow from their resting size of about 1 mm to a large, preovulatory size of about 14–15 mm. Courtship ends when the female lays her clutch of 2 eggs.

Both parents incubate the eggs for 14–15 days until the young hatch. The parents feed their young crop "milk." This substance derives from the lining of the crop sac and is produced under the influence of the hormone prolactin. Approximately 14 days after hatching, the squabs are able to peck for seeds themselves, and by the time they are 21 days of age, they are able to feed themselves. At this time, the parents begin to court anew and another breeding cycle begins.

The hormonal correlates of the behaviors that occur during the breeding cycle have been the subject of intense study (Silver, 1978; Cheng, 1979). As can be seen in Figure 5.2, high levels of luteinizing hormone (LH) from the pituitary and testosterone from the gonads occur during courtship and nest building. Progesterone levels do not show any systematic changes during the breeding cycle in males. In females, pituitary LH and gonadal estrogen and progesterone increase steadily during courtship and fall to baseline levels during incubation. Note that the temporal pattern of these hormone changes is strikingly similar to that described in wild species (see Chapter 6).

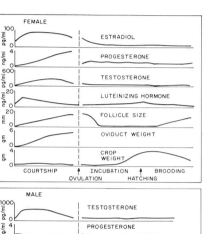

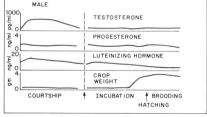

Figure 5.2. Changes in hormone secretion during the reproductive cycle of male and female ring doves. In the female, ovarian growth and secretion of LH, estrogen, and progesterone show a clear relationship to the state of the oviduct and ovary. In the male, there is an increase in LH and androgens during courtship. These hormones return to baseline levels during incubation and brooding. In both sexes, prolactin stimulates crop growth starting at about mid-incubation and ending around the time the young are able to feed themselves at 8–10 days. (Modified from Silver, 1978)

Crop-sac development reaches its peak during the parental phase of the cycle in both males and females. Prolactin stimulates crop-sac development and maintains incubation behavior. Plasma levels of this hormone begin to rise during the second half of the incubation and peak just after the young hatch.

When they are incubating and brooding their young, doves express dramatic daily rhythms in parental behavior. Each day the male sits on the eggs or newly hatched young for a block of time in the middle of the day, while the female sits the rest of the time. This shared parental care begins the day the eggs are laid and ends when the young are able to regulate their body temperature at about 8–10 days after hatching.

In order to understand this behavior, we have studied the internal and external stimuli that mediate sex differences in the timing of parenting. Questions of this type have been posed in the analysis of many different kinds of rhythmic responses in a variety of species. As we will see, this literature provides some clues on ways to search for and analyze timing mechanisms used by parent doves.

Though the work on other circadian rhythms is helpful, the circadian expression of parental behavior of ring doves differs in a significant way from that studied in other systems. In many studies of circadian rhythms, the response of an isolated individual animal is analyzed. In the analysis of sitting behavior of ring doves, we are concerned with how the mates are able to coordinate their responses so as to keep their young covered at all times. If oscillatory circadian timing mechanisms are operative, these presumably reside in two different individuals. Social organisms must adjust the time of expression of many of their behaviors to reflect the activities of other organisms. This leads to the broader question of how social factors influence circadian rhythms.

In this chapter, we review the work on the timing behavior of ring dove parents, explore the role of reproductive hormones and central neural mechanisms controlling timed responses, and show how the ring doves' behavior can be understood in the context of formal and physiological studies of circadian timing mechanisms in other species. To this end, we explore how circadian timing mechanisms serve as clocks providing information on time of day, and as calendars providing information on changing daylengths and seasons.

Timing Behavior of Parent Doves

When ring doves incubate their eggs, the male sits for a block of time in the middle of the day and the female sits the rest of the time. If we plot the parents' daily bout of sitting one day under the other, it is apparent that the onset (or termination) of incubation by each parent has a period of about 24 hours. To demonstrate this point, Figure 5.3 shows the timing of incubation by feral doves in Florida. How do the birds know whose turn it is to incubate? Are they responding to an environmental cue, or to an internal cue?

To approach problems of this type we can place ring doves in a constant environment which provides no external temporal cues, and analyze the resulting pattern of incubation. If ring doves use an internal clock, they should continue to express regular rhythms of incubation even in constant environmental conditions, and the period of the response should be close to 24 hours. If parent ring doves are responding to environmental cues in determining whose turn it is to sit, then they should be unable to maintain the species-typical pattern.

Breeding ring doves housed in constant dim illumination with uninterrupted access to food and water continue to show a regular pattern of incubation with a period somewhat shorter than 24 hours (Figure 5.4, upper panel). The drift observed in the timing of incubation under these conditions is an example of a free-run. In the example shown, the period of the free-run for the onset of each parent's sit bout is about 23.5 hours. Under normal

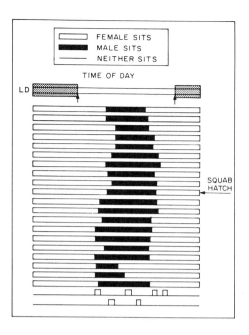

Figure 5.3. Timing of incubation by ring doves. The figure depicts the daily bouts of incubation by feral male (black bar) and female (open bar) ring doves breeding in Florida. Each day's data is plotted immediately beneath the data for the previous day. The male sits for a block of time in the middle of the day and the female sits the rest of the time until the young are about 8 days of age. The same temporal pattern of incubation is seen in laboratory-housed birds. Sunrise (6:46 hr) and sunset (20:30 hr) are indicated by arrows. The stippled area indicates night.

conditions of alternating light and darkness, the internal clock adjusts so that the animal is entrained to the photoperiod. Free-running activity rhythms in constant conditions are characteristic of a wide variety of responses that are thought to be regulated by circadian clocks (see Rusak, 1981, for review).

Given that two animals are involved in the timing of incubation by ring doves, we can ask whether one or both animals have endogenous circadian clocks, and how the two animals synchronize their behavior. To study the contribution of each partner to the timing of incubation, we can analyze when each bird approaches the nest to try to begin its bout of sitting. The animals are housed in a two-chambered cage (Figure 5.5). The chambers are connected by an L-shaped hallway. The identity of the parent sitting on the nest, and the approaches to the nest via the hallway by the nonsitting bird, are recorded by computer-monitored radio-telemetry. If only one of the partners were timing incubation bouts, then the "nontiming" bird should approach either randomly or after the "timing" bird gets off the nest.

In fact, neither partner waits for the sitting mate to leave the nest before going down the hallway to the nest chamber; each partner restricts its approaches to the nest to the interval just before nest exchange. In conditions of constant dim illumination described above, the timing of approaches to the nest area by each parent free-runs (Figure 5.4, lower panel). The ring doves' behavior in each of these conditions suggests that each mate has a circadian clock and that the circadian clock determines onset of incubation bout rather than its termination.

In natural conditions of alternating day and night, the endogenous clock is entrained to the day-night cycle. This was shown for parent ring

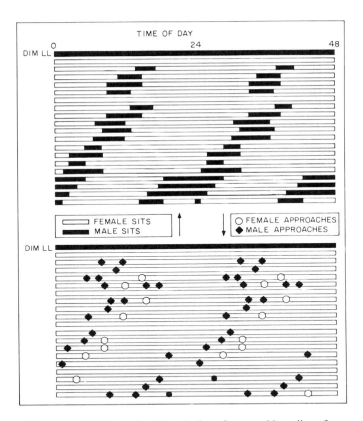

Figure 5.4. (Upper panel) Daily timing of incubation of eggs and brooding of young following egg laying. Birds are housed in a light-dark cycle of 14:10 until the female lays eggs. Once incubation begins, the lighting conditions are constant dim light (0.5 lux at cage floor). As in Figure 5.3, the black bar indicates sitting by the male, the open bar indicates sitting by the female. The figure is double-plotted to show 48 consecutive hours of activity, thereby permitting better visualization of the period of the activity. The determination of which mate is at the nest is made by computer-controlled telemetric monitoring of an antenna at the nest. (Lower panel) Approaches to the nest area by the pair of doves whose sitting behavior is depicted in the left panel. Approaches by the male (shown by a diamond) and by the female (shown by an open circle) are tracked by computer (see Figure 5.5). Note that the approaches to the nest area by both partners are largely limited to the time preceding nest exchange.

doves in an experiment where the light cycle was phase-shifted so that the middle of the day became the middle of the night (Figure 5.6). In response, the doves phase-shifted their sitting so that within a few days the male was sitting in the middle of the new day, and the female was sitting the rest of the time.

Evidence for Interval Timing

The foregoing evidence suggests that an endogenous oscillatory mechanism determines the onset of incubation bouts. We are still left with the

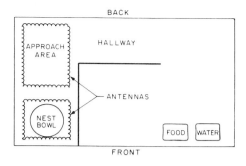

Figure 5.5. Diagram of two-chambered cage in which the nest area and the feeding chamber are separated by a connecting hallway. Antennas in the hallway and around the nest transmit the signal frequency of telemeters worn by each partner, allowing the computer to detect the presence of the parent ring doves in these areas.

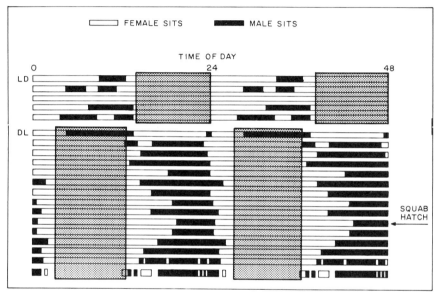

Figure 5.6. Effect of phase shift of the light-dark cycle on timing of incubation by parent doves. The timing of sitting by each partner is depicted as in Figure 5.3, and the data is double-plotted. The photoperiod is indicated on the bars labeled "LD" or "DL"; the stippled area represents the dark, while the open bar represents the light portion of the cycle. For the first five days of incubation, the doves are housed in a light-dark cycle of 14:10. On the sixth day the lights are adjusted so that the middle of the day becomes the middle of the night. The figure shows that the doves adjust the timing of their sitting so that the male again sits in the middle of the light period.

problem of how each mate decides when to quit each bout. One possibility is that the sitting bird is signalled to leave by the appearance of the nonsitting bird in the nest area. The other possibility is that the sitting (or nonsitting) bird measures the interval on (or off) the nest.

In an experiment where the male was prevented from starting his incubation bout at his usual time, we asked whether he would sit for his usual duration, or whether he would quit at the usual time of day (Gibbon et al., 1984). To this end, males of incubating pairs were prevented from approaching the nest for several hours by a gate placed in the hallway. Under these circumstances, the male stayed on the nest beyond his usual time, even though the female tried to get on the nest at her usual time (Figure 5.7). Videotape records of the mates' behavior strikingly document the vigor of their struggle for the nest. The results suggest that two different timing mechanisms are used to determine the time of the afternoon nest exchange: a circadian mechanism determines the onset of incubation by the female, and an interval mechanism influences the termination of incubation by the male. Studies are continuing to establish whether the female measures duration of incubation, and whether she times duration during nighttime as well as during daylight hours.

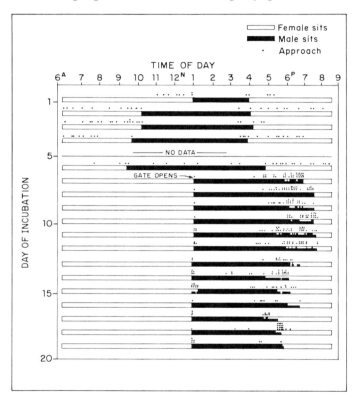

Figure 5.7. Timing of incubation on consecutive days by a pair of doves. The pair was permitted to nest-exchange without disturbance for the first 5 days of incubation. Starting on the sixth day, the gate in the hallway (see Figure 5.5) was closed after lights out, delaying the male from starting his sit bout by 3 hours. The dot signifying an approach to the nest sits above the bar which signifies incubation by the male (black bar), female (white bar), or both mates (half-black, half-white bar). (Modified from Gibbon et al., 1984)

Role of Gonadal Hormones in Sex-Typical Behavior

We have manipulated the hormone environment of adult birds in order to analyze whether gonadal hormones mediate sex differences in timing of incubation (R. Silver, unpublished data). A pair of intact adult male ring doves will not incubate eggs if they are provided. If the testes of one of the males are removed, and he is treated with the ovarian hormones estrogen and progesterone, he assumes the female's schedule of incubation. That is, the "feminized male" tends to sit during the evening, night, and morning hours, while its mate sits for the male-typical block of time in the middle of the day. Conversely, an ovariectomized, testosterone-treated female assumes the male's role when paired with a normal female and sits for the male-typical time in the middle of the day. These results suggest that sex hormones influence the expression of a circadian rhythm which is dependent on an endogenous clock. We do not yet know whether the hormones act on the clock itself or on the mechanisms coupling the clock to response systems.

Relation Between Various Circadian Responses

Is there a single master pacemaker that controls all (or several) circadian rhythms? In the case of seasonally breeding birds one might ask whether the clock that influences daily cycles of activity and incubation also serves as a "calendar" to determine seasonal cycles of gonadal growth. Studies on the possible relationship between the rhythms controlling locomotor activity and gonadal development have been done on avian species (see Murton and Westwood, 1977). Because the quality of light required to stimulate locomotor activity differs from that required for gonadal development, one can use dim light to entrain the behavioral response without stimulating the gonadal response. In one such experiment, a very dim green light (dimmer than a night light) was used to entrain the locomotor activity of house sparrows (*Passer domesticus*) without stimulating gonadal development (Menaker and Eskin, 1967). House sparrows, like most birds, are active during the light portion of the day (which in this case was 14 hours of dim green light), and inactive in the dark. The birds were then given a 75-minute pulse of white light either at the beginning or the end of the daily activity period. Such pulses have little effect on the phase (time of onset) of the activity rhythm, though they have markedly different effects on testis size. The light pulse does not produce gonadal growth when it is given early in the activity period, while it does produce gonadal growth when given at the end of the activity period. The results suggest that for gonadal stimulation by light, there is a restricted phase of sensitivity during the circadian cycle, and that there is a phase relationship between the behavioral and the gonadal response.

The evidence is very suggestive that a pacemaker with properties of a self-sustaining oscillator determines the phase of sensitivity of circadian-based responses. The fact that observed physiological and behavioral rhythms seem to obey the laws of oscillator theory remains to be explained in physiological terms. In the following sections we will examine the evidence that timing of seasonal breeding cycles is dependent on a circadian oscillatory mechanism. Next, we will explore the loci of neural oscillator(s).

PHYSIOLOGY OF BREEDING SEASONS

The Hypothalamo-Pituitary-Gonadal Axis

In order to examine how variation in daylength influences seasonal cycles of reproduction, we must understand how gonadal hormone secretion is regulated. Needless to say, a review of the vast literature on the anatomy and physiology of the reproductive system is beyond the scope of this chapter; the interested reader is referred to Crews and Silver (1985) and Nalbandov (1976). Our current understanding of the hierarchy of mechanisms controlling the gonads is as follows (Figure 5.8). Specialized peptides known as gonadotropin-releasing hormones (GnRH) are synthesized in the cell bodies of neurons in the hypothalamus. As discussed by Wingfield and Moore (see Chapter 6), it is not yet known whether there are one or two different forms of GnRH in birds. The cells that manufacture GnRH transport it via axons projecting to the median eminence. Here the GnRH is secreted into capillary beds that drain the portal

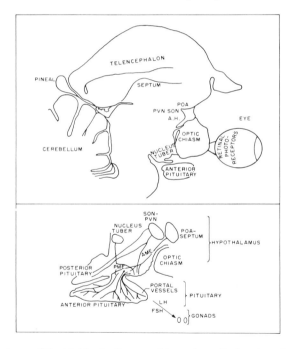

Figure 5.8. Anatomy of the bird brain. Top panel is a schematic drawing of a side view of the ring dove brain. Bottom panel represents the HPG. GnRH manufactured in the hypothalamus is released into portal vessels in the median eminence and is transported to the gonadotropin cells in the anterior pituitary. These cells release LH and FSH into the general circulation. The gonadotropic hormones stimulate the gonads to secrete steroid hormones and to produce gametes. Abbreviations are as follows: A.H., anterior hypothalamus; AME, anterior median eminence; POA, preoptic area; PME, posterior median eminence; PVN, paraventricular nucleus; SON, supraoptic nucleus. (The bottom panel is modified from Oksche and Farner, 1974.)

vessels that vascularize the anterior pituitary. Upon reaching the pituitary, GnRH stimulates the release of two pituitary gonadotropic hormones, luteinizing hormone (LH) and follicle-stimulating hormone (FSH). As suggested above, it is possible but not yet proven that two forms of GnRH act to release LH and FSH separately. The pituitary hormones travel via the general circulatory system. At the level of the gonads, LH and FSH stimulate the production of steroid hormones and gametogenesis. The steroids are released into the general circulatory system and subsequently are retained and concentrated in specific target tissue such as the vas deferens in the male and the oviduct in the female. The brain is also a target tissue with discrete steroid-hormone-concentrating areas that regulate the release of GnRH in both a positive and a negative feedback manner. This hierarchical regulatory system is known as the hypothalamo-pituitary-gonadal (HPG) axis.

One of the first studies indicating that daylength was involved in the determination of annual cycles came with Rowan's (1925) observations of migratory juncos (*Junco hyemalis*) as they flew south from Alberta. He captured some of these migrants and housed them in outdoor cages through the cold winter of Edmonton. He found that birds exposed to long days by means of light bulbs placed in the cages, had enlarged testes as though it were spring; those males kept in nearby cages and exposed to short days had small testes, as would be expected in wintering juncos. This experiment provided evidence that the daily duration of light was the cue to the seasonal regulation of testicular growth in juncos.

We now know that photoperiodic time measurement allows a variety of animals to anticipate breeding seasons. In temperate zones, spring is associated with increasing daylengths after the short days of winter. If birds that live in temperate zones are transferred from short to long days, there is an increase in the secretion of pituitary LH, FSH, and gonadal testosterone. In fact, in Japanese quail (*Coturnix coturnix japonica*) it has been shown that the rate of testicular growth reflects a direct relationship between the length of the photoperiod and the rate of gonadotropin secretion over the range from 11.5 to 14 hours (Follett et al., 1981).

Two types of experiments which manipulate light-dark schedules suggest that birds use a circadian system rather than absolute duration of light to measure critical daylength for gonadotropin release. In a resonance experiment, the amount of light is constant while the length of the dark period varies among experimental groups. White-crowned sparrows, *Zonotrichia leucophrys* kept in a light-dark schedule of 8 hours of light and 16 hours of darkness (LD 8:16) maintain small testes and low levels of plasma LH (Follett et al., 1974). If these individuals are placed in total darkness and exposed to an 8-hour light pulse at intervals from 2 to 100 hours, the light pulse induces LH secretion at approximately daily intervals, as can be seen in Figure 5.9. These results indicate that when the photoperiod is such that light falls at the photosensitive portion of the cycle, LH secretion is maximal. If the light pulses do not fall in the photosensitive phase, low levels of LH secretion are observed, as in short-day conditions.

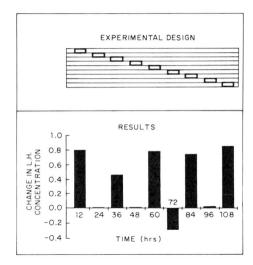

Figure 5.9. Illustration of the results of a resonance experiment with white-crowned sparrows. The effect is shown of an 8-hour test photoperiod on changes in plasma LH levels after variable periods of darkness. Each row in the top panel represents a different experimental group. In the bottom panel, the ordinate shows the change in plasma LH concentration between a blood sample taken in the last 8-hour light period before the onset of darkness and one taken 7–16 hours after the end of the various test photoperiods. The abscissa indicates time after the last real dawn. (Modified from Follett et al., 1974)

In the second type of experiment, known as a night-interruption experiment, brief periods of light during the dark phase are varied with respect to the onset of darkness across the experimental groups. In one such experiment (Follett and Sharp, 1969), quail were exposed to 6 hours of light daily; the dark period was interrupted by 15 minutes (0.25 hour) of light applied at various intervals after dark onset (Figure 5.10). Maximal gonadal size was obtained when the 0.25-hour light pulse was presented 12 hours after the onset of the longer light pulse. The 6.25-hour interrupted light duration produced testicular development similar to that seen during exposure to long days, even though the actual duration of exposure to light would normally result in atrophy of testes in short days. (See Turek and Campbell, 1979, and Follett, 1978, for review.)

Sites Underlying Seasonal Changes

The foregoing suggests that a pacemaker(s) with properties of a self-sustaining oscillator determines the phase of sensitivity of circadian-based responses. This hypothesis has led to many attempts to identify the mechanisms for transmitting information about light into functionally important changes in reproductive status (see Assenmacher, 1973, for review). Three candidate loci for these pacemakers are considered: the gonad, the pituitary, and the brain.

It is unlikely that seasonal changes in gonadal sensitivity to gonadotropins are responsible for gonadal recrudescence in long days. First, LH continues to be released in greater quantities during long days than short days in castrated Japanese quail (Gibson et al., 1975). Castrated white-crowned sparrows show increases in LH in the summer similar to what is observed in intact animals (Mattocks et al., 1976). Second, pituitary extracts elicit gonadal growth at times of the year when the testes are normally small (Benoit et al., 1950).

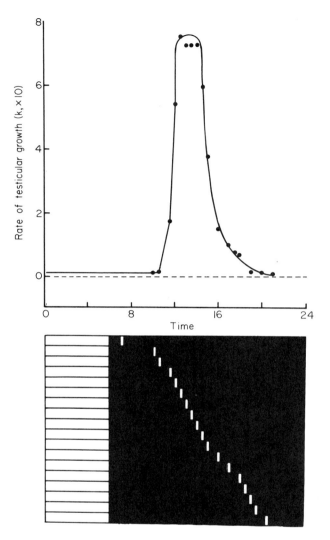

Figure 5.10. Illustration of an interrupted night experiment with Japanese quail. The effect is shown of 15-minute light-breaks on the rate of testicular growth in birds maintained under a photoperiod of 6 hours light and 18 hours of (interrupted) darkness. In the upper panel, the ordinate shows the rate of testicular growth; the time of the 15-minute light pulse is shown on the abscissa. The experimental design is shown in the bottom panel. Each row depicts a different experimental group. The small white bars represent the interval after dark onset that the animals were exposed to the 15-minute light pulse. (Modified from Follett and Sharp, 1969)

The pituitary can also be eliminated as a candidate structure responsible for seasonal changes in reproductive status. Systemic injections of GnRH cause the release of LH under photoperiods that are normally associated with low levels of LH release (Wingfield et al., 1979). Also, the response of the pituitary to GnRH is the same under different lighting schedules (Davies and Bicknell, 1976). The isolation of the pituitary from the brain hormones, however, disrupts seasonal changes in breeding (Yokoyama, 1976), suggesting that although an intact anterior pituitary is necessary for the occurrence of seasonal changes in gonadal status, the locus of seasonal changes lies outside the pituitary.

Several lines of evidence suggest that the brain itself is the site of seasonal changes. General aspects of the negative feedback system between steroid hormones and GnRH secretion by the brain were described above. If this negative feedback system is functional in the spring, how is it that plasma levels of both gonadotropin and steroid hormone increase in the spring? One hypothesis is that during spring there is a decrease in sensitivity of the hypothalamus to negative feedback by steroid hormones. An alternative hypothesis is that GnRH secretion occurs despite negative feedback from steroid hormones. Evidence for this latter hypothesis comes from experiments with castrated tree sparrows, *Passer montanus* (Wilson, 1985). One group of birds was maintained in short days while the other group was transferred to long days. If androgen feedback was solely responsible for changes in GnRH secretion in different lighting schedules, then one would expect the concentration of LH in the plasma to be the same in the two groups of birds. In fact, the birds transferred to long days had substantially higher concentrations of LH in their plasma than birds left in short days. This is confirmed and extended in studies of starlings (*Sturnus vulgaris*), where direct assays indicate a transient increase in GnRH content of the hypothalamus at the time of LH secretion and gonadal growth following exposure to long daylengths (Nicholls et al., 1984). The results support the notion of an androgen-independent mechanism in the hypothalamus that is driven by exposure to light.

Brain Areas Regulating Gonadal Status

Three major hypothalamic pathways that project to the median eminence have been analyzed with respect to their potential role in controlling seasonal changes in reproductive status: (1) the supraoptico-hypophysial, (2) the tubero-hypophysial, and (3) the preoptico-hypophysial tracts (Figure 5.8, lower panel).

The supraoptico-hypophysial tract originates in the supraoptic (SON) and paraventricular (PVN) nuclei and projects to the external layer of the anterior median eminence and the posterior pituitary. Early studies indicated a correlation between activity in the supraoptico-hypophysial system and reproductive status in birds. Attempts to identify the hypothalamic substance that causes seasonal changes in pituitary gonadotropin release focused on an unidentified substance called the neurosecretory substance (NSS) found in the SON and PVN. These studies suggest a correlation between the presence of NSS in the supraoptic-hypophysial system and reproductive status. Later work, however, indicates that there is no GnRH in this system; thus it probably is not directly responsible for the release of gonadotrophins. Instead, the hormone vasotocin, which is the neurosecretory substance released into the anterior median eminence by the supraoptico-hypophysial system (Goossens et al., 1977), may be related to nongonadal changes that occur seasonally in some birds. A discussion of the role of the NSS found in the external layer of the anterior median eminence during the different seasons can be found in Oksche and Farner (1974).

The nucleus tuber of the hypothalamus sends fibers through the supraoptico-hypophysial tract to the external layer of both the anterior and posterior median eminence (Wingstrand, 1951). The possible role of the tubero-hypophysial system was explored by Wilson (1967) in the white-crowned sparrow. Lesions in the medial basal portion of the nucleus tuber result in small testes even if males are maintained under a favorable LD schedule, suggesting that the nucleus tuber is important in regulating pituitary secretion of LH. If these lesion effects are due to destruction of cells that control gonadotropin directly, rather than due to damage to fibers of passage, then one would expect to find GnRH-containing cells in this region. The precise function of this nucleus is unclear, because some researchers find GnRH neurons in the tuberal region while others do not (see Mikami and Yamada, 1984, for discussion).

Immunocytochemical evidence indicates that the preoptic area (POA) of the hypothalamus and the septum contain GnRH perikarya and that the fiber bundle formed by the axons of these cells projects to the median eminence (see Mikami and Yamada, 1984, for discussion). Lesions of the POA block photoperiodically induced gonadotropin release and testicular recrudescence (see Sharp, 1983, for a review). If this is indeed the pathway whereby GnRH controls LH secretion, then the circadian clock must modulate neurosecretion by this system. Further research will determine whether this modulation is neural or hormonal.

PHYSIOLOGICAL MECHANISMS OF CIRCADIAN RHYTHMS

In this section we explore the neural basis for circadian and seasonal rhythms. Circadian rhythms are produced by an endogenous self-sustaining oscillator or a population of oscillators. The circadian system can be conceptualized as having several components: photoreceptive, oscillator, and coupling mechanisms whereby the output of the oscillator acts on effector response systems. In birds, several photoreceptive (eye, pineal, encephalic photoreceptor) and oscillatory (eye, pineal, suprachiasmatic nuclei [SCN]) elements have been identified. However, the mechanisms whereby the oscillator output is coupled to other neural and endocrine systems are poorly understood.

Photoreceptive Elements

Eye. The light-dark cycle, serving as a driving oscillator, acts on photoreceptors to entrain endogenous oscillators. The eye is one of the known photoreceptive elements in the circadian system. The eyes have a role in entrainment of locomotor activity. Removal of the eyes (enucleation) does not prevent pigeons (*Columba livia*) from entraining to dim light of 90–100 lux (Ebihara et al., 1984). Blind house sparrows are still able to entrain in LD at 500 lux, but only about 50% entrain in LD at 0.1 lux; about 20% of the birds will exhibit a free-run in the latter conditions (Menaker, 1968). In enucleated quail, some animals are arrhythmic in LD, while others show variable entrainment patterns (Underwood and Siopes, 1984; Konishi et al., 1985). Thus, there is strong evidence for the existence of another, possibly redundant entrainment system.

The role of the eyes in photoperiodically induced testicular growth has been investigated in several species of birds (see Oliver and Baylé, 1982, for review). In the white-crowned sparrow, house sparrow, quail, duck (*Anas platyrhynchos*), chicken (*Gallus domesticus*), and canary (*Serinus serinus*), the testicular growth cycles of photoperiodically stimulated blind and intact subjects are very similar.

Pineal. In mammals, the sole source of photic information appears to be the eyes. In nonmammalian vertebrates, extraretinal photoreceptors have been demonstrated. Opsin is the protein mediating the response of retinal photoreceptors to light. Immunocytochemical evidence indicates the presence of opsin in the pineal of a number of different avian species (Vigh et al., 1982). Its presence in the pineal, along with morphological similarities between photoreceptors of the retina and pinealocytes, suggests that the avian pineal can respond to light.

The role of the pineal in entrainment may be subtle. Pinealectomy alone has no effect on entrainment in pigeons (Ebihara et al., 1984) or quail (Underwood and Siopes, 1984). While controls become active at light onset, pinealectomized, blinded pigeons entrain, but show anticipatory activity before lights on (Ebihara et al., 1984). Two-thirds of blinded, and all blinded-pinealectomized quail are arrhythmic in LD (Underwood and Siopes, 1984).

Removal of the pineal does not appear to affect gonadal growth in normal LD cycles (Takahashi et al., 1979). However, when these pinealectomized birds are put in a skeleton LD schedule that would normally be photostimulatory, gonadal growth is inhibited. These investigators suggest that the pineal may exert its effect on the gonadal response to light indirectly via its role as a circadian pacemaker. Other researchers (Simpson et al., 1983) find no effect of pinealectomy on LH secretion in a variety of different photoperiods. Thus, the role of the pineal in birds is enigmatic. It will probably be better understood when the dynamics of avian melatonin secretion are better known (see below).

Encephalic photoreceptors. There is good evidence that in vertebrates other than mammals there are photoreceptors within the brain itself. While the precise morphology and location of these encephalic photoreceptors have not yet been discovered, several lines of evidence argue for their existence. Enucleated-pinealectomized house sparrows and pigeons are capable of entraining to an LD cycle. Photoperiodically induced gonadal growth does not require either the eyes or the pineal. Indeed, 50 years ago Benoit demonstrated that direct illumination of the hypothalamus will induce testicular growth in ducks. This pathbreaking research has been confirmed in a number of different avian species by other researchers (see Oliver and Baylé, 1982, for review). The current consensus is that brain photoreceptors are located in the medial basal area of the hypothalamus.

Oscillator Elements

Eye. The eyes are involved in circadian rhythms both in their role as photoreceptors and as oscillators in and of themselves. One piece of evidence suggesting that the eye is a circadian oscillator can be found in a study of N-acetyltransferase (NAT) activity in chick retina (Hamm and Menaker, 1980). This enzyme is necessary for the synthesis of melatonin, an indoleamine whose synthesis and/or secretion is entrained by the light-dark cycle such that high levels occur at night. The activity of NAT is highest during the night and lowest during the day. Furthermore, this rhythm of retinal NAT activity persists in DD, and in pinealectomized chicks housed in DD or constant light (LL), indicating that the retina itself exhibits a circadian rhythm of activity. Functional studies also point to a role of the eye in generating circadian rhythms in birds. Blinded quail are arrythmic in DD or dim LL (Underwood and Siopes, 1984; Konishi et al., 1985). In pigeons, combined pinealectomy and enucleation totally eliminates activity rhythms, while enucleation or pinealectomy alone is not sufficient (Ebihara et al., 1984).

Pineal. In some avian species, the pineal has both photoreceptor and oscillator components. When the chick pineal gland is maintained in a flow-through superfusion system, NAT continues to be released in a circadian rhythm both during a light-dark schedule and constant darkness (Kasal et al., 1979). Furthermore, if the pineal gland of chickens is cut into eight pieces, each is capable of producing a circadian rhythm of melatonin release in constant darkness (Takahashi and Menaker, 1984). This suggests that the synchronized circadian rhythmicity in melatonin is an emergent property of coupled pineal cells.

Several types of studies implicate the pineal gland in the expression of circadian rhythmicity. Pinealectomy abolishes free-running locomotor rhythms in sparrow and house finch (Fuchs, 1983) but not in quail and chicken (see Menaker et al., 1981, for review). The most direct evidence of a role for the pineal in rhythmic responses derives from studies in which the pineal gland is transplanted into the anterior eye chamber of an arrhythmic pinealectomized host sparrow (Zimmerman and Menaker, 1979). This operation restores rhythmicity to the host animal. Furthermore, the phase of the donor bird's rhythm is transferred to the host.

Suprachiasmatic nuclei. In mammals, both the location and function of a hypothalamic circadian pacemaker have been well established. The strength of the evidence that these nuclei serve as endogenous oscillators derives from the convergence of anatomical and functional studies. The SCN are bilaterally symmetrical and are located in the anterior hypothalamus, above the optic chiasm and adjacent to the third ventricle. These nuclei receive direct retinal input from the eyes via the retinohypothalamic tract. Lesions of the SCN disrupt a number of circadian activities such as locomotor activity. The SCN exhibit a circadian rhythm in metabolic activity; when isolated from the rest of the brain, these nuclei continue to show circadian rhythms of electrical (multiunit) activity. (See Moore-Ede et al., 1982, for a readable textbook describing this work.)

There is suggestive evidence that birds also have a circadian pacemaker in the anterior hypothalamus. This region of the hypothalamus receives direct retinal input (see Cooper et al., 1983, and Panzica, 1985, for discussion). There is confusion as to the precise location(s) of the retinorecipient area in birds, as it is reported to lie medially, adjacent to the third ventricle in some studies, and laterally, near the lateroventral geniculate nucleus, in others. Lesions of the medial region of the anterior hypothalamus disrupt circadian activity in some species but not in others (see Menaker et al., 1981, and Cassone and Menaker, 1984, for review). Unlike the situation in mammals, SCN-lesioned birds whose locomotor activity is disrupted still entrain to light-dark cycles. Furthermore, the lesions do not block photoperiodic control of gonadal activity (quail— Simpson and Follett, 1981). Strong evidence that the avian SCN serves as an endogenous oscillator awaits further functional studies such as have been done in mammals.

Coupling Elements

Melatonin.   The hormone melatonin has received a lot of attention as a candidate hormone which might affect expression of circadian rhythmicity and serve to couple photoreceptive and oscillatory components. As noted above, there are circadian rhythms in melatonin in both the pineal and the eye. These tissues contribute to diurnal rhythms of melatonin in the general circulation in the quail (Underwood et al., 1984). Following pinealectomy there is a 54% drop in serum melatonin, while a 33% drop occurs after enucleation. Melatonin has been implicated in the control of the overt activity rhythm in house sparrows (Turek et al., 1976). When capsules containing melatonin are placed in animals kept in constant darkness, either the free-running period is shortened or constant activity is induced. Also, daily injections of melatonin can entrain the activity rhythms of starlings (Gwinner and Benzinger, 1978). As in mammals, pinealectomy affects the rate of gonadal maturation, with melatonin having both stimulatory and inhibitory effects on the gonad (see Sharp, 1983).

In mammals, knowledge of the temporal parameters of melatonin secretion has contributed to our understanding of timing mechanisms. In Djungarian hamsters (*Phodopus sungorus*) and sheep (*Ovis aries*), it has been shown that the duration of melatonin secretion/synthesis is proportional to the duration of night in entrained conditions (see Bittman, 1984, for review). Timed melatonin replacement experiments in pinealectomized animals indicate that short melatonin infusions imitate the effects of short nights while long melatonin infusions imitate the effects of long nights irrespective of the photoperiod in which the animals are housed. The data are consistent with the hypothesis that a melatonin signal drives the photoperiodic response and that the *duration* of a circadian-based melatonin signal encodes night length (see Silver and Bittman, 1984, for further discussion).

The nature of the mechanism which decodes the melatonin duration signal is not yet known. If melatonin plays a role in birds, the suggestion might apply that seasonal cycles of gonadal growth involve a circadian system at one level and a different timing mechanism for decoding the duration of the melatonin signal at another level. Thus far the evidence is suggestive: The duration of pineal melatonin synthesis in quail is dependent on the duration of night (Cockrem and Follett, 1985). Timed melatonin replacement studies remain to be done.

Though we are lacking some of the necessary information, we can assume that in birds there are photoreceptors and that these provide information to an endogenous oscillator (or oscillators) which affect the expression of responses with circadian periodicity. There may be differences among species in the relative importance and functional roles of various oscillators and in their coupling mechanisms.

WHY OSCILLATORS?

Though interest in rhythms is fairly recent, it seems that circadian rhythms are a very ancient form of biological timekeeping. Pittendrigh (1966) suggests that circadian oscillations occur in all eukaryotes and probably arise from a single cell type. It is interesting to speculate why organisms use oscillators for chronometry. What advantage do oscillators confer over hourglass timers? Oscillations allow anticipatory responses or "planning," not only for the next day or days but also for the next month or months, as we have shown in the above examples. In a paper directed at the analysis of concatenated circadian and interval-timing mechanisms, we (Silver and Bittman, 1984) have argued that in various reproductive systems an oscillator at one level in the hierarchy of neural organization is coupled with other types (i.e., nonoscillatory) of timing mechanisms at other levels. Thus, a single oscillator might be coupled to one or more interval-timing processes, allowing the single circadian pacemaker to drive multiple outcomes independently and in appropriate temporal order. For example, a variety of seasonal changes such as alterations in fat stores, plumage, migratory activity, and readiness to breed may all be driven by the changes in daylength that are measured by the circadian system. Each of these responses may be executed at a different critical photoperiod. Alternatively, the critical photoperiod, measured by the oscillator, may trigger a second timed event with a duration characteristic of each response. While circadian timing processes are characterized by their properties of accuracy and temperature compensation, interval timers to which they might be linked are likely subject to modulation by a wide variety of factors, including temperature.

The order of linkage of oscillatory and nonoscillatory timers may also be critical. An interval timer can determine *whether* permissive conditions have been met. The circadian timer determines *when* the outcome will occur. Thus the two timing processes are independent functionally. In conjunction, they provide a mechanism that allows the response to occur at the appropriate time and sequence. The use of concatenated multiple timers may allow relevant but unpredictable environmental cues to bias different seasonal responses so that they occur earlier or later in the year. It is possible that nonphotoperiodic environmental cues have no direct access to the circadian oscillator. Rather, the former may influence the timing of reproductive activities (such as those discussed in Chapters 2 and 6) by acting on interval-timing processes whose rate can be modulated by a range of permissive conditions. In this way, thermal, social, and nutritional factors may act on interval timers to alter the influence of photoperiodic cues without accessing oscillators directly.

Future Directions

We have suggested that the formal analysis of properties of circadian systems has outpaced the understanding of the underlying physiological mechanisms. Oscillations in biochemical parameters occur at every level of circadian organization. Obviously, only some of these biochemical events oscillate with a circadian period. Other biochemical parameters may not oscillate or reset automatically. Much effort is currently being directed at understanding how these potential timing processes at various levels of the neuraxis are coordinated and coupled.

In birds, the search for physiological mechanisms has led to the discovery of photoreceptor elements in the eyes, the pineal, and in an unspecified hypothalamic site. Oscillators controlling behavioral and/or physiological responses have been described in the eye, the suprachiasmatic nucleus, and the pineal gland. Several aspects of the avian circadian system remain largely unknown. For example, the loci of the encephalic photoreceptor and the SCN need to be identified. The functional relationships among various photoreceptors and their relationship(s) to each oscillator(s) should be clarified.

At the level of the oscillator, it is important to determine whether there is a "master clock" (e.g., SCN) with several "slaves" (e.g., pineal, eye), or whether there are several coupled clocks with no driving oscillator. Species differences in circadian systems remain to be documented. Finally, the nature of the coupling mechanism from the oscillator to the target responses remains to be determined, though evidence for a role of melatonin is starting to accumulate.

The earliest studies of circadian rhythms were purely descriptive and of ecological interest. Today, attempts to understand the physiological basis of these rhythms are the domain of experimental scientists. In birds, external stimuli from the mate and from biotic factors markedly influence the timing of reproduction and a large number of responses which must be temporally coordinated. Studies of circadian rhythms of avian species will likely contribute to our understanding coupling of multiple (oscillatory and interval) timing mechanisms, and how environmental information reaches these timing systems to alter overt responses.

ACKNOWLEDGMENTS

We wish to thank Drs. E. Albers, G. Ball, and D. Crews for their helpful comments on previous versions of this manuscript. Work from this laboratory appearing in the manuscript was supported by grants from NIMH 29380 and NSF BNS 06282.

REFERENCES

ASCHOFF, J. (1979) Circadian rhythms: Influences of internal and external factors on the period measured in constant conditions. Z. Tierpsychol. *49*:225–249.

ASSENMACHER, I. (1973) Reproductive endocrinology: The hypothalamo-hypophysial axis. In *Breeding Biology of Birds*. D.S. Farner, ed., pp. 158–208, National Academy of Science, Washington, D.C.

BENOIT, J., P. MANDEL, F.X. WALTER, and I. ASSENMACHER (1950) Sensibilité testiculaire aux hormones gonadotropes hypophysaires chez le canard domestique au cours de la périod de régression testiculaire saisonnière. C.R. Soc. Biol. Paris *144*:1400–1403.

BITTMAN, E.L. (1984) Melatonin and photoperiodic time measurement. Evidence from rodents and ruminants. In *The Pineal Gland*. R.J. Reiter, ed., pp. 155–192, Raven Press, New York.

CASSONE, V.M., and M. MENAKER (1984) Is the avian circadian system a neuroendocrine loop? J. Exp. Zool. *232*:539–550.

CHENG, M.F. (1979) Progress and prospect in ring dove research: A personal view. In *Advances in the Study of Behavior*. J.S. Rosenblatt, R.A. Hinde, E. Shaw, and C. Beer, eds., pp. 97–129, Academic Press, New York.

COCKREM, J.F., and B.K. FOLLETT (1985) Circadian rhythm of melatonin in the pineal gland of the Japanese quail (*Coturnix coturnix japonica*). J. Endocr. *107*:317–324.

COOPER, M.L., G.E. PICKARD, and R. SILVER (1983) Retinohypothalamic pathway in the dove demonstrated by anterograde HRP. Brain Res. Bull. *10*:715–718.

CREWS, D., and R. SILVER (1985) Reproductive physiology and behavior interactions in nonmammalian vertebrates. In *Handbook of Behavioral Neurobiology*, Vol. 7. N. Adler, D. Pfaff, and R.W. Goy, eds., pp. 101–182, Plenum Press, New York.

DAVIES, D.T., and R.J. BICKNELL (1976) The effect of testosterone on the responsiveness of the quail's pituitary to LH-RH during photoperiodically induced testicular growth. Gen. Comp. Endocr. *30*:487–499.

DESJARDINS, C., and M.J. LOPEZ (1983) Environmental cues evoke differential responses in pituitary-testicular function in deer mice. Endocr. *112*:1398–1406.

EBIHARA, S., K. UCHIYAMA, and I. OSHIMA (1984) Circadian organization in the pigeon, *Columba livia*: The role of the pineal organ and the eye. J. Comp. Physiol. *154*:59–69.

FARNER, D.S. (1985) Annual rhythms. Ann. Rev. Physiol. *47*:65–82.

FOLLETT, B.K. (1978) Photoperiodism and seasonal breeding in birds and mammals. In *Control of Ovulation*. D.B. Crighton, G.R. Foxcroft, N.B. Haynes, and G.E. Lamming, eds., pp. 267–293, Butterworths, London.

FOLLETT, B.K., and P.J. SHARP (1969) Circadian rhythmicity in photoperiodically induced gonadotrophin release and gonadal growth in the quail. Nature *223*:968–971.

FOLLETT, B.K., P.W. MATTOCKS, JR., and D.S. FARNER (1974) Circadian function in the photoperiodic induction of gonadotrophin in the white-crowned sparrow, *Zonotrichia leucophrys gambelii*. Proc. Nat. Acad. Sci. USA *71*:1666–1669.

FOLLETT, B.K., J.E. ROBINSON, S.M. SIMPSON, and C.R. HARLOW (1981) Photoperiodic time measurement and gonadotrophin secretion in quail. In *Biological Clocks in Seasonal Reproductive Cycles*. B.K. Follett and D.E. Follett, eds., pp. 185–201, John Wiley & Sons, New York.

FUCHS, J.L. (1983) Effects of pinealectomy and subsequent melatonin implants on activity rhythms in the house finch (*Carpodacus mexicanus*). J. Comp. Physiol. *153*:413–419.

GIBBON, J.G., M. MORRELL, and R. SILVER (1984) Two kinds of timing in the circadian incubation rhythm of the ring dove. Am. J. Physiol. *247*:R1083–R1087.

GIBSON, W.R., B.K. FOLLETT, and B. GLEDHILL (1975) Plasma levels of luteinizing hormone in gonadectomized Japanese quail exposed to short or to long days. Endocr. *64*:87–101.

GOOSSENS, N., S. BLAHSER, A. OKSCHE, F. VANDESANDE, and K. DIERICKX (1977) Immunocytochemical investigation of the hypothalamo-neurohypophysial system in birds. Cell Tiss. Res. *184*:1–13.

GWINNER, E., and I. BENZINGER (1978) Synchronization of a circadian rhythm in pinealectomized European starlings by daily injections of melatonin. J. Comp. Physiol. *127*:209–213.

HAMM, H.E., and M. MENAKER (1980) Retinal rhythms in chicks: Circadian variation in melatonin and serotonin N-acetyltransferase activity. Proc. Nat. Acad. Sci. USA *77*:4998–5002.

HOFFMANN, K. (1960) Experimental manipulation of the orientation clock in birds. Cold Spring Harbor Symp. Quant. Biol. *25*:379–387.

KASAL, C.A., M. MENAKER, and J.R. PEREZ-POLO (1979) Circadian clock in culture: N-acetyltransferase activity of chick pineal glands oscillates *in vitro*. Science *203*:656–658.

KOBAYASHI, H., and M. WADA (1973) Neuroendocrinology in birds. In *Avian Biology*, Vol. III. D.S. Farner, J.R. King, eds., pp. 287–347, Academic Press, New York.

Konishi, H., H. Olta, and K. Homma (1985) Important role of the eyes controlling locomotor rhythm in quail. J. Interdisc. Cycle Res. *16*:217–226.

Mattocks Jr., P.W., D.S. Farner, and B.K. Follett (1976) The annual cycle in luteinizing hormone in the plasma of intact and castrated white-crowned sparrows, *Zonotrichia leucophrys gambelii*. Gen. Comp. Endocrinol. *30*:156–161.

Menaker, M. (1968) Extraretinal light perception in the sparrow, I. Entrainment of the biological clock. Proc. Nat. Acad. Sci. USA *59*:414–421.

Menaker, M., and A. Eskin (1967) Circadian clock in photoperiodic time measurement: A test of the Bunning hypothesis. Science *157*:1182–1185.

Menaker, M., D.J. Hudson, and J.S. Takahashi (1981) Neural and endocrine components of circadian clocks in birds. In *Biological Clocks in Seasonal Reproductive Cycles*. B.K. Follett and D.E. Follett, eds., pp. 171–183, John Wiley & Sons, New York.

Mikami, S., and S. Yamada (1984) Immunohistochemistry of the hypothalamic neuropeptides and anterior pituitary cells in the Japanese quail. J. Exp. Zool. *232*:405–417.

Moore-Ede, M.C., F.M. Sulzman, and C.A. Fuller (1982) The neural basis of circadian rhythmicity. In *The Clocks That Time Us*. M.C. Moore-Ede, F.M. Sulzman, and C.A. Fuller, pp. 152–200, Harvard University Press, Cambridge, Mass.

Murton, R.K., and N.J. Westwood (1977) Integration of gonadotrophin and steroid secretion, spermatogenesis and behavior in the reproductive cycle of male pigeon species. In *Neural and Endocrine Aspects of Behaviour in Birds*. P. Wright, P.G. Caryl, and D.M. Vowles, eds., pp. 51–89, Elsevier, Amsterdam.

Nalbandov, A.V. (1976) *Reproductive Physiology of Mammals and Birds*, 3rd ed. W.H. Freeman & Company, San Francisco.

Nicholls, T.J., A.R. Goldsmith, and A. Dawson (1984) Photorefractoriness in European starlings: Associated hypothalamic changes and the involvement of thyroid hormones and prolactin. J. Exp. Zool. *232*:567–572.

Oksche, A., and D.S. Farner (1974) Neurohistological studies of the hypothalamo-hypophysial system of *Zonotrichia leucophrys gambelii* (Aves, Passeriformes) with special attention to its role in the control of reproduction. Ergebn. Anat. *48/4*:1–136.

Oliver, J., and J.D. Baylé (1982) Brain photoreceptors for the photo-induced testicular response in birds. Experientia *38*:1021–1029.

Panzica, G.C. (1985) Vasotocin-immunoreactive elements and neuronal typology in the suprachiasmatic nucleus of the chicken and Japanese quail. Cell Tiss. Res. *242*:371–376.

Pittendrigh, C.S. (1966) The circadian oscillation in *Drosophila pseudoobscura* pupae: A model for the photoperiodic clock. Z. Pflanzenphysiol. *54*:275–307.

Rowan, W. (1925) Relation of light to bird migration and developmental changes. Nature *115*:494–495.

Rusak, B. (1981) Vertebrate behavioral rhythms. In *Handbook of Behavioral Neurobiology*, Vol. 4. J. Aschoff, ed., pp. 183–213, Plenum Press, New York.

Sharp, P.J. (1983) Hypothalamic control of gonadotrophin secretion in birds. In *Progress in Nonmammalian Research*, Vol. 3. G. Nisticò and L. Bolis, eds., pp. 123–176, CRC Press, Boca Raton, Fla.

SILVER, R. (1978) The parental behavior of ring doves. Amer. Sci. *66*:209–215.

SILVER, R., and E.L. BITTMAN (1984) Reproductive mechanisms: Interaction of circadian and interval timing. Ann. N.Y. Acad. Sci. *423*:488–515.

SIMPSON, S.M., and B.K. FOLLETT (1981) Pineal and hypothalamic pacemakers: Their role in regulating circadian rhythmicity in Japanese quail. J. Comp. Physiol. *144*:381–389.

SIMPSON, S.M., H.F. URBANSKI, and J.E. ROBINSON (1983) The pineal gland and the photoperiodic control of luteinizing hormone secretion in intact and castrated Japanese quail. J. Endocr. *99*:281–287.

TAKAHASHI, J.S., and M. MENAKER (1984) Multiple redundant circadian oscillators within the isolated avian pineal gland. J. Comp. Physiol. *154*:435–440.

TAKAHASHI, J.S., C. NORRIS, and M. MENAKER (1978) Circadian photoperiodic regulation of testis growth in the house sparrow: Is the pineal gland involved? In *Comparative Endocrinology*. P.J. Gaillard and H.H. Boer, eds., pp. 153–156, Elsevier, Amsterdam.

TUREK, F.W., J.P. MCMILLAN, and M. MENAKER (1976) Melatonin: Effects on the circadian locomotor rhythm of sparrows. Science *194*:1441–1443.

TUREK, F.W., and C.S. CAMPBELL (1979) Photoperiodic regulation of neuroendocrine-gonadal activity. Biol. Reprod. *20*:32–50.

UNDERWOOD, H., S. BRINKLEY, T. SIOPES, and K. MOSHER (1984) Melatonin rhythms in the eyes, pineal bodies, and blood of Japanese quail (*Coturnix coturnix japonica*). Gen. Comp. Endocr. *56*:70–81.

UNDERWOOD, H., and T. SIOPES (1984) Circadian organization in Japanese quail. J. Exp. Zool. *232*:557–566.

VIGH, B., I. VIGH-TEICHMANN, P. ROHLICH, and B. AROS (1982) Immunoreactive opsin in the pineal organ of reptiles and birds. Z. Mikrosk.-Anat. Forsch. *96*:113–129.

WILSON, F.E. (1967) The tubero-infundibular neuron system: A component of the photoperiodic control mechanism of the white-crowned sparrow, *Zonotrichia leucophrys gambelii*. Z. Zellforsch. *82*:1–24.

WILSON, F.E. (1985) An androgen-independent mechanism maintains photorefractoriness in male tree sparrows (*Spizella arborea*). J. Endocr. *107*:137–143.

WINGFIELD, J.C. (1983) Environmental and endocrine control of reproduction: An ecological approach. In *Avian Endocrinology: Environmental and Ecological Aspects*. S.I. Mikami, S. Ishii, and M. Wada, eds., pp. 265–288, Japanese Scientific Societies Press, Tokyo, and Springer-Verlag, Berlin.

WINGFIELD, J.C., J.W. CRIM, P.W. MATTOCKS, JR., and D.S. FARNER (1979) Responses of photosensitive and photorefractory male white-crowned sparrows (*Zonotrichia leucophrys gambelii*) to synthetic mammalian luteinizing hormone releasing hormone (Syn-LHRH). Biol. Reprod. *21*:801–806.

WINGFIELD, J.C., and M.C. MOORE (1986) Hormonal, social, and environmental factors in the reproductive biology of free-living male birds. In *Psychobiology of Reproduction: An Evolutionary Perspective*. D. Crews, ed., This volume.

WINGSTRAND, K.G. (1951) *The Structure and Development of the Avian Pituitary from a Comparative and Functional Viewpoint*. C.W.K. Gleerlup, Lund.

YOKOYAMA, K. (1976) Hypothalamic and hormonal control of the periodically induced vernal functions in the white-crowned sparrow, *Zonotrichia leucophrys gambelii.* I. The effects of hypothalamic lesions and exogenous hormones. Cell Tiss. Res. *174*:391–416.

ZIMMERMAN, N.H., and M. MENAKER (1979) The pineal gland: A pacemaker within the circadian system of the house sparrow. Proc. Nat. Acad. Sci. USA 76:999–1003.

SIX
Hormonal, Social, and Environmental Factors in the Reproductive Biology of Free-Living Male Birds

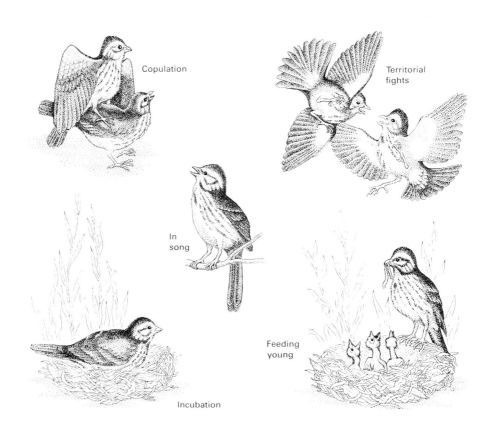

Copulation

Territorial fights

In song

Feeding young

Incubation

John C. Wingfield* and Michael C. Moore
Department of Zoology
University of Washington
Seattle, Washington
and Department of Zoology
Arizona State University
Tempe, Arizona

After a long and dreary winter, the bird songs of spring are greeted by most of us as the harbingers of warmer weather and the onset of summer. Less familiar, however, is the fact that those first songs also signal the beginning of a complex and well-coordinated series of behaviors and physiologic processes that make up the breeding season.

There are numerous variants on this cycle, but in many species of the passeriformes (perching birds), especially in migratory species, the males arrive on the breeding grounds before females and begin to establish breeding territories. Usually these territories are used exclusively by the male and his eventual mate throughout the breeding season. Typically, a male begins singing and patrolling the territory shortly after arrival. Agonistic interactions with neighboring or competing males are frequent and fights are not uncommon, but only occasionally are the combatants severely injured. A few days or weeks later the females arrive and pair formation is rapid. A period of courtship follows, culminating in construction of a nest, copulations, and egg-laying. This period is also marked by an increase in aggressive behavior in the male as he *mate-guards* his now sexually receptive female. The function of mate-guarding by the male is to reduce the possibility that neighboring males may gain a chance to copulate with his mate. In other words he *protects* his paternity of the clutch of eggs.

Once egg-laying is completed, or sometimes a day or two before the female begins incubation, she is no longer sexually receptive. Depending on the species, the incubation period lasts about 10–20 days. After the young hatch, usually both the male and female feed young in the nest, although in some species males provide little parental care. However, in many finches, males may feed the young for a further two weeks after they leave the nest (*fledge*) and before they become independent. During this time the females may begin building a second nest and produce a second clutch of eggs (*multiple brooding*). Multiple brooding is common at lower latitudes, and three or even four broods may be raised in a single season. However, reproduction is not continuous in any species studied so far, and nesting is terminated usually in mid or late summer. Many species then abandon their breeding territories for the winter and return the following spring—if they survive.

In species nesting at northern latitudes, the breeding season begins and ends with remarkable regularity each year. Birds arrive at about the same time, plus or minus a few days, and nesting begins within the same 2–3 week

---

* This chapter was prepared while John C. Wingfield was Associate Professor at The Rockefeller University, Field Research Center, Millbrook, New York.

period year after year. Why do birds have such well-defined breeding seasons? How are they able to achieve this remarkable precision in timing, as well as to organize the complex temporal pattern of reproductive behaviors within a nesting cycle? The answer to the first question is relatively simple. The production of eggs and feeding of young requires a large amount of food, much more than that needed for self-maintenance during the winter (Lack, 1968). Clearly there is much more food during the spring and summer, and that food tends to be more rich in protein and nutrients. In addition, the vernal growth of vegetation provides shelter for the nest, and increasing temperatures provide a more amenable environment for the young (Perrins, 1970) that, in many species, are born naked and helpless (altricial). Obviously, those individuals that reproduce when food supplies increase, and environmental conditions ameliorate, will leave more offspring and contribute more genes to future generations (Lack, 1968). Thus natural selection favors individuals that begin breeding in spring. The environmental factors that provide the selection pressure (food, cover, etc.) are known as *ultimate factors* (Baker, 1938).

The answer to the second question, or rather questions, is much more complex. Individuals use *proximate* environmental factors (Baker, 1938) to predict or signal changes in the environment. These environmental stimuli thus provide cues for the onset and termination of breeding, as well as integrating the temporal sequence of events once the nesting cycle is initiated. The literature on the role of proximate factors is very extensive, perhaps reflecting the large number of bird species and the wide variety of habitats in which they live. Nevertheless, it is possible to classify proximate factors into four major groups based on how each factor affects the timing of the reproductive cycle (Wingfield, 1983). These groups are: (1) *initial predictive information*, which provides the stimulus for the onset of gonadal growth, development of secondary sex characters, and reproductive behavior. Since development of a functional reproductive system requires several weeks, individuals must predict the ensuing reproductive period and begin maturation well in advance so that the gonads are near functional when environmental conditions become favorable. (2) *Supplementary information* provides cues on the state of the local environment and fine-tunes the onset of breeding with year-to-year differences in phenologic progression. Usually the variation in the onset of breeding is 2–3 weeks from one year to the next. (3) *Synchronizing and integrating information* constitutes a further set of environmental cues that synchronizes the reproductive effort of the pair, such as the transition from sexual to parental behavior. (4) Finally, *modifying factors*, such as inclement weather or nest predators, interrupt breeding. Usually, a pair will renest once conditions become favorable again.

It is not possible in a single review to cover all of the mechanisms by which environmental factors regulate the reproductive process. In this chapter we will focus specifically on the regulation of sexual and territorial behavior of the male throughout the breeding cycle. We will also concentrate on two species that are common breeders in north temperate latitudes of

North America, the white-crowned sparrow (*Zonotrichia leucophrys*) and the song sparrow (*Melopsiza melodia*). Both are closely related, have migratory and sedentary forms, and can raise two or more broods in a single season (although northern forms tend to be exclusively single-brooded). Over the past decade or so we have learned much of their reproductive physiology, both in the laboratory and field, and thus they are ideal subjects for investigations on the interactions of hormones and behavior.

HORMONAL CONTROL OF GONADAL GROWTH AND REPRODUCTIVE BEHAVIOR IN MALE BIRDS

Most birds maintain their reproductive organs in a completely regressed and nonfunctional state during the nonbreeding season. This saves on the energy that would be required to maintain fully functional reproductive structures when they are not needed and, for migratory forms, reduces the cost of transporting large reproductive organs during long migratory flights. The testis of a fully mature sparrow can weigh over 600 mg, whereas in the nonbreeding season the same organ weighs only 1–2 mg. Before the breeding season can begin, the male must activate the reproductive system and develop a fully functional gonad. This means completing a nearly 600-fold increase in the weight of the testis that requires at least four weeks. The need to complete most of this growth prior to the beginning of the breeding season is one of the main reasons why migratory birds must respond to environmental cues that predict the beginning of the breeding season. They respond to these cues by activating hormonal systems that will bring about the full development of the reproductive system.

As in mammals, the development of the avian testis is controlled by two glycoprotein hormones secreted from the anterior pituitary gland located at the base of the central part of the brain. These hormones, usually called gonadotropins, are follicle-stimulating hormone (FSH), which acts primarily on the sperm-producing structures (seminiferous tubules) within the gonad, and luteinizing hormone (LH), which acts on the interstitial cells of the testis (cells of Leydig), causing them to secrete the steroid hormone testosterone. The secretion of LH and FSH are controlled by one, possibly two, decapeptides called gonadotropin-releasing hormones (avian GnRH-1 and avian GnRH-2; e.g., Millar and King, 1984). Both are synthesized in the hypothalamus (the region of the brain just dorsal and anterior to the pituitary gland), and there is evidence that at least GnRH-1 is released from a region of the hypothalamus called the median eminence. This hormone is transported in the blood via the hypophysial portal vein system to gonadotroph cells within the anterior pituitary, where it stimulates secretion of FSH and LH (see Figure 6.1). Secretion of GnRH is regulated by neurotransmitters within the brain, by negative feedback from secretion of androgen, and possibly also by short-loop feedback from the gonadotropins themselves.

Plasma levels of testosterone tend to increase as the gonad develops, and in synergy with FSH, promote sperm production. Testosterone also has

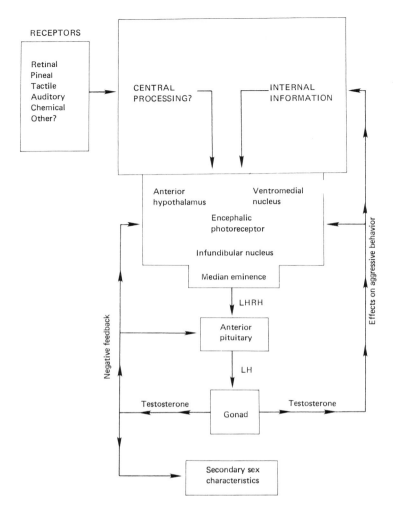

RECEPTORS

Retinal
Pineal
Tactile
Auditory
Chemical
Other?

CENTRAL
PROCESSING?

INTERNAL
INFORMATION

Anterior
hypothalamus

Ventromedial
nucleus

Encephalic
photoreceptor

Infundibular nucleus

Median eminence

LHRH

Anterior
pituitary

LH

Testosterone

Gonad

Testosterone

Secondary sex
characteristics

Negative feedback

Effects on aggressive behavior

Figure 6.1. A schematic diagram of the relationship between the central nervous system (brain) and reproductive system of male birds. Also included are the hypothesized receptors for environmental information, and an indication that this information is transduced in the central nervous system in conjunction with internal information such as endogenous rhythms. Note that testosterone secreted from the testis acts not only on sperm production but also on secondary sex characteristics, secretion of gonadotropins by negative feedback, and reproductive behavior.

profound stimulatory effects on the development of secondary sex characteristics such as wattles, combs, and spurs (found in many gallinaceous birds such as the domestic fowl), the cloacal protuberance (a copulatory organ), and in some species, development of bright nuptial colors of bills, legs, and plumage. These secondary sex characteristics are used extensively in sexual and aggressive displays.

Classical experiments conducted on mammals and birds some decades ago showed that if the testes, the primary source of testosterone, are removed, then the frequency and intensity of aggressive and sexual behaviors declines. Such behaviors include singing, threat postures, courtship, and copulation. If testosterone is given to these castrates, then the frequency of reproductive behaviors increases again (e.g., Balthazart, 1983). However, the extent to which aggressive and sexual behaviors decline after castration, or increase after administration of exogenous testosterone, varies greatly from species to species, and in some they are independent of hormonal control (Moore and Kranz, 1983; Crews and Moore, 1986). For example in mammals, adult male cats show only a slight decline in territorial aggression and scent marking following castration, whereas other species, such as many rodents and most of the few species of birds that have been studied, show very marked declines. Similarly, castration can reduce courtship and copulatory behavior in a variety of mammals and a few birds such as quail. However, in at least one species, the white-crowned sparrow, the male will copulate normally when presented with a sexually receptive female, even if castrated in the first year before any sexual experience (Moore and Kranz, 1984).

These observations have led to two hypotheses for the mode of action of testosterone on aggressive and sexual behavior. One hypothesis suggests that testosterone has *organizational* effects early in life, often just after birth (see Chapter 9). The neural circuits involved in aggressive and sexual behavior become *hard-wired* at this time and are subsequently independent of testosterone in the adult. The second hypothesis claims *activational* effects of testosterone in which the expression of a certain behavior requires the constant and immediate presence of testosterone. In many species it is likely that testosterone has both organizational and activational effects on behavior, although in some species, one or the other may predominate. In birds, activational effects appear to be very important, although even in the absence of testosterone, aggressive behaviors do not disappear entirely.

TEMPORAL PATTERNS OF REPRODUCTIVE BEHAVIOR AND SECRETION OF TESTOSTERONE

Since it is clear that testosterone is intimately involved in the development and expression of reproductive behavior, the next logical question is, how do seasonal changes in plasma concentrations of testosterone correlate with changes in territorial aggression and sexual behavior through the complex sequence of events that make up the breeding cycle? This question has been answered by characterizing changes in hormone levels in free-living male sparrows throughout a breeding season. Two subspecies of white-crowned sparrows were studied on their breeding grounds near Puget Sound in Washington State (*Z. l. pugetensis*, from here on referred to specifically as the Puget Sound sparrow), and near Fairbanks, Alaska (*Z. l. gambelii*, from here on called Gambel's sparrow). Additionally, male song sparrows, *M. m. melodia*, were investigated in natural populations breeding in the mid-Hudson Valley of New York State. Previous investigations on the seasonal breeding and behavior of these species are extensive, and thus they are ideal subjects for field study.

How can changes in circulating levels of hormones be determined in natural populations? Males are first captured in *mist* nets or in traps baited with seeds. Immediately after capture, a small blood sample (approximately 200–300 μl) is collected from a wing vein. Plasma harvested from this sample can be assayed later for LH and testosterone. In addition to collection of a blood sample, each bird is marked with a U.S. Fish and Wildlife Service aluminum leg band with a specific number, and a unique combination of colored plastic leg bands for subsequent identification of each individual in the field. All birds are then released. Capture and sampling does not seriously harm the sparrows, and frequently some males sing within 15–30 minutes of release (Wingfield and Farner, 1976). Extensive data also show that these birds reproduce quite normally, despite being captured and sampled 5–10 times within a single breeding season! This hardiness obviously makes these sparrows ideal subjects for investigations in *field endocrinology*.

The results of the field studies are summarized in Figure 6.2. In general, all three forms show a close correlation between peak levels of male territorial behavior and maximum levels of testosterone. During breeding there are two periods when defense of the territory by the male is most intense: initial establishment of the territory, and mate-guarding when the female is egg-laying and sexually receptive. All three species have the highest circulating levels of testosterone at these times. However, plasma concentrations of testosterone during other phases of the cycle are not basal but are maintained at intermediate levels that correspond with the reduced intensity, but continuing maintenance, of territorial defense. Curiously, plasma levels of testosterone do not increase in multiple-brooded forms when females become receptive for production of the second clutch. Males, of course, copulate freely with their receptive mates at this time but do not appear to mate-guard, at least not so intensely as for the first clutch. Possible reasons for this will be discussed after we examine the hormone cycles of males of the three forms in more detail.

Gambel's sparrows are single-brooded, owing to the rather brief summer on their Alaskan breeding grounds. Males arrive with circulating titers of LH and testosterone already elevated well above basal winter levels. Because of the brief breeding season, females arrive shortly after males have established territories and while initial territorial interactions among males are still intense. Females become receptive and begin egg-laying within a few days, and plasma levels of LH and testosterone in males increase even further as they initiate mate-guarding. After all the eggs are laid, females cease soliciting copulations from males and begin incubation. At the same time there is a precipitous drop in testosterone levels in the males. Intermediate levels of testosterone are maintained by males throughout the parental phase and reach basal as young fledge and the breeding season terminates (Figure 6.2).

The populations of Puget Sound and song sparrows we studied breed at lower latitudes (48°N and 42°N, respectively), where the longer summers

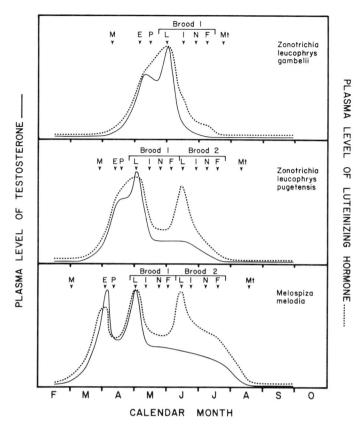

Figure 6.2. Changes in circulating levels of luteinizing hormone (LH) and testosterone during a breeding cycle of free-living male Gambel's sparrows (*Zonotrichia leucophrys gambelii*), Puget Sound sparrows (*Z. l. pugetensis*), and song sparrows (*Melospiza melodia*). The data are organized as to stage in the breeding cycle and spaced according to the average time required for each stage. M = vernal migration; E = establishing a territory; P = pair formation; L = egg-laying period; I = incubation; N = feeding nestlings; F = feeding fledglings; Mt = postnuptial molt. In the middle and lower panels note that two broods are depicted and the laying to fledgling stages are repeated. (Compiled from Wingfield and Farner, 1980; and Wingfield, 1984a)

allow significantly earlier breeding and production of two and sometimes three and even four broods. As in the Gambel's sparrow, males of both these forms arrive on the breeding grounds with plasma levels of LH and testosterone elevated well above basal concentrations found in winter. Male-male agonistic interactions are frequent as males establish territories. Females arrive shortly after territories are established, and pairing occurs immediately. In Puget Sound sparrows, females quickly become receptive, and egg-laying begins 7–10 days after pairing. As in the Gambel's sparrow, levels of testosterone appear to increase further in males as they begin mate-guarding their sexually receptive mates (Figure 6.2).

In contrast, female song sparrows often wait 4–5 weeks after pairing before becoming receptive and beginning egg-laying. During this interim, plasma concentrations of LH and testosterone in males decline to intermediate levels and then return to maximum when females become receptive (Figure 6.2). This correlates with a resurgence in the intensity of territorial defense associated with mate-guarding.

As in the Gambel's sparrow, testosterone levels in males of both the multiple-brooded forms decline precipitously to intermediate concentrations as soon as the female ceases soliciting copulations and begins incubating. The rate of singing, patrolling, and agonistic interactions among males also declines in parallel with this decrease in testosterone. As pointed out above, males maintain these intermediate concentrations of testosterone throughout the remainder of the breeding season, even though plasma levels of LH increase during subsequent periods of female receptivity for subsequent clutches of eggs (Figure 6.2).

Thus, there is good evidence for the three species and subspecies of sparrows that plasma levels of testosterone wax and wane in parallel with changing patterns of male territorial aggression. The correlation with periods of male sexual behavior, however, is less precise. During the first period of courtship and copulation, males have maximum levels of testosterone, but in multiple-brooded forms, males court and copulate for subsequent broods while their testosterone levels remain relatively low. Before examining these differences further, we must turn to the question of how this complex pattern of testosterone is regulated. Successful reproduction requires that an organism coordinate its reproductive activities with a variety of events in its physical and social environment, and these vary from one stage of reproduction to another. It is not surprising, then, that the pattern of testosterone secretion is the result of complex responses to a variety of different cues whose importance varies at each stage of the breeding cycle.

As mentioned earlier, each individual must anticipate the onset of favorable breeding conditions by at least several weeks so that development of the gonads and behavior can begin in readiness for the ensuing breeding season. What are the environmental cues available that predict the onset of favorable breeding conditions, especially for migratory species that may over-winter at a site far removed from the breeding grounds, and how do they affect the pattern of secretion of testosterone? One of the most reliable, and therefore useful, cues is the increase in daylength that occurs in the spring. It has been shown at least since the 1920s that long, summerlike days can stimulate reproductive development in a variety of organisms including birds. The effects of daylength on LH and testosterone secretion are summarized below.

EFFECTS OF DAYLENGTH ON PLASMA LEVELS OF LH, TESTOSTERONE, AND GONADAL GROWTH

It is well known that birds have a *biological clock* within the central nervous system that allows them to measure daylength precisely to within a few minutes (see Chapter 5). Birds use this clock to respond to the vernal increase in daylength by initiating development of the gonads and secondary sex characters. This effect can be demonstrated dramatically in laboratory experiments. If adult male white-crowned or song sparrows are held on a winterlike daylength of 8 hours of light and 16 hours dark (8L 16D) and then transferred to a long summerlike daylength of 20 hours of light (20L 4D), they respond with rapid testicular growth accompanied by increases in LH and testosterone (Figure 6.3). Sperm production is completed, secondary sex characters develop fully, and the entire repertoire of reproductive behavior develops. In Gambel's sparrows, there is a spontaneous decline in testis size as well as a marked decrease in plasma levels of LH and testosterone after approximately 60 days of photostimulation (about 100 days in the song sparrow), despite the fact that days remain long. This spontaneous *switching off* of the reproductive system is known as photorefractoriness. This process terminates the breeding season so that individuals do not initiate another nesting attempt, and also have time to molt while food supplies are still abundant.

The mechanisms by which daylength is perceived are still not understood, but it is quite clear that the eyes are not the primary photoreceptor (see Chapter 5). Numerous experiments, including localized destruction of

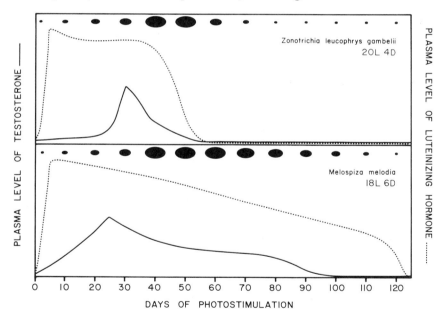

Figure 6.3. Plasma levels of luteinizing hormone (LH) and testosterone in photostimulated male Gambel's sparrows (*Zonotrichia leucophrys gambelii*) and song sparrows (*Melospiza melodia*). The solid ovals at the top of each panel give an indication of relative testis size throughout the experiment. Note that testis size and plasma levels of LH and testosterone do not change in males held on short days as controls (not shown), at least for the duration of the experiment. (Compiled from Follett et al., 1975; Lam and Farner, 1976; J.C. Wingfield, unpublished)

neuronal tissue (lesions) and the use of minute light-pipes placed in the brain, indicate clearly that the photoreceptors are localized within the central nervous system, probably lying in the infundibular region of the basal hypothalamus (e.g., Yokoyama et al., 1978).

Several hypotheses attempt to explain how birds respond to increased daylength with enhanced secretion of reproductive hormones. In the white-crowned sparrow, it has been proposed that exposure to long days initiates an internal *program* or *programs* of events (molt, migration, gonadal growth, and photorefractoriness). Full expression of this program requires continued exposure to long days, and it does not repeat until it has been *reset* by exposing the birds to winterlike short days for several weeks (e.g., Moore et al., 1982). Because this program is not expressed in the absence of long-day stimulation, long days can be said to *drive* reproductive development and associated events. Another widely held theory suggests that some species have an internal, continuously repeating annual rhythm of migration, molt, gonadal growth and regression that oscillates with a period of about one year under any environmental conditions. These are usually called *circannual rhythms* (see Gwinner, 1981). In this case, the seasonal changes in daylength act only to adjust the timing and duration of this internal rhythm so the events occur at the proper time during the seasonal progression of the natural 365-day year. Because the events proceed even in the absence of photostimulation, long days are said in this case to act only as a *Zeitgeber* or *time-giver* for the internal rhythm.

The proposed mechanisms by which photoreceptors respond to change in daylength, or how time is measured in these birds (and indeed all photoperiodic organisms), are complex and beyond the scope of this review. However, the following references may be of interest to the reader wishing to learn more about them: Gwinner (1981), Farner (1985), and Farner and Gwinner (1980).

Thus it appears that simple exposure of the male to long days is a sufficient stimulus to attain complete reproductive development. However, if we compare the temporal pattern of testosterone on long days in the laboratory (Figure 6.3) with the pattern in free-living males (Figure 6.2), it can be seen that there are dramatic differences. In general, levels of testosterone measured in laboratory experiments are lower (Figure 6.4), and the pattern of secretion is much less complex than those observed under natural conditions. In the free-living song sparrow there are two distinct peaks of testosterone before declining to a maintenance level, and finally to basal in July and August. In Puget Sound and Gambel's sparrows there are also hints of two peaks of testosterone, although the vernal events in these forms are very short-lived and the two peaks appear compressed together. Like the song sparrow, however, plasma testosterone levels decline to maintenance levels before reaching basal later in summer. These data suggest strongly that other environmental stimuli in addition to daylength can influence the secretion of testosterone. These additional environmental cues must stimulate not only increases in testosterone secretion above that induced by long days, but also superimpose these peaks on the basic

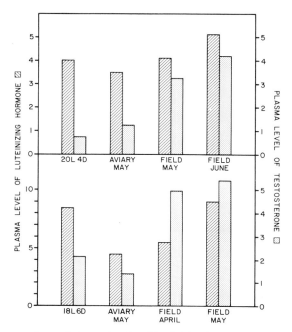

Figure 6.4. A comparison of plasma levels of luteinizing hormone (LH) (hatched bars) and testosterone (stippled bars) in captive and free-living male Gambel's sparrows (*Zonotrichia leucophrys gambelii*) (top panel), and song sparrows (*Melospiza melodia*) (bottom panel). 20L 4D = males held on artificial long days of 20 hours light and 4 dark, and 18L 6D = males held on artificial long days of 18 hours light and 6 dark. Aviary May = captive males exposed to natural daylength and sampled in May when plasma levels of LH and testosterone are maximal. Field May and Field June = free-living males sampled in May and June when mate-guarding. (Compiled from Wingfield and Farner, 1980; Wingfield 1984a; and J.C. Wingfield, unpublished)

photoinduced cycle (note that the maintenance levels in free-living birds are very similar to the highest levels measured under laboratory conditions).

Since the peaks of testosterone in free-living birds are associated with periods of heightened aggression (during establishment of territory) and mate-guarding activity, it is logical to suggest that the stimulus for these surges in testosterone levels might involve social interactions both among males and between mates. These cues can be included as synchronizing and integrating information in the classification of proximate factors described above. The experimental evidence for a role of social interactions in the regulation of reproductive function and behavior will be discussed next.

TESTOSTERONE SECRETION AND MALE-MALE INTERACTIONS

Male song and white-crowned sparrows arrive on their breeding territories with elevated levels of circulating testosterone that are correlated with high frequencies of agonistic interactions over territory boundaries. Are these high levels of testosterone associated with increased levels of aggressive behavior (see Chapter 2)? To test this, adult male Gambel's sparrows were castrated, one group given empty implants as controls, and another group given implants of testosterone. Sparrows were housed one per cage and the aggressive behaviors as they interacted with each other (frequency of songs, threats, and wing flutters) recorded for a period of 13 days after implant. Surprisingly, frequencies of aggression increased in both groups, even though one had a very low plasma level of testosterone and the other a very high level. There was a tendency for the testosterone-implanted castrates to show greater frequencies of aggression, but this was not significant (Wingfield, 1985a). After 13 days the levels of aggression declined markedly in both groups, probably a reflection of habituation to their neighbors. However, if a novel male, which the subject birds had never interacted with or even seen before, was placed in a neighboring cage, there was an immediate increase in levels of aggression in both groups. In this case, however, the testosterone-implanted males displayed significantly higher frequencies of aggression than did the controls (Wingfield, 1985a). Thus, it appears that increases in testosterone level are correlated with elevated aggression, but this relationship is only apparent if the individual is challenged by another male. Under more stable conditions, there may be no apparent correlation of testosterone and aggression because social relationships have already been established. If this social stability is challenged, then frequencies of aggression correlate well with testosterone levels (see also Wingfield and Ramenofsky, 1985).

The laboratory experiment described above is somewhat artificial, since we cannot be sure that a male in a small cage is *territorial* and regards a novel male placed in a cage alongside as an *intruder*. Therefore, a field experiment was conducted using free-living, territorial male song sparrows. Male sparrows were given subcutaneous implants of testosterone to maintain maximum plasma levels. In a separate area, other males were given empty implants as controls. The aggressive territorial behavior of all males was tested in late May and June when plasma levels of testosterone in the controls had declined to maintenance levels (Figure 6.2). Thus, one group (implanted with testosterone) had a very high level of testosterone and the other a much lower level (control). Do they show the same degree of territorial aggression? To test this each subject male was exposed to a simulated territorial intrusion by placing a conspecific male in a cage within the subject's territory and then playing conspecific songs through an adjacent speaker. The territory owner responds to the simulated intruder and attempts to drive him away. The behavioral responses of experimental and control males can then be recorded easily by a nearby observer. Both groups of males responded to the intrusion, but those with the implants of testosterone displayed more frequent and intense territorial aggression than the controls (Wingfield, 1984b). For example, testosterone-implanted males approached the intruder more closely, spent more time within 5 meters, and performed more *flutter flights* (regarded as being highly aggressive in context). Thus, it appears that the maximum levels of testosterone in spring are involved, at least in part, with heightened expression of territorial aggression.

Since long days of spring are sufficient to increase plasma levels of testosterone only partially, what additional environmental stimuli cause increased secretion of testosterone? The first peak of testosterone in song sparrows is coincident with establishment of territory. Thus there are two possible stimuli: (1) obtaining a territory *per se*, or (2) interacting with other males as the boundary is established, or (3) a combination of both hypotheses. To investigate these possibilities territorial male song sparrows were captured in April (after territories had been established and plasma levels of testosterone had waned) and held in captivity. Other males, who either have been unable to obtain a territory or who have one of poor quality, will move in and take over the vacant spot within 12–72 hours. If no replacement male appears, then the neighbors will expand their boundaries to take over the territory instead. In both cases a period of increased agonistic interactions follows as new territory boundaries are formed. During this period blood samples were collected from both the replacements and their neighbors. Control samples were collected from adult territorial males that were captured and immediately returned to their territories (i.e., an area in which territory boundaries were stable). Both replacement males and their neighbors have plasma levels of testosterone that are elevated over those of controls (Figure 6.5). Since the neighbors and controls already have a territory, and the latter have significantly lower levels of testosterone, this suggests that ownership of a territory per se is not a major stimulus for increased secretion of testosterone. Rather it suggests that the interaction with the replacement male as new boundaries are established is the cue.

To test this further, changes in hormone levels in territorial male song sparrows following simulated territorial intrusions were examined. Males were allowed to interact with the apparent intruder for ten minutes or so, then captured in mist nets, and a blood sample collected for measurement of testosterone levels. Foraging control males, not involved in an encounter, were captured in traps baited with seeds. One experiment was conducted in June and July and another in April (during the nadir between the two peaks

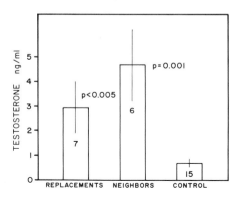

Figure 6.5. Plasma levels of testosterone in free-living male song sparrows (*Melospiza melodia*) after removal of a territorial male. Replacements are those males that took over the vacant territory, and neighbors are those males with territories adjacent to the replacements. Controls were captured in a separate area in which territory boundaries were known to be stable. Histograms represent the means, and vertical bars are the standard errors. Figures within the histograms are sample sizes. (From Wingfield, 1985b, with permission of Academic Press)

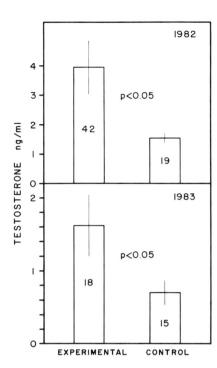

Figure 6.6. Plasma levels of testosterone in free-living male song sparrows (*Melospiza melodia*), after exposure to a simulated territorial intrusion (experimental), and controls (captured while foraging). One experiment was conducted in April 1983, the other in late May–July 1982. Histograms represent means, and vertical bars are the standard errors. Figures within histograms are sample sizes. (From Wingfield, 1985b, with permission of Academic Press)

of testosterone in Figure 6.2). In both experiments, plasma levels of testosterone were significantly higher in birds exposed to intrusions than in controls (Figure 6.6). These results support the hypothesis that agonistic interactions between males, and more specifically the stimuli emanating from a challenging male, are the cues for increased secretion of testosterone. That this response can be elicited both early and late in the season may be of adaptive significance. Although most agonistic interactions occur in early spring as territories are set up, males with an established territory are occasionally challenged at all stages of the breeding season.

There is a third line of evidence for the role of male-male interactions in promoting the secretion of testosterone. Adult male song sparrows with implants of testosterone remain very aggressive throughout the breeding season. If male-male interactions result in elevations of testosterone, then plasma levels in neighbors of testosterone-implanted males should be higher than in neighbors of controls. Males with territories next to testosterone-implanted subjects have significantly higher testosterone levels in blood than neighbors of control birds in April (Figure 6.7). However, in May and June this effect is not seen, possibly because of overriding stimuli such as presence of young. Toward the end of the season (July) the relationship appears once again.

It is important to emphasize here that males with territories one or two removed from a testosterone-implanted male do not have elevated levels of testosterone even though they can see and hear the interactions between

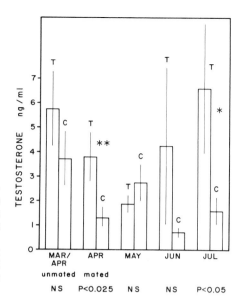

Figure 6.7. Plasma levels of testosterone in free-living male song sparrows (*Melospiza melodia*) that had territories next to testosterone-implanted males (T) or control-implanted males (C). NS = not significant. Histograms represent means, and vertical bars are the standard errors. (From Wingfield, 1984b, with permission of Academic Press)

immediate neighbors and implanted males (Wingfield, 1984b). This observation raises the fascinating possibility that the observance of a challenging male is not sufficient to increase testosterone secretion, but that the challenge must be directed at a specific individual to get the full response. This mechanism may prevent generalized responses that might otherwise result in severe disruption of the breeding effort.

The experiments summarized above indicate clearly that challenges from conspecific males can increase the secretion of testosterone. But why not maintain plasma levels of testosterone at a maximum and always be ready? Since male white-crowned and song sparrows feed young and, after fledging, may do so without much help from the female, it is possible that high levels of testosterone and resulting heightened levels of aggression are incompatible with parental behavior. This has been well demonstrated in another species, the pied flycatcher (*Ficedula hypoleuca*) of Europe. If males are given implants of testosterone just before the young hatch, they begin singing and patrolling the territory and spend little time, if any, feeding young (Silverin, 1980). As a result an individual's reproductive success is reduced dramatically. Thus it appears that in species in which the male provides a significant amount of parental care, plasma levels of testosterone are kept at the minimal level required to maintain the gonad, secondary sex characters, and low levels of territorial behavior, without interfering with the expression of parental behavior. However, mechanisms do exist whereby the plasma levels of testosterone can be increased if the need arises—as is the case if a male is challenged by an intruder. The heightened levels of testosterone in turn increase the frequency and intensity of aggression, especially if the interaction lasts for hours, or even a day or more. Once the intruder has been repelled, the stimulus for increased secretion of testosterone is removed and plasma levels decline, allowing the male to return to feeding young. Such finely tuned responses to social cues may increase the reproductive success over an entire season or several seasons.

Although plasma levels of testosterone are elevated in response to a challenge by another male, there appears to be no consistent increase in LH, the hormone that promotes secretion of testosterone (Wingfield, 1984b, 1985b). There is a trend for increased levels of LH, but this is not always significant. It is possible that our assay for avian LH is not sufficiently sensitive to discern slight increases that may be sufficient to elevate testosterone secretion, or that other mechanisms, thus far unknown, may also be operating. Clearly, more experimentation is required to clarify this issue.

ENDOCRINE RESPONSES OF MALES TO THEIR SEXUALLY RECEPTIVE MATES

Male white-crowned and song sparrows also have elevated levels of LH and testosterone during the egg-laying stage for the first brood (see Figure 6.2). These high levels are correlated with increased aggression as males mate-guard their sexually receptive females. Elevated levels of aggression are directed at conspecific males in an attempt to reduce the risk of cuckoldry by neighbors. The possibility of cuckoldry is quite high because neighboring males are opportunistic and will usually copulate with any female should they get a chance. The stimulus for continued high levels of LH and testosterone in white-crowned sparrows, or a second surge of LH and testosterone in song sparrows, is thought to be related to stimuli emanating from the sexual behavior of the female. Such effects of females on the neuroendocrine and endocrine systems of males have been well documented in mammals, but until recently similar documentation in birds was lacking.

Captive male Gambel's sparrows held on long days to stimulate a gonadal cycle (see Figure 6.3) show further increases in LH and testosterone (Figure 6.8) if exposed to a female implanted with estradiol-17β (a hormone that promotes sexual behavior in the female). In a complementary field study, female Puget Sound sparrows were given implants of estradiol during the egg-laying stage of the first brood. These implants maintained plasma levels of estradiol at a maximum and thus prolonged the period of sexual behavior, particularly the female's solicitation of copulation, into the parental phase of the breeding cycle. The decline of plasma levels of LH and testosterone that normally accompanies onset of parental behavior did not occur in males with estrogenized females (Figure 6.9; Moore, 1982b). This supports the hypothesis that female sexual behavior stimulates secretion of LH and testosterone.

Curiously, the parental behavior of females implanted with estradiol does not appear to differ from that of controls. Incubation progresses normally, young are hatched and fledged, despite the continued expression of sexual displays. This is an important point, since it suggests that the onset

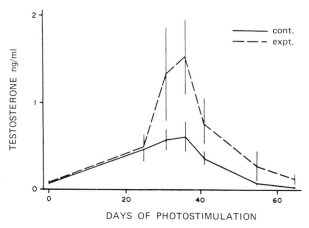

Figure 6.8. Plasma levels of testosterone in photostimulated male Gambel's sparrows (*Zonotrichia leucophrys gambelii*), exposed to estradiol-treated (expt.), or control (cont.) females. Values are means plus or minus standard errors. (From Moore, 1982a, 1983, with permission of the Zoological Society of London)

of parental behavior (i.e., incubation by the female) is not a stimulus for decreased secretion of LH and testosterone in male sparrows, but rather a direct effect of reduced sexual behavior of the female.

The responses of males to sexual behavior of females has also been demonstrated in the song sparrow with essentially identical results. Indeed, male song sparrows can maintain relatively high plasma levels of LH and testosterone throughout the breeding season if females are treated continuously with estradiol (Wingfield et al., manuscript).

Because the relatively low levels of testosterone in photostimulated males in captivity are sufficient to cause full development of the testis, secondary sex characters, and the full repertoire of reproductive behaviors, the further increase in testosterone levels in free-living males at the time of egg-laying is probably involved only in maintaining a high frequency and intensity of aggressive displays while mate-guarding. This suggestion is

Figure 6.9. Plasma levels of testosterone (T in panel A) in free-living male Puget Sound sparrows (*Zonotrichia leucophrys pugetensis*), during courtship (COURT.) and incubation (INCUB.), including a comparison of incubation levels in control males (CON), whose untreated mates had ceased soliciting copulations, and in experimental males (EXP), whose estradiol-treated mates continued to solicit copulations. Plasma levels of luteinizing hormone (LH in panel B) from the same males. Histograms represent means, and vertical bars are standard errors. (From Moore, 1982a)

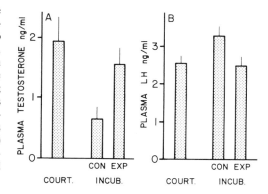

reinforced by the observation that male Puget Sound sparrows implanted with testosterone during the parental phase respond far more aggressively to a simulated intruding male than do controls that have a much lower level of testosterone (Moore, 1984). Very similar observations have been made in male song sparrows implanted with testosterone and exposed to a simulated territorial intrusion (Wingfield, 1984c; see also above).

MULTIPLE-BROODING AND RENESTING

Many avian species that breed at lower latitudes take advantage of the long summers and raise two or more broods within a single breeding season. In Puget Sound sparrows and song sparrows, females begin to prepare for a second clutch soon after young of the first brood fledge. The fledglings are fed primarily by the male until they become independent at about 30 days of age. By this time the female has produced a second nest and clutch of eggs and may be incubating. Thus, throughout the postfledging period the male is feeding young and also must copulate with his mate when the second clutch is produced. In Figure 6.2 it can be seen that although there is an increase in plasma levels of LH in males whose mates are producing a second clutch, there is no parallel increase in testosterone. This differs from the pattern during egg-laying for the first clutch and raises some interesting questions. Since one would expect the male to mate-guard for the second clutch, why is there no increase in testosterone? Also, since LH is known to stimulate secretion of testosterone, why is there an increase in LH and no effect on testosterone secretion?

Let us consider the first question concerning why there is no second peak of testosterone. Throughout the fledging period the male is feeding the young while the female prepares for the second clutch. Although we would expect the male to mate-guard as intensively for the second clutch as he does for the first, there may actually be a potential for reduced nesting success if he does. It is known that survivability of young from the first clutch is better than that for subsequent broods (Perrins, 1970). Also, a male with fledglings has a genetic investment *in hand*, and it would be advantageous to ensure that the first brood reaches independence. Mate-guarding may take away time that the male could invest more profitably in parental care for the first brood. Furthermore, the high levels of testosterone that accompany mate-guarding behavior may inhibit parental behavior such that the young of the first brood may not reach independence at all. Clearly then, there appears to be a compromise here—the male feeds young of the first brood and plasma levels of testosterone remain low. Note that he is still able to copulate with the female, although full paternity of the second clutch may be lost due to reduced levels of mate-guarding. Nevertheless, the net reproductive success for the male at the end of the breeding season may still be higher than if he ensured full paternity of that second clutch. Indeed, the independence of male copulatory behavior from hormonal control in the white-crowned sparrow may have evolved to meet this need for independent expression of copulatory behavior and testosterone-dependent territorial aggression (Moore, 1984; Crews and Moore, 1986).

This concept of incompatibility of mate-guarding with male parental care is also supported by observations that both plasma levels of LH *and* testosterone increased during the egg-laying stage for a replacement clutch, after the previous brood had been lost to a predator or a bad storm (see Figure 6.10). In this case, since the young were lost, the male was no longer burdened with feeding young and could thus benefit from mate-guarding as intensively as he did for the first clutch. This explains an increase in testosterone during renesting versus no increase during the second brood after *successful* raising of the first. The data also point out that it is important to consider multiple-brooding and renesting separately, since the endocrine mechanisms involved may be different.

We are still left with the endocrinologic problem as to why there is an increase in plasma levels of LH during the egg-laying stage of the second brood, but no parallel increase in testosterone. It appears that the response of the testes to LH is somehow blocked. It is well known that elevated levels of another pituitary hormone, prolactin, are associated with parental behavior (e.g., Goldsmith, 1983), and that prolactin can inhibit secretion of gonadotropins (e.g., Camper and Burke, 1977a,b). Since LH secretion increases at this time, it is possible that prolactin may be acting at the

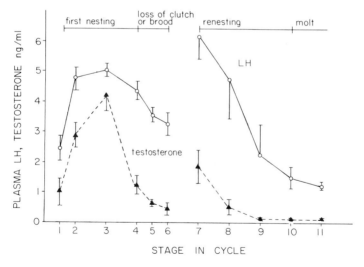

Figure 6.10. Plasma levels of luteinizing hormone (LH) and testosterone during renesting in male Gambel's sparrows (*Zonotrichia leucophrys gambelii*). Stage 1 = vernal migration; 2 = arrival on breeding grounds; 3 = egg-laying; 4 = early incubation; 5 = late incubation; 6 = feeding nestlings; 7 = renesting (egg-laying); 8 = incubation of replacement clutch; 9 = feeding nestlings of replacement brood; 10 = feeding fledglings of replacement brood; 11 = postnuptial molt. Each point represents the mean and vertical bars are standard errors. (From Wingfield and Farner, 1979, with permission of Academic Press)

testicular level to inhibit androgen secretion (Moore, 1984; Wingfield, 1985c). Moreover, if the nest and young are lost, then it seems reasonable that prolactin levels would decrease, since it is well known that the stimulus for secretion of prolactin involves presence of the nest and young (Lehrman, 1965; Goldsmith, 1983). As prolactin levels decline, the inhibition on secretion of testosterone is removed, resulting in a resurgence of this hormone as LH levels increase during the egg-laying stage for the renesting attempt. This would explain the curious dichotomy in temporal patterns of testosterone secretion in multiple-brooding and renesting.

Recent reports lend some support to this hypothesis in other species in which prolactin levels increase as incubation begins, and reach a peak as the young hatch (e.g., Goldsmith, 1983; El Halawani et al., 1984). Removal of the nest results in a decline of prolactin that can be reversed if the nest is restored (e.g., Goldsmith, 1983; El Halawani et al., 1980). Thus the decline in prolactin following nest loss and prior to renesting seems to be a reasonable hypothesis. The temporal patterns of prolactin in relation to multiple-brooding and renesting in free-living sparrows are currently under investigation.

TERMINATION OF THE BREEDING SEASON

In July and August, white-crowned and song sparrows cease reproductive activity and begin the postnuptial (*prebasic*) molt. This apparent premature termination of breeding while food is still abundant and weather is fair appears to be related to extremely low survivability of young raised late in the season (Perrins, 1970) and also to the high metabolic requirements of molt (e.g., Farner and Follett, 1979). Reproductive activity and molt are usually regarded as mutually exclusive, and thus reproduction is terminated early enough so that feather replacement can be completed while food is still abundant. Further, in those species that migrate, preparations such as premigratory fattening are most efficiently accomplished during periods of food abundance and before the first autumnal storms, which at high latitudes may be very severe.

Termination of reproduction in these sparrows clearly involves development of a photorefractory state in which individuals no longer respond to long days with increased secretion of gonadotropins (e.g., Farner and Follett, 1979; Nicholls et al., 1984). A spontaneous decline in plasma levels of LH and testosterone follows, causing subsequent gonadal involution (see Figure 6.3). Onset of photorefractoriness occurs fairly synchronously among individuals held on artificial long days in the laboratory, but in the field there may be a difference of up to four weeks in termination of reproduction (Wingfield and Farner, 1979). This variation is invariably linked to the stage in the nesting phase. For example, it would be clearly disadvantageous if the onset of photorefractoriness terminated the breeding effort while adults were incubating the last clutch, or while feeding young. Rather, it appears that although photorefractoriness may develop fairly synchronously in all individuals within a population, additional factors (supplementary) appear to delay the overt effects of photorefractoriness (rapid gonadal involution, declines of reproductive hormones to basal, and the waning of reproductive behaviors) until the final brood has been raised to independence, or has at least fledged (Wingfield and Farner, 1979). Thus photorefractoriness prevents the initiation of further clutches but allows completion of a nesting attempt already underway.

What are the supplementary factors that delay the effects of photorefractoriness in sparrows? In females it is possible that stimuli from the nest and eggs during incubation are effective, but this is less likely for males who do not incubate. Since males respond to sexual stimuli from the female, at least during the egg-laying stage of the first brood, and during renest attempts, it is possible that stimuli from the late-nesting female may also provide the environmental cue that delays the effects of photorefractoriness until the young hatch. Since the male does feed young, it is also possible that stimuli from the nest and young are effective later in the final nesting attempt.

To test the hypothesis that prolonged sexual behavior of the female delays termination of breeding in males, free-living female song sparrows were given implants of estradiol in July (mostly during the early parental phase of the last brood, Runfeldt and Wingfield, 1985). These implants of estradiol maintained the female in a breeding state for up to two months longer than controls which were given an empty implant. Furthermore, the onset of molt was delayed by 1–2 months in estrogenized females. Males mated to estrogenized females also delayed onset of molt by 1–2 months, and 6 of 8 males were still on their breeding territories in October. In contrast, males mated to control females ceased reproductive activity and began molting in July and August, as is normal (Runfeldt and Wingfield, 1985).

Further experimentation on the effects of estrogenized females on their male mates indicate that the territorial behavior (as assessed by simulated territorial intrusion) of control and experimental males did not differ in July, when all pairs were still breeding. However, by August and September, when all controls had ceased reproduction, the experimental males showed clear territorial responses to intrusion that were higher than the few control males that responded. Furthermore, the plasma levels of testosterone in experimental males were significantly higher than controls that were presumably photorefractory (Figure 6.11, Runfeldt and Wingfield, 1985). Note that these plasma levels of testosterone are similar to the intermediate levels measured during the parental stages (Figure 6.2). They are above basal, but not as high as the vernal maxima.

In the converse experiment, free-living male song sparrows were given implants of testosterone to delay the effects of photorefractoriness. These males remained territorial (8 of 9) through October, and onset of molt was delayed again by 1–2 months compared with controls. However, females mated to testosterone-implanted males did not delay the effects of photorefractoriness.

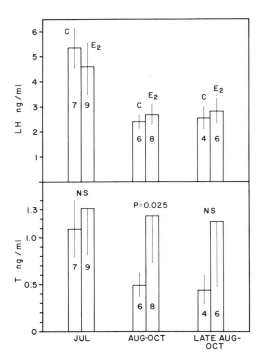

Figure 6.11. Plasma levels of luteinizing hormone (LH) and testosterone (T) in free-living male song sparrows (*Melospiza melodia*) mated to estradiol-implanted (E2) or control-implanted (C) females, and sampled late in the breeding season and beyond (July–October). Histograms represent means, and vertical bars are standard errors. Figures within the histograms are sample sizes. (From Runfeldt and Wingfield, 1985, with permission of Balliere Tindall)

They ceased breeding activity and began the postnuptial molt at the same time as females mated to control males (Runfeldt and Wingfield, 1985). Thus, it appears that the female may fine-tune the termination of reproduction and the male synchronizes his reproductive activity to that of his mate. One would expect that males would remain in breeding condition as long as there are females accessible for matings. In contrast, since the production of a clutch of eggs incurs a great energetic cost, it is reasonable to suggest that females would not delay termination of reproduction in response to availability of active males, but rather cease at a time when it would no longer be an advantage to produce more young.

These findings emphasize how behavioral interactions between mates can fine-tune the temporal progression of the breeding season, including its termination.

CONCLUDING REMARKS

The progress of the breeding cycle of these small birds under natural conditions is a model example of the complex interplay between an organism's external environment and its internal physiologic state. Such interrelationships are essential if an individual is to survive and reproduce successfully. Natural selection, through the differential survival and reproduction of more successful genotypes, has honed this extraordinarily sophisticated system to exquisite precision. Males successfully integrate information about the nature of their environment, the state of neighboring male competitors, the reproductive status of their female, and the success of their own reproductive effort.

This complex array of information is received by the central nervous system, which in turn regulates secretion of hypothalamic hormones and thus the physiologic state of the reproductive system. As a result, plasma levels of testosterone fluctuate, with direct consequences on male behavior. Both male-male and male-female interactions act to keep testosterone levels, and thus frequency of territorial behavior, high during the initial phases of the breeding cycle. However, high levels of testosterone appear to be incompatible with parental behavior. Therefore, plasma levels of testosterone are maintained at lower, intermediate, levels that sustain the reproductive apparatus and minimum territorial behavior but do not interfere with parental care. Nevertheless, male-male interactions at this time can result in an increase in testosterone, possibly to maintain a high level of aggression for the duration of the challenge. In contrast, male-female interactions, specifically the onset of receptivity by the female, affect testosterone levels of males only in the absence of young. Thus it appears that increased aggressiveness in response to direct challenges by other males is adaptive during the parental-care period, whereas the general increased vigilance of mate-guarding is not.

Males do not respond endocrinologically to these behavioral cues, whether from another male or female, unless the individual is directly involved. Males do not respond when their neighbors are challenged, or when their neighbor's mate is receptive. This suggests that in addition to processing the visual and auditory information that make up the behavioral stimulus, there is some additional screening by the central nervous system that provides the correct context of the stimulus. In other words, the challenge must be directed at the resident male, or the displaying female must be his mate, before an endocrine response is elicited.

These observations also provide insight into the evolutionary forces that have shaped the male's response to the hormonal signal. Territorial aggressive behavior, which is initiated by the male and must be expressed in varying frequencies and intensities at different stages of the reproductive cycle, is tightly linked to the socially and environmentally induced variations in plasma levels of testosterone. In contrast, male copulatory behavior is a simple all-or-none response to the occurrence of an external stimulus— female solicitation displays. Male copulatory behavior also must be expressed independently of aggressive behavior during the overlapping periods of parental care and production of subsequent clutches. This conflict, and the availability of an external triggering stimulus, has apparently resulted in the evolutionary emancipation of male copulatory behavior from control by testosterone (Moore, 1984; Crews and Moore, 1986).

Although we now have much evidence to back up the ideas and hypotheses outlined above, it is clear that much work remains to be done. All of the hypotheses presented here are testable. Our ability to understand

and unravel at least part of this complex series of interdependent events has been greatly enhanced by the fact that is was possible to carry out rigorously controlled studies under naturalistic field conditions. Laboratory investigations alone can yield limited and sometimes misleading answers. For example, it is well known that a male's aggressive responses vary depending whether he is on his home territory or not. We do not know whether a captive male in a small cage considers that to be his territory. This fact, however, will greatly affect both his behavioral and hormonal response to intruders. In the field it is easy to separately examine the responses of intruders, residents, and neighbors—concepts that have no clear meaning in simple laboratory settings. As a second example, earlier laboratory studies tended to overemphasize the role of the male in stimulating female ovarian development. Field investigations reveal that females respond more to the presence of sufficient food for egg production, and that males, after the initial establishment of a territory, adjust their physiology and behavior to match the female's activities and essentially *track* the female's reproductive cycle. Thus, in addition to controlled laboratory studies, it is clear that *holistic* investigations under natural conditions are crucial to the complete elucidation of mechanisms and their significance to the individual.

Finally, what relationship do these kinds of investigations have to current research and thought in the life sciences? There is no doubt that we live in an era preoccupied with reductionistic and molecular approaches to biological problems, but it must not be forgotten that even the fundamental molecular mechanisms of, for example, cellular metabolism evolved in response to a need to survive and reproduce successfully in a complex and sometimes capricious environment. While it is certainly important to understand the specifics of biochemical mechanisms, we cannot claim to understand those processes fully until we gain a clearer picture of the suite of environmental factors that caused them to evolve, and the nature of their functioning when exposed to the complex fluctuations of a natural environment.

ACKNOWLEDGMENTS

Preparation of this manuscript was aided by grant number DCB-8316155 from the National Science Foundation, a Charles H. Revson Foundation Fellowship in Biomedical Research, and an Irma T. Hirschl Foundation Research Career Development Award to J.C.W., and a Presidential Young Investigator Award DCB-8451641 from the National Science Foundation to M.C.M. We also extend many thanks to Christine Levesque, who drafted the figures.

REFERENCES

BAKER, J.R. (1938) The evolution of breeding seasons. In *Evolution*. G.R. deBeer, ed., pp. 161–177, Oxford University Press, London.

BALTHAZART, J. (1983) Hormonal correlates of behavior. In *Avian Biology*, Vol. 7. D.S. Farner, J.R. King, and K.C. Parkes, eds., pp. 221–365, Academic Press, New York and London.

CAMPER, P.M., and W.H. BURKE (1977a) The effect of prolactin on the gonadotropin induced rise in serum estradiol and progesterone of the laying turkey. Gen. Comp. Endocrinol. *32*:72–77.

CAMPER, P.M., and W.H. BURKE (1977b) The effect of prolactin on reproductive function in female Japanese quail (*Coturnix coturnix japonica*). Poultry Sci. *56*:1130–1134.

CREWS, D., and M.C. MOORE (1986) Evolution of mechanisms controlling mating behavior. Science *231*:121–125.

EL HALAWANI, M.E., W.H. BURKE, J.R. MILLAM, S.C. FEHRER, and B.M. HARGIS (1984) Regulation of prolactin and its role in gallinaceous bird reproduction. J. Exp. Zool. *232*:521–529.

FARNER, D.S. (1985) Annual rhythms. Ann. Rev. Physiol. *47*:65–82.

FARNER, D.S., and B.K. FOLLETT (1979) Reproductive periodicity in birds. In *Hormones and Evolution*. E.J.W. Barrington, ed., pp. 829–872, Academic Press, New York and London.

FARNER, D.S., and E. GWINNER (1980) Photoperiodicity, circannual, and reproductive cycles. In *Avian Endocrinology*. A. Epple and M.H. Stetson, eds., pp. 331–366, Academic Press, New York and London.

FOLLETT, B.K., D.S. FARNER, and P.W. MATTOCKS, JR. (1975) Luteinizing hormone in the plasma of white-crowned sparrows, *Zonotrichia leucophrys gambelii*, during artificial photostimulation. Gen. Comp. Endocrinol. *26*:126–134.

GOLDSMITH, A.R. (1983) Prolactin in avian reproductive cycles. In *Hormones and Behaviour in Higher Vertebrates*. J. Balthazart, E. Pröve, and R. Gilles, eds., pp. 375–387, Springer-Verlag, Berlin.

GWINNER, E. (1981) Circannual systems. In *Handbook of Behavioral Neurobiology*, Vol. 4, *Biological Rhythms*. J. Aschoff, ed., pp. 391–410, Plenum Press, New York and London.

LACK, D. (1968) *Ecological Adaptations for Breeding in Birds*. Chapman and Hall, London, 409 pp.

LAM, F., and D.S. FARNER (1976) The ultrastructure of the cells of Leydig in the white-crowned sparrow (*Zonotrichia leucophrys gambelii*) in relation to plasma levels of luteinizing hormone and testosterone. Cell Tiss. Res. *169*:93–109.

LEHRMAN, D.S. (1965) Interaction between the internal and external environments in the regulation of the reproductive cycle of the ring dove. In *Sex and Behavior*. F.A. Beach, ed., pp. 355–380, John Wiley & Sons, New York.

MILLAR, R.P., and J.A. KING (1984) Structure-activity relations of LHRH in birds. J. Exp. Zool. *232*:425–430.

MOORE, M.C. (1982a) Behavioral endocrinology of reproduction in white-crowned sparrows, *Zonotrichia leucophrys*. Ph.D. Thesis, University of Washington, 114 pp.

MOORE, M.C. (1982b) Hormonal responses of free-living male white-crowned sparrows to experimental manipulation of female sexual behavior. Horm. Behav. *16*:323–329.

MOORE, M.C. (1983) Effect of female sexual displays on the endocrine physiology and behavior of male white-crowned sparrows, *Zonotrichia leucophrys*. J. Zool. (London) *199*:137–148.

MOORE, M.C. (1984) Changes in territorial defense produced by changes in circulating levels of testosterone: A possible hormonal basis for mate-guarding behavior in white-crowned sparrows. Behaviour *88*:215–226.

MOORE, M.C., and R. KRANZ (1983) Evidence for androgen independence of male mounting behavior in white-crowned sparrows (*Zonotrichia leucophrys gambelii*). Horm. Behav. *17*:414–423.

MOORE, M.C., R.S. DONHAM, and D.S. FARNER (1982) Physiologic preparations for autumnal migration in white-crowned sparrows. Condor *84*:410–419.

NICHOLLS, T.J., A.R. GOLDSMITH, and A. DAWSON (1984) Photorefractoriness in European starlings: Associated hypothalamic changes and the involvement of thyroid hormones and prolactin. J. Exp. Zool. *232*:567–572.

PERRINS, C.M. (1970) The timing of birds' breeding seasons. Ibis *112*:242–255.

RUNFELDT, S., and J.C. WINGFIELD (1985) Experimentally prolonged sexual activity in female sparrows delays termination of reproductive activity in their untreated mates. Anim. Behav. *33*:403–410.

SILVERIN, B. (1980) Effects of long-acting testosterone treatment on free-living pied flycatchers, *Ficedula hypoleuca*, during the breeding period. Anim. Behav. *28*:906–912.

WINGFIELD, J.C. (1983) Environmental and endocrine control of reproduction: An ecological approach. In *Avian Endocrinology: Environmental and Ecological Aspects*. S.-I. Mikami, S. Ishii, and M. Wada, eds., pp. 265–288, Japanese Scientific Societies Press, Tokyo, and Springer-Verlag, Berlin.

WINGFIELD, J.C. (1984a) Environmental and endocrine control of reproduction in the song sparrow, *Melospiza melodia*. 1. Temporal organization of the breeding cycle. Gen. Comp. Endocrinol. *56*:406–416.

WINGFIELD, J.C. (1984b) Environmental and endocrine control of reproduction in the song sparrow, *Melospiza melodia*. II. Agonistic interactions as environmental information stimulating secretion of testosterone. Gen. Comp. Endocrinol. *56*:417–424.

WINGFIELD, J.C. (1985a) Environmental and endocrine control of territorial behavior in birds. In *The Endocrine System and the Environment*. B.K. Follett, S. Ishii, and A. Chandola, eds., pp. 265–277, Japanese Scientific Societies Press, Tokyo, and Springer-Verlag, Berlin.

WINGFIELD, J.C. (1985b) Short-term changes in plasma levels of hormones during establishment and defense of a breeding territory in male song sparrows, *Melospiza melodia*. Horm. Behav. *19*:174–187.

WINGFIELD, J.C. (1985c) Influences of weather on reproductive function in male song sparrows, *Melospiza melodia*. J. Zool. (London) *205*:525–544.

WINGFIELD, J.C., and D.S. FARNER (1976) Avian endocrinology—field investigations and methods. Condor *78*:570–573.

WINGFIELD, J.C., and D.S. FARNER (1979) Some endocrine correlates of renesting after loss of clutch or brood in the white-crowned sparrow, *Zonotrichia leucophrys gambelii*. Gen. Comp. Endocrinol. *38*:322–331.

WINGFIELD, J.C., and D.S. FARNER (1980) Control of seasonal reproduction in temperate-zone birds. Prog. Reprod. Biol. *5*:62–101.

WINGFIELD, J.C., and M. RAMENOFSKY (1985) Testosterone and aggressive behavior during the reproductive cycle of male birds. In *Neurobiology*. R. Gilles and J. Balthazart, eds., pp. 92–104, Springer-Verlag, Berlin.

YOKOYAMA, K., A. OKSCHE, T.R. DARDEN, and D.S. FARNER (1978) The sites of encephalic photoreception in photoperiodic induction of the growth of testes in the white-crowned sparrow, *Zonotrichia leucophrys gambelii*. Cell Tiss. Res. *189*:441–467.

SEVEN
A Functional Approach to the Behavioral Endocrinology of Rodents

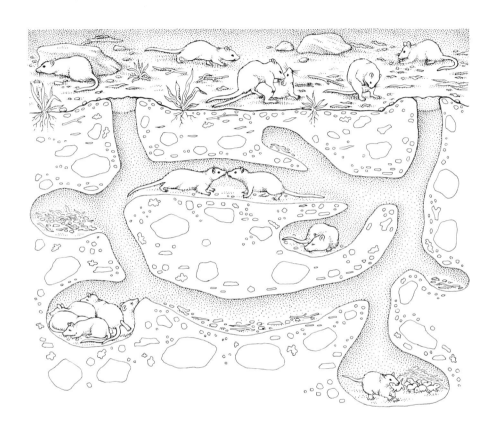

Martha K. McClintock
Department of Behavioral Sciences
The University of Chicago

Traditionally, behavioral endocrinology has focused on the study of stereo-typed behaviors in simple artificial environments. This has proved to be a powerful strategy, because it (1) greatly simplifies the task of measuring behavior and (2) creates a stable dependent variable that can be used to quantify the effects of an endocrine manipulation. In this way, many endocrine mechanisms of behavior have been effectively analyzed. In the past six years of the journal *Hormones and Behavior*, over 90 percent of the articles have taken this approach. Thus we know a great deal about the role of hormones, neurotransmitters, and cell nuclear receptors in the regulation of such reproductive behaviors as the lordosis reflex, copulation, and nursing (Adler, 1981; Pfaff, 1980).

However, the simplicity of traditional testing environments ignores the evolutionary function of behavior. Behavior evolved as a means for moving about a complex environment to ensure successful reproduction and sur-vival. It is the interface between an animal's external physical and social environment and its internal physiological state that permits an animal to select and even alter microhabitats to serve this function. Therefore, knowledge of the natural consequences and evolutionary function of behav-ior provide essential information and guidance in the analysis of the relationship between behavior and physiology. Such information may not be obtainable in an environment that is simplified artificially and lacks essential features of the animal's natural environment.

An appreciation of the function of behavior in a natural environment has affected behavioral endocrinology in two ways. First, it has increased interest in the reciprocal nature of the interaction between behavior and physiology. Not only do hormonal events produce both a fertile state and reproductive behavior, but hormonal events are, in turn, modulated by changes in behavior and the environment. This reciprocal interaction doubly ensures coordination of fertility with a social and physical environment that can support successful reproduction.

Second, there has been increased use of techniques developed by ethologists for studying behavior in complex environments. Traditional testing environments have been designed to artificially restrict the range of behaviors to the simple behaviors that are the focus of a particular study. However, a functional approach permits an animal to regulate its own behavior in a complex environment in coordination with its hormonal state. Ethological techniques permit identification of stable patterns in complex streams of behavior. These stable patterns reflect the natural consequences of behavior and can be used in a functional analysis of its hormonal mechanisms.

The purpose of this chapter is therefore twofold. The first is to describe ways in which behavior regulates physiology by examining the social regulation of fertility and mating behavior. This provides an understanding of the different pathways by which information is transduced from the social and physical into neuroendocrine events. The second purpose is to demonstrate the use of behavioral units of analysis that are based on functional consequences of behavior in a complex environment. These functional units of analysis are powerful tools which elucidate the lawful and reciprocal relationship among behavior, the environment, and physiology.

DIVERSITY IN THE SOCIAL REGULATION OF FERTILITY

These goals can be illustrated by considering the relationship between sociality and fertility in different species of small mammals. Among rodents, social behavior plays a variety of roles in the regulation of female fertility, ranging from complete determination to minor modulation of endogenous neuroendocrine mechanisms (see Chapter 8 for a discussion of the environmental and social regulation of male fertility).

Determination

Naked mole rats of East Africa (*Heterocephalus glaber*) represent one extreme of this continuum. This colonial species has a mating system that resembles the eusocial insects (Jarvis, 1981, and personal communication). Only one female in the group breeds, even in colonies with over 250 members, and the other females in the colony have immature ovaries with only primordial and primary follicles. Because female naked mole rats in established colonies become fertile and breed only if they occupy a unique social position, they are an excellent example of a species in which the capacity to become fertile and breed is determined by social organization (see Chapters 1 and 2 for similar examples in fish).

Naked mole rats live entirely underground, subsisting on roots, bulbs, and tubers. Their burrow system is complex and can have as many as 3 kilometers of foraging tunnels. The burrow also contains communal toilet areas, where colony members both defecate and urinate, and a communal nest site, where colony members sleep piled on each other (see Figure 7.1). The breeding female is the largest female, almost double the others in weight, with fully developed ovaries, a perforate vagina, and prominent teats. None of the other females reproduce; they are in castes which forage, repair tunnels, protect the colony, and care for the young. All are reproductively quiescent, suppressed by some social signal from the breeding female. Similarly, only a few of the males mate with the breeding female; the rest are workers or sentinels.

Pheromones in the breeding female's urine or feces are one likely source of female social suppression, particularly because all colony mem-

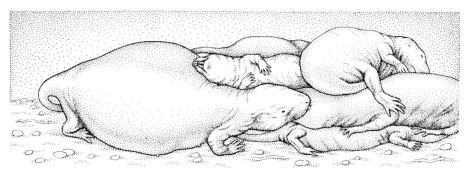

Figure 7.1. The breeding female of a laboratory colony of naked mole rats (*Heterocephalus glaber*). (Drawing from photographs by J.U.M. Jarvis)

bers contact the pheromones while using the common toilet area. They also sleep in a communal nest, piled on top of each other along with the breeding female. In addition, the breeding female patrols the burrow system and frequently passes other colony females. Dominance interactions may occur during passing, reinforcing reproductive suppression of the nonbreeding females.

If the breeding female is removed or prevented from interacting with the other females, the reproductive system of only one of the reproductively quiescent females matures. Within several weeks, this female is reproductively active and becomes the breeding female. She is always one from the worker caste that digs and forages, rather than the larger caretaking and sentinel caste. She is also a female that works only infrequently and is already growing rapidly. Thus there are additional social and endogenous factors that determine which individual replaces the breeding female.

Induction

In female prairie voles (*Microtus ochrogaster*), the reproductive system of all of the females develops and is maintained in a more fully developed state than does that of the naked mole rat. Nonetheless, fertility does occur spontaneously in the prairie vole; social interactions with a male are necessary for stimulating final maturation of the reproductive system, inducing mating behavior and triggering ovulation.

Young female prairie voles that remain in their natal nest are reproductively suppressed by social signals from their mother (Carter and Getz, 1985), although their ovaries do develop secondary follicles. Young females become fertile only when they emigrate, when their mother dies, or when strange males enter their nest area. After only brief (1 hour) direct contact with a male, particularly with pheromones in his urine, the female's uterus doubles in weight within 48 hours (Figure 7.2). If physical contact with the male continues, she comes into heat and mates within six days. Only then, in response to the stimulation of mating, does she ovulate (Carter and Getz, 1985).

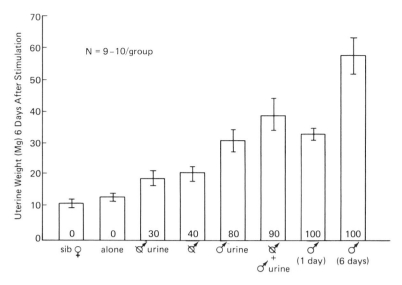

Figure 7.2. Uterine weights of female prairie voles (*Microtus ochrogaster*) exposed to various stimuli and autopsied 6 days after the onset of treatment. Numbers shown within bars indicate the percentage of females with uterine weights greater than 20 mg. (Carter et al., 1980)

At low population densities, the male and female remain together after mating and are monogamous as long as both are alive. They share a home nest and attack intruders of either sex, defending their territory and offspring. The daughters that remain in the natal nest do not come into heat, even though urine from the father or their brothers is capable of triggering their reproductive maturity. They remain reproductively suppressed, and incest is avoided. This is because young females in established families do not sniff or anogenitally groom their brothers or fathers. They only sniff and anogenitally groom strange males or males from whom they have been separated for at least one to two weeks. They thereby behaviorally avoid reproductive activation. In addition, even if daughters do become reproductively activated, their mothers directly suppress their mating behavior. Daughters that have been activated artificially by direct applications of male urine on the nose do not mate with family members provided that they continue to live with their mothers.

Thus, in the prairie vole, both the social environment and individual behavior regulate fertility. However, the mating system is more facultative than obligatory. For example, at high population densities, fewer females are found living in monogamous pairs, and females can be found living in multifemale groups. Furthermore, particular social behaviors are not prerequisites for the basic development of the reproductive system as they are in the naked mole rat. They only trigger or induce the final maturation of a partially developed reproductive system, including uterine growth, mating behavior, and ovulation.

Modulation

Female Norway rats (*Rattus norvegicus*) spontaneously come into heat and ovulate, whether they live alone or in social groups with other females and males. Under laboratory conditions, where food is plentiful and the environment is optimal for reproduction, rats come into heat and ovulate every four to six days in a pattern termed the estrous cycle. Although the rat's estrous cycle is primarily controlled endogenously by the neuroendocrine system, social signals can alter its length, thereby modulating the timing of fertility. For example, when females live together, cycles change in length until estrus is synchronized within the social group; as a consequence, females tend to come into heat and ovulate on the same day (McClintock, 1983a). When the females are separated and live alone, estrous synchrony is no longer maintained (Figure 7.3).

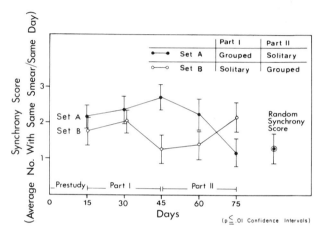

Figure 7.3. Estrous synchrony among female Norway rats (*Rattus norvegicus*) is significantly greater when they live in groups than when they live alone. (McClintock, 1978)

Estrous synchrony develops among females that simply share a recirculated air supply, indicating that the timing of fertility in the rat can be modulated by airborne chemosignals or pheromones. (See Chapter 2 for pheromones in aquatic environments.) The synchrony is achieved by the coordinated action of at least two different pheromones which have opposing effects on the timing of estrus: one that shortens the cycle and enhances the probability of coming into estrus and ovulating and another that lengthens the cycle and suppresses estrus and ovulation (Figure 7.4).

Given that females in the wild are likely to spend time in a birth cycle of pregnancy, delivery, and lactation (Davis and Hall, 1951; McClintock, 1981a), it is noteworthy that pheromones from females undergoing a birth cycle also affect the timing of fertility. Pheromones from pregnant rats shorten and regularize the estrous cycle, increasing the probability of ovulation. Pheromones from lactating rats and their pups have the opposite

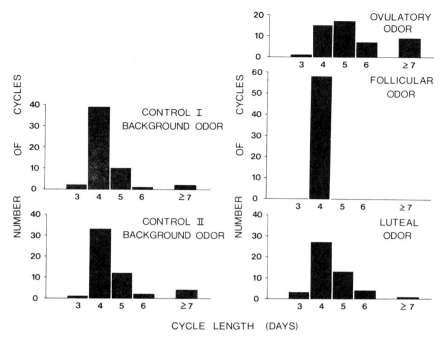

Figure 7.4. Odors from female Norway rats (*Rattus norvegicus*) at various phases of the estrous cycle have opposing effects on the estrous cycle length of other females exposed to these odors. (McClintock, 1983b)

effect; they lengthen the estrous cycle, increase its variability, and reduce the probability of ovulation (McClintock, 1983b). Thus the effects of birth and estrous cycle pheromones are similar: preovulatory and pregnancy odors enhance fertility, while ovulatory and lactation odors suppress fertility.

However, the female rat does not have spontaneous estrous cycles in all physical environments. Females become acyclic and stop ovulating spontaneously if they live in an environment without circadian cues (e.g., with constant illumination). Females also become acyclic if they have insufficient food and they become underweight. Under these conditions, the rat is similar to the prairie vole; contact with a male triggers estrus and ovulation (Cooper and Hayes, 1967; Johns et al., 1978). Furthermore, direct nasal contact with the male's urine is the most effective stimulus for inducing ovulation, suggesting that the rat may have a vomeronasal system which mediates the induction of ovulation by social interactions with a male. This same system also operates, although in an attenuated form, when conditions do permit spontaneous estrous cycles; a female housed in a colony room with males is more likely to have shorter estrous cycles than a female housed only with females (Aron, 1979).

Thus, the mechanisms of regulating fertility in the rat are facultative. In some environments, the rat ovulates spontaneously, and social behavior only modulates the timing of fertility. In other environments, social stimuli are prerequisite for inducing ovulation and estrus.

Fine Tuning

The golden or Syrian hamster (*Mesocricetus auratus*) represents the other end of the continuum. Females ovulate spontaneously, and their estrous cycles are precisely four days long with minimal variation. The striking regularity of the hamster's cycle depends not only on endogenous ovarian mechanisms, but on the integrity of endogenous circadian mechanisms as well. The ovarian cycle in this species is a quadruple multiple of the circadian cycle. For example, when the circadian cycle is lengthened artificially, either by living in constant dim illumination without periodic cues or by consuming deuterium oxide (heavy water), the estrous cycle is also lengthened to a period that is four times that of the circadian cycle (Fitzgerald and Zucker, 1976). Furthermore, the estrous cycle is disrupted by lesioning the suprachiasmatic nucleus of the hypothalamus, an area which is necessary for normal circadian rhythmicity (Rusak and Groos, 1982).

Nonetheless, even these very stable cycles can be mutually entrained by social interactions among females, creating estrous synchrony within the social group (Handelmann et al., 1980). The subordinate female has a few irregular cycles until synchrony is established, while the dominant female continues unperturbed with regular 4-day cycles. Thus, synchrony in the golden hamster represents only slight modulations of a very stable rhythm which is primarily regulated by endogenous mechanisms linked to photoperiod. This particular balance of endogenous, environmental, and social regulation could function well in the environment in which the golden hamster evolved. Presumably, they live underground in the desert and are a solitary species (Murphy, 1971). Therefore, they are likely to live with other females only in family groups when young. More importantly, their fertility and mating behavior must be precisely timed with nocturnal burrow emergence in order to be coordinated with finding a mate (Lisk et al., 1983).

TRANSDUCTION PATHWAYS

In order for social behavior to regulate fertility, social interactions must be transduced into physiological information that can affect neuroendocrine mechanisms of reproduction. The specific sequence of social interactions and neuroendocrine responses that mediate the aforementioned phenomena illustrates the variety of pathways by which social behavior is transduced into physiological information. This information in turn affects the final maturation of the reproductive system, induces ovulation, and stimulates mating behavior. These transduction pathways are essential to the reciprocal interactions integrating behavior, the environment, and physiology.

Social dominance may mediate both reproductive suppression and synchrony within a group. In the naked mole rat, the breeding female is socially dominant. Other females in the colony are suppressed even in odor-free colonies, suggesting that behavioral interactions with the dominant female may contribute to their reproductive suppression (J.U.M. Jarvis and R. Brett, personal communication). In the prairie vole, when two unrelated estrous females mate in a group with a male, only one bears a litter, while reproduction in the other is suppressed. This suppression is due to the agonistic and stressful interactions between the females. However, if the two females are familiar with each other, agonistic encounters are less frequent and both are likely to reproduce successfully (Carter et al., 1986). In the golden hamster, the estrous cycles of pairs of females become synchronized. The socially dominant female maintains regular ovarian cycles, while the socially subordinate female has variable cycles which entrain to those of her dominant partner (Handelmann et al., 1980).

The endocrine responses to social subordination may be the pathway by which dominance regulates the neuroendocrine mechanisms of reproductive suppression and synchrony. For example, when groups of wild house mice (*Mus musculus*) live in a seminatural environment, subordinate females are less likely to mate and become pregnant than dominant females (Franks and Lenington, 1986). When the males of this species fight, the pituitary-adrenal function of the loser, not the winner, is markedly altered; gonadal function is also altered in the loser and not the winner (Leshner, 1978). The resultant hormonal changes affect their future aggressive and submissive behavior (Roche and Leshner, 1979). If females have a similar endocrine response to the experience of defeat and subordination, this transduction pathway could affect the hormonal mechanisms of ovulation and pregnancy, thereby mediating the observed reproductive suppression. Similarly, dominance may mediate ovarian synchrony within a group (McClintock, 1983a).

The social environment can also affect fertility by a more direct pathway. Pheromones from a conspecific group member can trigger a specific neuroendocrine response, mediated by the primary or accessory olfactory system (Vandenbergh, 1983). Pheromones regulate fertility at different points of the reproductive lifespan in a wide variety of species, including reproductive maturation in naked mole rats, puberty in mice, induction or synchronization of estrus in adult rats, voles and hopping mice, and even such pathological conditions as constant estrus in rats (J.U.M. Jarvis, personal communication; Bronson and MacMillan, 1983; Carter et al., 1986; McClintock, 1983a; and Vandenbergh, 1983).

In prairie voles, a single drop of male urine can trigger the release of luteinizing hormone-releasing hormone (LHRH) and norepinephrine in olfactory bulb tissue (Dluzen et al., 1981). This response to the pheromone is very specific. LHRH and norepinephrine change only in the posterior and not the anterior portion of the olfactory bulb; furthermore the dopamine system is unaffected (Figure 7.5). These neuroendocrine events result in a dramatic rise in circulating luteinizing hormone (LH) (Ramirez et al., 1984).

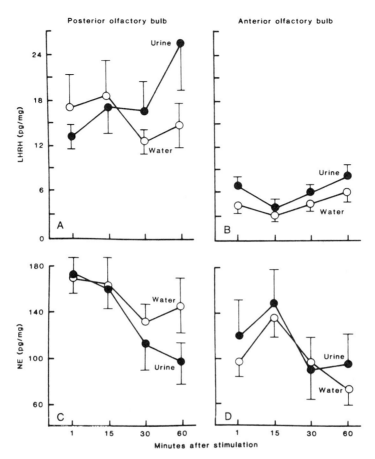

Figure 7.5. Mean concentrations of LHRH and NE in posterior and anterior olfactory bulb extracts from female prairie voles (*Microtus ochrogaster*). Animals were exposed to either male urine or to water and autopsied at 1, 15, 30, or 60 minutes after exposure. (Dluzen et al., 1981)

The surges in the circulating concentrations of LH are an endocrine stimulus for increased estrogen production by the ovary. When female prairie voles have prolonged exposure to male urine (e.g., 75 minutes), circulating concentrations of estrogen in the plasma rise; 18 hours later, there is a significant increase in estrogen binding by nuclei of uterine and pituitary cells and an increase in uterine weight. Although the short exposure to males is not sufficient to bring females into heat, it does increase estrogen binding in the cell nuclei of the brain as well, a response which may mediate the activation of female sexual behavior when exposure is prolonged even more (Carter et al., 1986).

The pathway by which male pheromones trigger the LH surge may include neuroendocrine stimulation of the hypothalamus, which is known to regulate pituitary LH release via the hypothalamic-pituitary portal system (see Chapters 2 and 11). It is also possible that the pathway includes olfactory neurons that project directly to the portal system and affect the pituitary directly without hypothalamic mediation. If so, this pheromonal system would demonstrate both a multiplicity of levels of neuroendocrine regulation and a diversity of transduction pathways by which social stimuli influence reproduction.

Most rodents live in a seasonal or periodically fluctuating physical environment and therefore benefit by modulating their fertility in response to these fluctuations. Light and temperature are probably the best-studied environmental cues. The golden hamster evolved in the desert where food is limited to specific seasons. Males are likely to be solitary, rarely living with other males and only briefly with females during mating. The male hamster's testicular function is exquisitely sensitive to daylength (photoperiod). In the short days of winter (less than 11 hours of light per day), the testes shrink dramatically and spermatogenesis ceases altogether (Reiter, 1973).

In contrast, photoperiod does not have a strong effect on testicular function of intact male Norway rats. Rats are a species that often breeds in groups (Calhoun,1962; Telle, 1966), and the olfactory bulbs mediate the olfactory social cues that affect their mating behavior (McClintock, 1984). However, if the olfactory bulbs are removed, a responsiveness to photoperiod is unmasked. Males who have had their olfactory bulbs removed and are exposed to only 8 hours of light per 24-hour day experience a drop in testicular weight, atrophy of the seminal vesicles, decrease in plasma testosterone, and difficulty in ejaculating during mating (Nelson and Zucker, 1981). This demonstrates that the rat has a pathway for transducing photoperiodic information into a form that affects reproductive function in addition to a pathway for transducing social information. Thus, even within a single species, there are multiple pathways which transduce both environmental and social information. The relative importance of each pathway appears to depend on the particular environment in which the species evolved.

VERIFICATION IN THE NATURAL ENVIRONMENT

These examples illustrate the central role in both the present and evolutionary time-frames of the physical and social environment in the regulation of physiological mechanisms of behavior. An essential step in establishing the generality of these and any laboratory results is verification that the same relationship between behavior and the neuroendocrine system exists under natural or seminatural conditions.

It had been well established in the laboratory that urine from adult female house mice would delay puberty of immature females (Vandenbergh, 1983). Furthermore, it had been established that adult females had to have intact adrenals in order to produce the pheromone (Drickamer and McIntosh, 1980). Nonetheless, it was still possible that this pheromonal effect might be an epiphenomenon, manifest only in a laboratory environment (Bronson, 1979; McClintock, 1981a).

The house mouse (*Mus musculus*) lives and breeds in a wide variety of environments, demonstrating remarkable reproductive adaptability (Bronson, 1979). Furthermore, there is enormous variability in the social organization of mouse populations. Nonetheless, when food supply is plentiful and stable and the physical environment is moderately complex, house mice live in groups containing a single breeding male, several breeding females, their offspring, as well as a few subordinate and presumably nonbreeding males. The breeding male, and occasionally pregnant females, defend this territory against intruders. Female offspring often emigrate as they approach maturity, traveling long distances away from their natal nest. While still in the natal nest, their reproductive system is suppressed, presumably by the presence of their mothers and sisters. Thus, they are not inseminated by the males in the territory and do not incur the additional metabolic demands of pregnancy during their emigration. Female reproductive suppression becomes even more crucial when the opportunity for emigration is limited, as it is on an island. The population can increase, outstripping food resources if there is no mechanism for population regulation.

Massey and Vandenbergh (1980) conducted an elegant test of the role of pheromonal communication in natural populations of mice. Taking advantage of the natural island created by the cloverleaf of a highway interchange, they established that pheromonal regulation of puberty is dependent on the population density of the island. They studied two feral highway island populations through seasonal cycles of high and low density. Female urine collected during high population density was effective in delaying puberty of subadult females; urine collected when the population density was low did delay puberty (Table 7.1).

TABLE 7.1. Age in days (mean ± standard error) at first estrus of juvenile female laboratory mice exposed to the urine of wild female house mice (Massey and Vandenbergh 1980)

		Living conditions of urine donor females			
		Natural populations			
	Laboratory Population (N = 4 per cage)	Low density (spring)		High density (winter)	
Treatment		Population 1	Population 2	Population 1	Population 2
Female urine	45.4 ± 1.4 (N = 20)	39.7 ± 1.2 (N = 19)	41.4 ± 1.3 (N = 20)	39.9 ± 1.5 (N = 19)	46.8 ± 1.7 (N = 20)
Control	38.7 ± 1.1 (N = 19)	39.2 ± 1.5 (N = 20)	39.9 ± 1.5 (N = 20)	38.1 ± 1.2 (N = 19)	39.2 ± 1.6 (N = 20)
	P < .05*				P < .05*

*Mann-Whitney U test

A later study demonstrated that female puberty-delaying pheromones could be induced in adult feral females by large acute increases in population density (Coppola and Vandenbergh, 1986). This was done experimentally in the field by introducing over 40 interlopers to the highway islands and collecting urine from the same resident females before and after the density increase. Both adrenal size and gonadal function were affected by population density. Therefore, the adrenal may be essential for transducing information about population density into an endocrine form that can regulate phero-mone production. In any event, the density-dependent nature of the puberty-suppressing pheromone indicates that it may be one of the ways that an individual can coordinate its fertility with the availability of resources in a natural population, resulting in population regulation.

THE PHYSICAL ENVIRONMENT AND BEHAVIOR

Behavior that can be measured reliably in an artificial testing environment of a laboratory may not even occur in the environment in which the species evolved. Even behaviors that are robust, i.e., that can be measured with a variety of different measurement techniques (von Békésy, 1961), may be epiphenomena and not serve the function of coordinating the animal's physiological state and natural environment.

Traditionally, studies of the neuroendocrine mechanisms of rodent behavior have used environments which limit behavior to the simple motor pattern being studied. For example, when an investigator wishes to study the neuroendocrine mechanisms of mating in the Norway rat, a stud male and a hormone-primed female are taken from different parts of the laboratory colony and put together into a small glass enclosure. Often the testing arena is no more than a 1–2 foot square devoid of anything but sawdust. This environment ensures that mating behavior is stable and predictable and that the animal is not distracted by other activities. Mating behavior can be easily quantified, while the endocrine and nervous systems can be manipulated using increasingly sophisticated techniques.

Nonetheless, under these conditions, the animal is deprived of the environment that normally controls its behavior. Thus, the behavioral aspect of the traditional protocol is essentially a deprivation paradigm. Results from any deprivation experiment need to be interpreted with caution, because deprivation can distort the system under study so much that valid general-izations to normal function are precluded (Gregory, 1968). That is, the behavior that occurs in artificial environments is not necessarily behavior that was selected to coordinate physiology with the normal social and physical environment.

An alternative research strategy focuses on the functions of behavior in a complex environment and defines behavior in terms of its functional consequences, not just specific motor patterns. By studying the animal in a complex physical and social environment, the experimenter reduces the constraints imposed on behavior. Thus, it is the animal, not the experimenter, that selects the features of the environment with which the animal interacts. This often requires that the experimenter give up a great deal of direct control over the behavior being studied. However, if the testing environment contains some features of the animal's natural environment, its behavior will be functionally organized, generating stable and quantifiable units of analysis which reflect a predictable relationship between behavior and physiology (McClintock, 1981b).

In the small barren arenas traditionally used to study rat mating behavior, copulation is initiated by the male; his approaches and chases are striking and predictable. However, when rats mate in a large seminatural environment with the large open areas, burrows, and runways typical of the natural environment, it is the female that often initiates copulation.

The female paces the timing of copulation by soliciting the male (McClintock, 1984). After approaching the male, the female may nose or sniff him and groom his head or anogenital area. This is termed the orientation component of the solicitation or coupling (Hedricks and McClintock, 1985). She then abruptly orients away from the male and runs away, sometimes with a dart-hopping gait. The male follows, chasing the female until he mounts and has an intromission. The pair then separate and come together again. There is a series of intromissions that finally culminates with the male's ejaculation and a period of post-ejaculatory quiescence. When the pair is familiar with each other, most intromissions are preceded by a female solicitation, and, if the male is receptive, most solicitations result in copulation.

Females can modify the basic form of solicitation in a large variety of ways which accommodate their particular situation (Hedricks and McClintock, 1985; McClintock, 1984). For example, if a female is already within a body length of the male and oriented away from him, she may simply glance over her shoulder at the male, substituting this behavior, which is called a touch back, for the approach and orientation, before running away (Figure 7.6). All three components of the solicitation (approach, orientation, and runaway) are not necessary for eliciting a mount and intromission from the male; partial solicitations can be equally effective. Therefore, the solicitation cannot be considered a fixed action pattern.

Although the components of female solicitation were noted previously during mating in small cages (e.g., approaches and the dart-hop gait), they were not recognized as an integrated behavior with functional consequences. This is undoubtedly because the small testing arena keeps the female within one or two body lengths of the male and traps her in the orientation component of her solicitation. From the male's perspective, it probably appears that she is constantly soliciting him. The traditional testing environment thereby minimizes the female's contribution to the pace of mating, the male's behavior becomes the dominant factor in determining when copulation occurs, and it is impossible to observe the natural consequences and function of female solicitation.

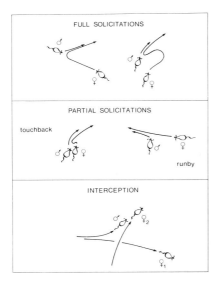

Figure 7.6. Examples of the variety of solicitations made by female Norway rats (*Rattus norvegicus*) during mating. (McClintock, 1984)

The testing environment can also have a dramatic influence on the neuroendocrine consequences of mating. Female rats need stimulation from the male's intromissions to trigger progesterone production, a prerequisite for successful implantation of the developing blastocysts (Adler, 1969). The female's neuroendocrine system is exquisitely sensitive to the timing of intromissions, with an optimal interval and number for triggering the progestational state. Because the optimal pattern is specific to each species of rodent, it has been termed "the vaginal code" (Diamond, 1970). Despite having such a code, rats are highly adaptable; they can mate in small cages in a suboptimal pattern which eventually triggers a progestational state. However, this mating pattern is not necessarily the most efficient one; indeed, the frequency of intromissions observed in traditional testing arenas are more rapid than the physiological optimum. If mating takes place in a large seminatural environment that permits female solicitation, and hence a slower mating pace, intromissions are paced in a pattern which is closer to the physiological optimum (McClintock, 1984).

In seminatural environments, a female may also alter the pace of solicitation and mating in response to a change in her neuroendocrine system. For example, female rats can mate immediately after delivering a litter; this is called a postpartum estrus. Because the preceding pregnancy alters the parturient female's endocrine system, the stimulus requirements for inducing a progestational state are different during a postpartum estrus than those found during estrous cycles. The rate of mating in postpartum females is increased substantially, presumably in response to her altered hormonal state, and perhaps in response to an altered "vaginal code" (Hedricks and McClintock, 1985).

Females can even pace mating within a small space if the environment gives her a way to control interactions with the male. For example, if the test cage has a lever which raises a partition and frees the male or her own compartment which lets her escape from him, the female can slow the pace of copulation. This results in the female requiring significantly fewer intromissions to trigger the progestational state than are required in a traditional testing environment (Gilman et al., 1979). Furthermore, the female terminates the mating session sooner than she does when she does not have the opportunity to pace copulation, presumably because mating is more effective in fulfilling her stimulus requirements (Figure 7.7) (Erskine, 1985).

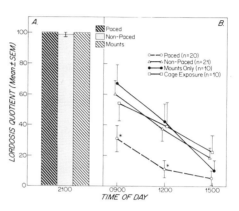

Figure 7.7. Termination of sexual receptivity of female Norway rats (*Rattus norvegicus*) in natural estrus following the indicated types of mating stimulation (* = p ≤ .05). Sexual receptivity was measured by the lordosis quotient (no. of lordosis responses / no. of male mounts during mating; Erskine, 1985)

These experiments demonstrate that female solicitation is an integral part of mating in the Norway rat and that the neuroendocrine consequences of mating are markedly different when the environment gives females the opportunity to pace copulation. The observation that female pacing has similar neuroendocrine consequences in a diversity of environments emphasizes that the form or motor pattern of solicitation is not the functional aspect of the behavior. Any behavior that allows the female to pace copulation, whether by soliciting, running into an escape compartment, or pressing a lever, has a similar relationship to the neuroendocrine system. Therefore, the motor pattern is not the most powerful unit of analysis for studying female sexual behavior. Instead, the most appropriate unit must include pacing, which is the functional aspect of solicitation.

Unfortunately, little is known about the neuroendocrine mechanisms of solicitation in the female rat. Most investigators have studied only one of the simplest and most reflexive components of the behavior, the dart-hop gait, the unique darting and hopping movements which the female rat uses to move away from the male. While it is true that dart-hopping can be part of a solicitation, it is not necessary. It is primarily a gait and most probably integrated on a spinal or subcortical level, whereas the pacing and diversity which are the essential functional characteristics of solicitation undoubtedly have more encephalized controls (McClintock, 1984).

As the testing environment approximates the natural environment, the relationship between behavior and neuroendocrine function becomes more regular or stable (McClintock, 1981b). This same principle holds for many species. When rhesus monkeys mate in a small cage, copulation does not vary with the hormonal fluctuations of the female's menstrual cycle and often occurs when the female is not fertile. However, in a larger compound which provides space for social interactions, the female solicits the male and affects the frequency of ejaculation (see Chapter 6). Furthermore, her solicitations and her attractiveness do vary during her menstrual cycle, as measured by the amount of time that she spends sitting close to the male with her back towards him and the frequency with which she is approached (Wallen, 1982). Solicitations, female attractiveness, and copulation are most likely in the preovulatory or follicular phase of the cycle. These behaviors show a marked decline in the postovulatory or luteal phase (Figure 7.8). Consequently, mating in a large environment that permits female solicitation is better coordinated with the time of maximum fertility than mating in the confines of a small laboratory cage.

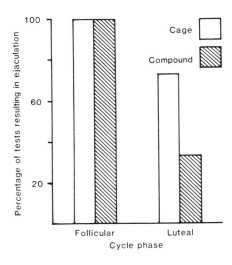

Figure 7.8. Percentage of tests resulting in ejaculation for 15 pairings of three male and five female rhesus monkeys (*Macaca mulatta*) tested in two types of environments during the follicular and luteal phases of the female's ovarian cycle. (Wallen, 1982)

This study parallels some aspects of human sexual behavior. In contrast with rodents, sexual activity can occur throughout a woman's menstrual cycle, and the frequency with which couples have sexual intercourse is not affected significantly by the menstrual cycle (Spitz et al., 1975). However, female initiation of intercourse has been reported to increase at the time of ovulation (Adams et al., 1978). This pattern is not robust. That is, many other aspects of libido do not rise around ovulation, such as arousal by erotic films (Morrell et al., 1984). Furthermore, the pattern has not been detected by all investigators (Persky et al., 1978). Nonetheless, it is found in lesbian couples, where fear of conception does not confound female sexual initiation (Matteo and Rissman, 1984).

Traditional experimental designs have artificially simplified the social as well as the physical environment. Typically, when a male Norway rat is paired with a single female in heat, copulation is rapid and continues until both individuals are sexually exhausted. However, domestic Norway rats do not necessarily mate in pairs (McClintock, 1984). Many strains have been selected for an ability to produce a large number of offspring when they mate in groups with sex ratios ranging from 1:5 to 4:15. And, although wild rats have been found living alone or in pairs, it is more common to find them living in large burrows, reproducing in groups ranging from 7 to 100 or more individuals (Robitaille and Bouvet, 1976; Telle, 1966). Furthermore, Calhoun (1962) observed that wild rats also produce substantially more litters when they live in multifemale groups than they do when living alone or in pairs. Thus, a group of males and females is one of the social environments in which the Norway rat's mating behavior and neuroendocrine system coevolved.

Rats mating in pairs fail to mate in the optimal pattern from the perspective of both the male and the female neuroendocrine systems. As indicated earlier, the female's progestational state is triggered readily if she has 10–15 minutes between intromissions. In contrast, the optimal interval for the male is significantly shorter; males ejaculate after the fewest intromissions and with a low cost as measured in time and effort, if there are 2–3 minutes between intromissions (McClintock, 1984). Nonetheless, when rats mate in traditional testing cages, they mate at 1-minute intervals, an interval that is neither the optimum for either sex nor a compromise between the two.

This paradox was resolved by observing rats mating in groups with several males and several females. In these groups, Norway rats change partners repeatedly during copulation and even before the male ejaculates for the first time. This type of mating is called a *panogamous* system; the animals are more than promiscuous, because they copulate with several partners within a single mating session (McClintock, 1984). Under some conditions, rats may also take turns mating. Males are likely to take turns mating after they have ejaculated, and females take turns mating after they receive intromissions. Thus, mating in groups with several males and females frees them from the constraints imposed by mating in pairs. Females and males do not have to mate with identical intervals between intromissions. By changing partners and taking turns, each sex can mate at a different pace, fulfilling the different requirements of their respective neuroendocrine systems (McClintock, 1984).

In panogamous mating systems, social behavior is an integral part of successful copulation and must be taken into account when analyzing its neuroendocrine mechanisms and consequences. For example, the sequence of behavior is not the same for the two sexes. From the male perspective, the ejaculatory series (i.e., multiple intromissions before ejaculation) is robust. It occurs in both pair and group mating and is an appropriate unit of analysis for studying the neuroendocrine mechanisms and function of male sexual behavior. However, when females mate in groups, they do not always receive intromissions and ejaculations together in an ejaculatory series, as they must when they mate with a single male in a pair. Instead, they may receive two ejaculations in a row before receiving any intromissions, or 20 intromissions before receiving an ejaculation (Figure 7.9). Therefore, from the female perspective, the ejaculatory series is not a robust unit of analysis and is inappropriate for studying the neuroendocrine mechanisms and consequences of her mating behavior.

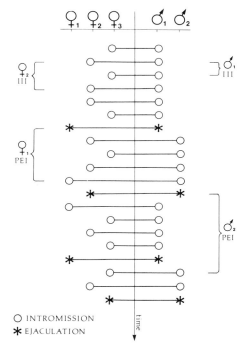

Figure 7.9. A schematic of the sequence of copulation by Norway rats (*Rattus norvegicus*) during mating in a group with a 2:3 sex ratio. The male and female sharing a copulatory event are connected by a horizontal line. To see the sequence of copulation from the perspective of one of the individuals, follow down that individual's column. The time line indicates only the order of events, not the actual intervals between them. (McClintock, 1984)

These same principles are also illustrated by reproductive behavior of rhesus monkeys. When they mate in pairs, there is no clear peak in her sexual behavior at the time of ovulation, although it is lower in the luteal phase. However, when rhesus monkeys mate in a group with one male and several females, there is a dramatic ovulatory peak in female-initiated behavior (Figure 7.10) (Wallen and Winston, 1984). Ejaculation is also more likely to occur around ovulation when the female is most fertile. Therefore, the impact of the social environment on the coordination of mating behavior and hormonal state is as dramatic in rhesus monkeys as it is in Norway rats.

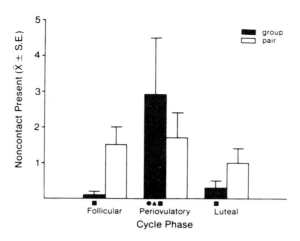

Figure 7.10. Mean frequency of solicitations (noncontact presents) by the female rhesus monkey (*Macaca mulatta*) during either group or pair tests and as a function of the phase of her ovarian cycle. (Wallen and Winston, 1984, reprinted by permission of Pergamon Press, Ltd.)

TEMPORAL FEATURES OF THE ENVIRONMENT AND BEHAVIOR

New aspects of the relationship between behavior and physiology are revealed when a testing protocol simulates temporal features of the natural environment. A female golden hamster that is not in heat fights intruders, defending her territory and food supply. As she comes into heat, she becomes less aggressive, marks her territory with attractive vaginal secretions, and adopts a tail-up posture that signals her willingness to mate (Lisk et al., 1983). In a seminatural environment, a female entices a male to enter her burrow, perhaps reducing competition from other females for a mating partner. After an hour of mating, however, the female becomes aggressive once again, ousts the male from her territory, and even takes his food supply for herself.

This relationship between the ovarian cycle and the female's social and mating behavior can only be observed if the female has had time to interact with her physical and social environment for a few hours before she comes into heat. Lisk and co-workers (1983) have estimated the amount of time that is both necessary and sufficient for the natural pattern of behavior to occur. If a female is introduced to the male after the onset of heat, without the opportunity for nonmating interactions, mating occurs wherever she first encounters the male; her mating behavior and conception are no longer coordinated with her own territory or food supply. However, if the female interacts with the male for as little as two hours before coming into heat, the normal functional pattern emerges. The pair mates in the female's territory and their behavior is indistinguishable from that of pairs that have lived together for over four days.

Time in a mating environment may also affect the mating behavior of female Norway rats. As stated before, when mating takes place in a seminatural environment permitting female solicitation, the pace of mating is slower, and males have fewer preejaculatory intromissions than they do during mating in a standard testing cage. This pattern is seen when a female has 3–4 days for adaptation to the male and the seminatural environment before she comes into heat. When a female has only 5 minutes to adapt to a large testing environment, the mating pattern is more similar to that of a small testing cage than that of a seminatural environment with comparable square footage (Figure 7.11) (Price, 1980).

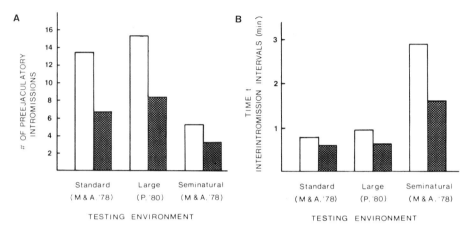

Figure 7.11. The effect of adaptation to a complex testing environment on the mating pattern of Norway rats (*Rattus norvegicus*). After 5 minutes of adaptation to a large but barren environment (Price, 1980), copulatory behavior is more similar to behavior in a small standard testing arena than it is when the animals have had 3 days to adapt to a seminatural environment. This effect is seen when domestic females mate with either a domestic male (open columns) or a wild male (filled columns). (McClintock, 1984)

NEUROENDOCRINE UNITS OF ANALYSIS

Behavioral disruption is not always the source of a mismatch between physiology and behavior; the laboratory environment may also distort the normal timing of the neuroendocrine system, while the temporal organization of behavior remains stable. For example, in the field, female yellow baboons (*Papio cynocephalus*) remain amenorrheic for a year after giving birth if their infants survive. Once they resume their menstrual cycles, it takes an average of four months for them to conceive. Thus, they usually experience almost a two-year interval between births of their infants (Altmann et al., 1978). The neuroendocrine mechanisms that temporarily suppress ovulation neatly coordinate the mother's fertility with the amount of time that it takes to successfully raise an infant baboon to independence. However, when female baboons reproduce in captivity, where resources are readily available, the length of their postpartum amenorrhea is cut in half, and the mother is physiologically capable of a second pregnancy within one year. Nevertheless, the amount of time that it takes to raise her infant to physical, emotional, and cognitive independence remains the same. Therefore, the laboratory environment disrupts the temporal coordination of neuroendocrine function and maternal behavior by altering the mother's neuroendocrine system and making her fertile when it is inappropriate, given the behavioral demands of her first infant.

The problem of functional units of analysis must also be addressed at the neuroendocrine level. Traditionally, hormone measurements in behavioral endocrinology have been limited to a single sample of hormone levels in plasma. Such studies can yield results which are highly variable and inconsistent, precluding identification of a lawful or stable relationship with behavior. Variability is more than a bothersome artifact. It is a functional aspect of the neuroendocrine system underlying functional consequences. This natural variability must be incorporated into the units of analysis used to measure neuroendocrine function.

There is growing evidence that the temporal pattern of hormone secretion may be a better predictor of its effects than is the absolute concentration in the blood. Luteinizing hormone-releasing hormone (LHRH) must be given in a pulsatile fashion mimicking the natural pattern of release to trigger luteinizing hormone (LH) release from the pituitary; sustained constant levels of LHRH desensitize the pituitary and will not stimulate LH production (Rabin and McNeil, 1980). Another requirement for the ovulatory LH surge is that estrogen must fluctuate in a temporal pattern characteristic of the ovarian cycle (Figure 7.12) (Fox and Smith, 1985). Estrogen is also more effective in increasing estrogen receptors in the brain and inducing behavioral receptivity in female rats if it is injected in a pulsatile pattern that more closely resembles the physiological release pattern (Clark and Roy, 1983). Many of these findings are species specific (Ramirez et al., 1984). Nonetheless, they demonstrate that the episodic pattern of hormone secretion must be quantified and used to study neuroendocrine mechanisms (Merriam and Wachter, 1982).

The external environment can modulate the temporal pattern of neuroendocrine function with dramatic consequences, particularly for the development of behavior. For example, the sexual behavior of male rats is demasculinized if their mothers are stressed during the first trimester of pregnancy; as adults, these animals have difficulty mating and ejaculating (Ward and Ward, 1985) (see Chapter 9). Development of normal adult male sexual behavior requires a rise in testosterone that organizes the brain in a male pattern on days 17–19 post conception, when the fetus is still *in utero*. The temporal pattern of fetal testicular function is disrupted when the mother is stressed, either behaviorally by physical restraint or physiologically by increased body temperature. The rise in testicular enzyme activity and plasma testosterone does not occur between days 17 and 19 as it normally does. Instead, levels are high both before and after this critical period. Thus, prenatal stress disrupts the normal ontogenetic pattern of

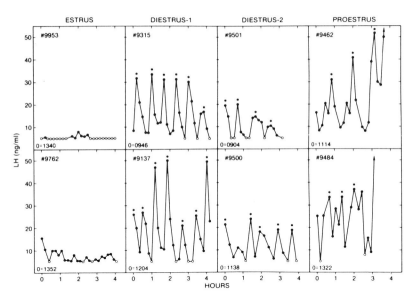

Figure 7.12. The temporal pattern of LH secretion during the 4-day estrous cycle of the Norway rat (*Rattus norvegicus*). The pattern is shown by two representative animals for each day of the cycle. The animal's number appears in the upper left-hand corner of each graph. (Fox and Smith, 1985)

hormone secretion, which organizes the brain in a male pattern, with long-term consequences for adult behavior.

The organizational effects of prenatal hormones can be modified by the postnatal environment. Males that are reared with a female from the time they are weaned are more likely to have normal sexual behavior as adults than are males raised in social isolation. In fact, the male's postnatal environment has a larger impact on his potential for normal adult male sexual behavior than does the amount of prenatal stress (Figure 7.13) (Ward and Reed, 1985).

CONCLUSION

Environments used in behavioral tests that omit features of the normal physical and social environment can distort behavior if these features are essential for the function of behavior. Although such environments may be useful for enhancing subtle species-typical behavior, they preclude an accurate description of functional organization of behavior and its neuroendocrine mechanisms. Similarly, experimental designs that severely restrict the time that animals have to interact with one another and their environment can also distort behavior, obscuring a regular relationship with its hormonal mechanisms. It is not just time per se that is important to the integration of behavior and neuroendocrine function, but the opportunity to interact with the social and physical environment in different endocrine states.

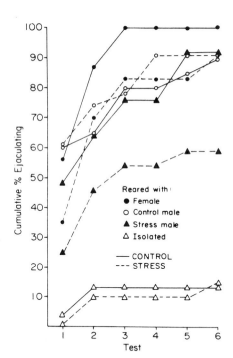

Figure 7.13. Cumulative percentage of adult male Norway rats (*Rattus norvegicus*) that can mate until they ejaculate. Prenatally stressed and control animals had been reared from 16 days of age onward with either a female, a control male, another prenatally stressed male, or in isolation. (Ward and Reed, 1985)

Behavior and neuroendocrine mechanisms evolved together in specific environments. This has several implications for the study of behavioral endocrinology. It highlights the reciprocal interaction between endocrinology and behavior. In the present time-frame, endocrine mechanisms are regulated both by the individual's behavior and by its social, physical, and biotic environment. In an evolutionary time-frame, endocrine mechanisms are selected as a consequence of an organism's behavioral interaction with its internal and external environments. This is a specific example of a way in which the function of a behavior or trait can shape its neuroendocrine mechanisms over the course of evolution (Mayr, 1958; Simon, 1969).

By focusing on behaviors that serve the same function under similar conditions, an appropriate basis for cross-species comparison of physiological mechanisms is established. Therefore, units of analysis based on function are essential for the comparative study of the interaction between behavior and physiology, and will enable meaningful comparisons across species.

> The central task of a natural science is to make the wonderful commonplace; to show that complexity, correctly viewed, is only a mask for simplicity; to find pattern hidden in apparent chaos. . . . [A]nd when we have explained the wonderful, unmasked the hidden pattern, a new wonder arises at how complexity was woven out of simplicity.
>
> H.A. Simon, *The Sciences of the Artificial*

ACKNOWLEDGMENTS

This work was supported by National Science Foundation Grant BNS 80 19496 and Biomedical Research Support Grant PHS 2SOR-07029-20.

REFERENCES

ADAMS, D.B., A.R. GOLD, and A.D. BURT (1978) Rise in female-initiated sexual activity at ovulation and its suppression by oral contraceptives. N. Engl. J. Med. *299*:1145–1150.

ADLER, N.T. (1969) Effects of the male's copulatory behavior on successful pregnancy of the female rat. J. Comp. Physiol. Psychol. *69*:613–622.

ADLER, N.T. (1981) *Neuroendocrinology of Reproduction*. Plenum Publishing Corporation, New York.

ALTMANN, J., S. ALTMANN, G. HAUSFATER, and S.A. MCCUSKY (1977) Life history of yellow baboons: Physical development, reproductive parameters, and infant mortality. Primates *18*:315–330.

ARON, C. (1979) Mechanisms of control of the reproductive function by olfactory stimuli in female mammals. Physiol. Rev. *59*:229–282.

BRONSON, F.H. (1979) The reproductive ecology of the house mouse. Q. Rev. Biol. *54*:265–299.

BRONSON, F.H., and B. MACMILLAN (1983) Hormonal response to primer pheromones. In *Pheromones and Reproduction in Mammals*. J.G. Vandenbergh, ed., pp. 175–199, Academic Press, New York.

CALHOUN, J.B. (1962) *The Ecology and Sociology of the Norway Rat*. U.S. Public Health Service Publication No. 1008, U.S. Government Printing Office, Washington, D.C.

CARTER, C.S., L.L. GETZ, L. GARISH, J.L. MCDERMOTT, and P. ARNOLD (1980) Male-related pheromones and the activation of female reproduction in the prairie vole (*Microtus ochrogaster*). Biol. Reprod. *23*:1038–1045.

CARTER, C.S., and L.L. GETZ (1985) Social and hormonal determinants of reproductive patterns in the prairie vole. In *Proceedings of the Invited Lectures of the First International Comparative Physiology and Biochemistry Conference, Hormones and Behavior Symposium*. R. Giles and J. Balthazart, eds., pp. 18–36, Springer-Verlag, Berlin.

CARTER, C.S., L.L. GETZ, and M. COHEN-PARSONS (1986) Relationships between social organization and behavioral endocrinology in a monogamous mammal. In *Advances in the Study of Behavior*, Vol. 16. J.S. Rosenblatt, C. Beer, M.-C. Bushnell, P.J.B. Slater, eds., pp. 109–145, Academic Press, New York.

CLARK, A.S., and E.J. ROY (1983) Behavioral and cellular responses to pulses of low doses of estradiol-17β. Physiol. Behav. *20*:561–565.

COOPER, K.J., and N.B. HAYES (1967) Modification of the estrous cycles of the underfed rat associated with the presence of the male. J. Reprod. Fertil. *14*:317–324.

COPPOLA, D.M., and J.G. VANDENBERGH (1986) Induction of a puberty regulating chemosignal in wild mice populations. J. Mammal. (in press).

Davis, D.E., and O. Hall (1951) The seasonal reproductive conditions of female Norway (Brown) rats in Baltimore, Maryland. Physiol. Zool. *24*:9–20.

Diamond, M. (1970) Intromission pattern and species vaginal code in relation to induction of pseudopregnancy. Science *169*:995–997.

Dluzen, D.E., V.D. Ramirez, C.S. Carter, and L.L. Getz (1981) Male vole urine changes luteinizing hormone-releasing hormone and norepinephrine in female olfactory bulb. Science *212*:573–575. Copyright 1981 by the AAAS.

Drickamer, L.C., and T.K. McIntosh (1980) Effects of adrenalectomy on the presence of a maturation-delaying pheromone in the urine of female mice. Horm. Behav. *14*:146–152.

Erskine, M.S. (1985) Effects of paced coital stimulation on estrus duration in intact cycling rats and ovariectomized-adrenalectomized hormone-primed rats. Behavioral Neuroscience *99*:151–191.

Fitzgerald, K.M., and I. Zucker (1976) Circadian organization of the estrous cycle of the golden hamster. Proc. Natl. Acad. Sci. USA *73*:2923–2927.

Fox, S.R., and M.S. Smith (1985) Changes in the pulsatile pattern of luteinizing hormone secretion during the rat estrous cycle. Endocrinology *116*:1485–1492.

Franks, P., and S. Lenington (1986) Dominance and reproductive behavior of wild house mice in a seminatural environment correlated with T locus genotype. Behav. Ecol. Sociobiol. *18*:395–404.

Gilman, D.P., L.F. Mercer, and J.C. Hitt (1979) Influences of female copulatory behavior on the induction of pseudopregnancy in the female rat. Physiol. Behav. *22*:675–678.

Gregory, R.L. (1968) Models and the localization of function in the central nervous system. In *Key Papers: Cybernetics*. C.R. Evans and A.D. Robertson, eds., pp. 90–102, Butterworth, London.

Handelmann, G., R. Ravizza, and W.J. Ray (1980) Social dominance determines estrous entrainment among female hamsters. Horm. Behav. *14*:107–115.

Hedricks, C., and M.K. McClintock (1985) The timing of mating by postpartum estrous rats. Z. Tierpsychol. *67*:1–16.

Jarvis, J.U.M. (1981) Eusociality in a mammal: Cooperative breeding in naked mole-rat colonies. Science *212*:571–573.

Johns, M.A., H.H. Feder, B.R. Komisaruk, and A.D. Mayer (1978) Urine-induced reflex ovulation in anovulatory rats may be a vomeronasal effect. Nature (London) *272*:446.

Leshner, A. (1978) *An Introduction to Behavioral Endocrinology*, pp. 78–113, Oxford University Press, New York.

Lisk, R.D., L.A. Ciaccio, and C. Catanzaro (1983) Mating behaviour of the golden hamster under seminatural conditions. Anim. Behav. *31*:659–666.

Massey, A., and J.G. Vandenbergh (1980) Puberty delay by a urinary cue from female house mice in feral populations. Science *209*:821–822.

Matteo, S., and E.F. Rissman (1984) Increased sexual activity during the midcycle portion of the human menstrual cycle. Horm. Behav. *18*:249–255.

Mayr, E. (1958) Behavior and systematics. In *Behavior and Evolution*. A. Roe and G.G. Simpson, eds., pp. 341–362, Yale University Press, New Haven, CT.

McClintock, M.K. (1978) Estrous synchrony and its mediation by airborne chemical communication (*Rattus norvegicus*). Horm. Behav. *10*:264–276.

McClintock, M.K. (1981a) Simplicity from complexity: A naturalistic approach to behavior and neuroendocrine function. In *New Directions for Methodology of Social and Behavioral Science*, Vol. 8. I. Silverman, ed., pp. 1–19, Jossey-Bass, San Francisco.

McClintock, M.K. (1981b) Social control of the ovarian cycle. Am. Zool. *21*:243–256.

McClintock, M.K. (1983a) Pheromonal regulation of the ovarian cycle: Enhancement, suppression and synchrony. In *Pheromones and Reproduction in Mammals*. J.G. Vandenbergh, ed., pp. 113–149, Academic Press, New York.

McClintock, M.K. (1983b) Synchronizing ovarian and birth cycles by female pheromones. In *Chemical Signals in Vertebrates*, Vol. 3. D. Muller-Schwarze and R.M. Silverstein, eds., pp. 159–178, Plenum Publishing Corp., New York.

McClintock, M.K. (1984) Group mating in the domestic rat as a context for sexual selection: Consequences for the analysis of sexual behavior and neuroendocrine responses. In *Advances in the Study of Behavior*, Vol. 14. J. Rosenblatt, C. Beer, and R. Hinde, eds., pp. 1–15, Academic Press, New York.

Merriam, G.R., and K.W. Wachter (1982) Algorithms for the study of episodic hormone secretion. Am. J. Physiol. *243*:E310–E318.

Morell, M.J., J.M. Dixen, C.S. Carter, and J.M. Davidson (1984) The influence of age and cycling status on sexual arousability in women. Am. J. Obstet. Gynecol. *148*:66–71.

Murphy, M. (1971) A natural history of the Syrian golden hamster—A reconnaissance expedition. Am. Zool. *11*:632.

Nelson, R., and I. Zucker (1981) Photoperiodic control of reproduction in olfactory-bulbectomized rats. Neuroendocrinology *32*:178–183.

Persky, H., N. Charney, H.I. Lief, C.P. O'Brien, W.R. Miller, and D. Strauss (1978) The relationship of plasma estradiol level to sexual behavior in young women. Psychosom. Med. *40*:523–537.

Pfaff, D.W. (1980) *Estrogens and Brain Function*. Springer-Verlag, New York.

Price, E.O. (1980) Sexual behavior and reproductive competition in male wild and domestic Norway rats. Anim. Behav. *28*:657–667.

Rabin, D., and L.W. McNeil (1980) Pituitary and gonadal desensitization after continuous luteinizing hormone-releasing hormone infusion in normal females. J. Clin. Endocrinol. Metab. *51*:873–876.

Ramirez, V.D., H.H. Feder, and C.H. Sawyer (1984) The role of brain catecholamines in the regulation of LH secretion: A critical inquiry. In *Frontiers in Neuroendocrinology*, Vol. 8. L. Martini and W.F. Ganong, eds., pp. 27–84, Raven Press, New York.

Reiter, R.J. (1973) Pineal control of a seasonal reproductive rhythm in male golden hamsters exposed to natural daylight and temperature. Endocrinology *92*:423–430.

Robitaille, J.A. and J. Bouvet (1976) Field observations on the social behaviour of the Norway rat, *Rattus norvegicus* (Berkenhout). Biol. Behav. *1*:289–308.

Roche, K.E., and A.I. Leshner (1979) ACTH and vasopressin treatments immediately after a defeat increase future submissiveness in male mice. Science *204*:1343–1344.

RUSAK, B., and G. GROOS (1982) Suprachiasmatic stimulation phase shifts rodent circadian rhythms. Science 215:1407–1409.

SIMON, H.A. (1969) *The Sciences of the Artificial*. M.I.T. Press, Cambridge, MA.

SPITZ, C.J., A.R. GOLD, and D.B. ADAMS (1975) Cognitive and hormonal factors affecting coital frequency. Arch. Sex. Behav. 4:249–263.

TELLE, H.J. (1966) Beitrag zur Kenntnis der Verhaltenweise von Ratten, vergleichend dargestellt bei *Rattus norvegicus* und *Rattus rattus*. Z. Angew. Zool. 53:129–196.

VANDENBERGH, J.G. (1983) *Pheromones and Reproduction in Mammals*. Academic Press, New York.

VON BÉKÉSY, G. (1961) cited in TEITELBAUM, PHILIP, *Physiological Psychology*, p. 12, Prentice-Hall, Englewood Cliffs, NJ.

WALLEN, K. (1982) Influence to female hormonal state on rhesus sexual behavior varies with space for social interaction. Science 217:375–376. Copyright 1982 by the AAAS.

WALLEN, K., and L.A. WINSTON (1984) Social complexity and hormonal influences on sexual behavior in rhesus monkeys (*Macaca mulatta*). Physiol. Behav. 32:629–637.

WARD, I.L., and J. REED (1985) Prenatal stress and prepubertal social rearing conditions interact to determine sexual behavior in male rats. Behavioral Neuroscience 99:301–309. Copyright 1985 by the American Psychological Association. Reprinted by permission of the author.

WARD, I.L., and O.B. WARD (1985) Sexual behavior differentiation: Effects of prenatal manipulations in rats. In *Handbook of Behavioral Neurobiology*, Vol. 7. N.T. Adler, D. Pfaff, and R. Goy, eds., pp. 77–98, Plenum Publishing Corp., New York.

EIGHT
Environmental Regulation of Reproduction in Rodents

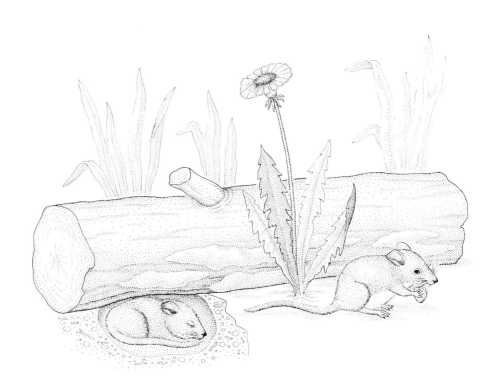

F.H. Bronson
Institute of Reproductive Biology
Department of Zoology
University of Texas
Austin, Texas

It is a biological truism that the production of offspring must occur in harmony with existing dietary, physical, and social conditions. To this end natural selection has provided vertebrates with a rich variety of signalling systems, each of which couples environmental variation of some kind with appropriate internal responses. Our general concern here will be with the ways in which these signalling systems act and interact to regulate reproduction in mammals. In particular we will be concerned with the ways that environmental factors regulate reproduction in mammals of small size.

Small size places great and complex constraints upon successful reproduction. To the author's mind at least, this makes the study of environmental regulation immensely more interesting in these animals than it would be in larger mammals. Furthermore, since the typical mammal on this planet is only about the size of a laboratory rat (Eisenberg, 1978), most of our mammals indeed are relatively small in stature.

Our model here will be the muroid rodent. This group contains most of the animals known generically as rats or mice. They occur on almost every land mass in the world, and as a group they account for over one-quarter of all living mammals. Importantly for our purposes here, more effort has been expended in the study of muroid rodents than for all other mammals combined.

Several research strategies have contributed to our knowledge of the ways in which environmental factors modulate reproduction (Sadleir, 1969). At one extreme is the study of wild animals in wild habitats, where general indices of reproduction are correlated with naturally occurring variation in environmental factors. At the other extreme is the study of fine physiological details in domesticated animals when they are subjected to discrete environmental manipulations in controlled confines. In between these extremes are other strategies involving the study of wild or semidomesticated mammals in controlled or seminatural conditions.

My research efforts have been limited largely to studying the impact of three or four environmental factors on the reproduction of wild and domestic rodents in a laboratory setting. Nevertheless, it has been my express intent to develop a total picture of the environmental regulation of reproduction in muroid rodents. I will use data from my laboratory studies wherever possible; where this is not possible, I will rely upon the contributions of other laboratory investigators. In both cases, however, I intend to view these laboratory findings within the framework of knowledge about natural populations that has been developed by ecologists. It is only within this larger context that much of our laboratory research has biological meaning.

ENVIRONMENTAL REGULATION: A BRIEF LOOK

The environmental factors known to influence reproduction in mammals as a whole are food availability, a variety of social cues, and four aspects of the physical environment: the day-night cycle, temperature, humidity, and rainfall. Food intake must be acknowledged as the most fundamental of these factors, since all facets of an animal's well-being are dependent ultimately upon it. For our purposes here only two major components of food will be considered: calories and nutrients.

The bioenergetic regulation of reproduction forms the core of the organization presented in Figure 8.1. All adult mammals must forage for their food; they must assimilate energy from that food, and then they must partition the use of that energy among many interacting and often competing demands, only one of which is to reproduce. The demands that must be satisfied first are cellular maintenance, thermoregulation, and the locomotor costs of obtaining food. Once these primary demands have been satisfied, whatever energy remains can be allocated to growth, or to the physiological and behavioral demands of reproduction, or it can be stored for emergencies in the form of fat. Ambient temperature determines a mammal's thermoregulatory demand, and thus it influences indirectly the amount of energy available for reproduction. Ambient humidity acts along this same pathway.

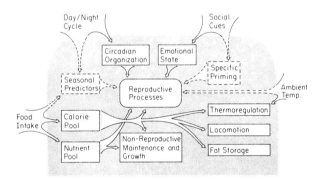

Figure 8.1. The major environmental factors known to influence reproduction in mammals, and the general pathways each follows. Solid lines indicate those pathways that are universally constant in mammals; dashed lines indicate those that occur in some but not all mammals. (Reprinted from Bronson, 1985)

Reproducing animals have a need for nutrients, such as amino acids, vitamins, etc., as well as energy. Nutrients also must be partitioned competitively among reproductive and nonreproductive needs.

Most mammals live in seasonally changing environments. Thus many are seasonal breeders, and traditionally this is the phenomenon that has garnered most of our interest. Some mammals use predictors that prepare themselves metabolically for a breeding season; others do not. Two factors known to be used by mammals as seasonal predictors are the annual cycle of daily photoperiod and some secondary plant compounds found in newly emerging vegetation. The day-night cycle also entrains the circadian organization that often permeates the reproductive processes of mammals.

A final point to keep in mind is that efficiency can vary both within and between breeding seasons, particularly in small mammals. The causes for this variation typically are the climatic and dietary factors that shape seasonal breeding in the first place. The social environment emerges here as a potent force as well, however. Some populations have evolved specific systems for priming particular reproductive processes by pheromonal, tactile, and/or auditory cues emanating from other members of the population. In addition, a variety of social conditions can evoke nonspecific emotional states that somehow depress reproduction. Usually we classify all such effects simply as "stress" or sometimes as "emotional stress." Although not shown in Figure 8.1, a complex relationship between social status, food availability, and emotional state can determine which individuals breed and which do not.

ANNUAL PATTERNS OF BREEDING

The most spectacular action of the environment on reproduction in any species relates to the phenomenon of seasonal breeding. Like other mammals, the typical small rodent often lives in a seasonally changing environment, and thus it usually breeds only at certain times of the year. Two characteristics greatly influence the annual patterns of breeding in these animals. First, they have relatively short life expectancies in the wild. Second, as noted earlier, small size places great constraints upon the dietary and physical conditions under which they can breed. Because of these characteristics, one expects small rodents to mature relatively fast and thereafter to continuously produce relatively large numbers of offspring, unless inhibited from doing so by adverse environmental conditions.

Two annual patterns of reproduction will be examined here in order to develop generalities: those of the ubiquitous house mouse (*Mus domesticus*), and those shown by the various members of the genus *Peromyscus*.

House mice evolved in southwestern Asia. Because they often live commensally with humans, they have been inadvertently transported and retransported by us throughout the world, often following the spread of wheat (Berry, 1982). Their reproduction is sufficiently flexible to allow them to invade natural habitats in most parts of the world to which they have been carried (Bronson, 1979). Thus this one species now exhibits an almost worldwide distribution, wherein individual populations can be found living in human structures or in totally feral habitats; in some cases individuals shift from one to the other seasonally. As shown in Figure 8.2 members of this species tend to breed continuously, year-around, when they reside in the more climatically constant environments of humans, and seasonally in natural habitats.

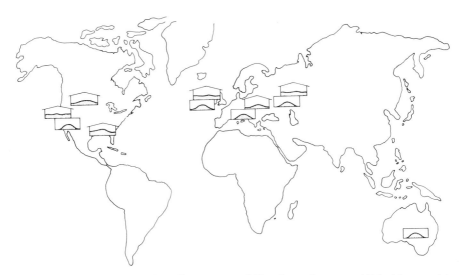

Figure 8.2. Reported annual breeding patterns of *Mus domesticus*, as published by a variety of investigators and summarized in Bronson (1979). Rectangles indicate feral populations; roofed boxes indicate populations living commensally in human buildings. In both cases a one-year period is represented with January on the left and December on the right. The stippled area between indicates changes in the proportion of females examined that were pregnant.

The genus *Peromyscus* includes a variety of small rodents in North America known variously as deermice, white-footed mice, beach mice, cactus mice, and so forth. In the laboratory these animals breed rapidly and continuously if given an appropriate environment. As suggested in Figure 8.3, they may or may not show seasonal inhibition of their reproduction in natural habitats (see also Millar, 1984). The overall impression here is one of great variation. While a breeding season limited to three summer months has been observed near Great Slave Lake, above 60° of latitude, a winter breeding season of six months has been recorded in central Texas at 30° latitude. Two hundred miles south in the Rio Grande River valley, a summer peak in breeding is seen with an occasional winter pregnancy occurring as well, and just west of here, in the state of Coahuila, Mexico, pregnant females may be found in all 12 months of the year.

Year-around breeding of *Peromyscus* also has been recorded at one time or another in Kansas, coastal South Carolina, Florida, eastern Washington, and southern Mexico. Bimodal patterns of spring and fall breeding are common near 40° latitude, as is a more simple 5- to 7-month spring and summer breeding season. Importantly, most of these patterns can be seen even within a single species of this genus, the deermouse (*P. maniculatus*).

The variation obvious in Figure 8.2 is apparent also when one examines the year-to-year variation in the reproduction of deermice living in the same locality. For three consecutive years Sadleir (1974) studied a population of these animals living on the Frazer River delta in British Columbia. As shown in Figure 8.4, the onset of breeding in this population varied by as much as

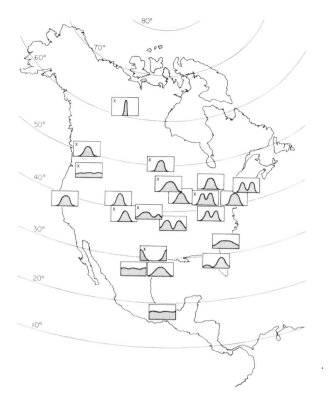

Figure 8.3. Observed breeding seasons (percent of females pregnant each month) in several populations of *Peromyscus*, as reported by many investigators and summarized in Bronson (1985). The left axis of each rectangle represents January, the right axis represents December, and the stippled area in between represents the annual breeding pattern observed over a 12-month period. The patterns noted with an × are those reported for a single species, the deermouse (*P. maniculatus*).

two months—a period of time almost equivalent to the length of the entire breeding season in one of the three years.

Several conclusions can be drawn from the annual patterns of reproduction shown by *Peromyscus* and house mice. Most of these conclusions probably are applicable to muroid rodents generally. First, when these small animals live in benign climates with a seasonally stable food supply, they will

Figure 8.4. Percentage of females pregnant in a population of deermice in British Columbia over a 3-year period. (Data extracted from Sadleir, 1974)

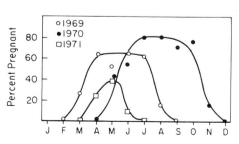

breed rapidly and continuously. Many habitats in which they dwell vary seasonally, however. Even in the tropics there often are pronounced seasonal patterns in rainfall which result in seasonal fluctuations in food availability. Thus small mammals may breed seasonally at all latitudes.

Second, the species is a poor unit of interest here. Climate and dietary factors vary from region to region and from year to year, and thus one expects great variation in patterns of breeding even within a single species. Likewise one expects to often find situations in which the annual patterns of reproduction of two populations of different species inhabiting the same locality are more similar to each other than they are to other populations of their own species living somewhere else.

Third, while one expects natural selection to have yielded great population-to-population variation in sensitivity to different environmental factors, the results may not always be what one might expect upon superficial appraisal. As shown in Figure 8.5, for example, deermice from south central Texas are well adapted to breed in cold temperatures, while their counterparts in Alberta are better adapted for warm-temperature breeding. This seeming paradox is not a paradox at all. This particular population of deermice in Texas is adapted to breed in the winter because of exceptionally harsh summer conditions. Thus natural selection has acted to assure success during the only part of the year when they could breed. The Alberta deermice breed in the summer, and failure can come here only by being too sensitive to heat.

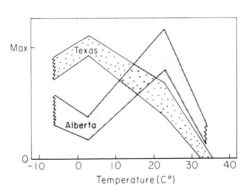

Temperature (C°)

Figure 8.5. Number of young born at different temperatures to pairs of deermice whose ancestors had been caught either in Texas or Alberta. Pairs were constituted when both the male and female were fully adult, and after each had been slowly conditioned to the temperature at which they were to be tested. Since average litter size varied markedly between these two populations at a control temperature, the left axis simply represents reproductive success between none and maximum, as the latter was characterized separately for each stock. The stippled area indicates the mean number of young born plus and minus one standard error. (From Bronson and Pryor, 1983)

THE ENERGETICS OF REPRODUCTION

As has been recognized for some time (Baker, 1938), the "ultimate" factors controlling seasonal breeding in mammals always are climate, caloric availability, and/or the nutrient quality of an animal's food. Following the lead of several ecologists, I tend to use the energetics of reproduction as a core for organizing principles about annual breeding. My reasons for doing so are threefold.

First, the energy available for reproduction is influenced by all but one of the "ultimate" factors of concern in natural habitats: caloric availability, rainfall, temperature, and humidity. Only nutrient availability cannot be encompassed within an energetic framework. Thus a bioenergetic core can act as a potent unifying force when considering ultimate factors. Second, the fact that body size is a major correlate of much of the variation seen in the annual breeding patterns of mammals is predicted on the basis of energetic theory (Bronson, 1985). Third, from a practical standpoint, we simply know very little about the nutritional requirements for the breeding of wild mammals, and we know little about the process by which nutrients are allocated to reproductive versus nonreproductive needs. Thus, viewing seasonal breeding in energetic terms is both rational and parsimonious.

The Energetics of Reproduction in Females

Generally the energetic constraints on reproduction are most obvious when one considers them in females. This is particularly true in the small rodents. As has been known for some time now, two characteristics of small females make them exceptionally susceptible to energetic constraint. First, their large surface-to-volume ratio results in increased thermoregulatory costs even at mildly low temperatures (Hart, 1971). This demand competes with reproduction, and either it must be countered by increased food intake or reproduction will suffer (Barnett, 1973). Second, the energetic costs of a small female's reproductive cycle are extremely high, both in relation to her ability to obtain food and in relation to her fat stores.

How these characteristics interact to shape reproductive activity has been a concern of my laboratory for some time now. In the wild, small mammals normally live in burrows that are thermally buffered. To obtain food they must emerge and forage in whatever conditions exist outside, usually at night. Prolonged foraging will be required whenever food is in short supply, and the energetic cost/gain ratio of foraging can become critical as temperatures decrease. Importantly the temperatures of concern here can be quite mild by human standards.

Perrigo and Bronson (1985), for example, studied this problem in a caging system in which peripubertal female house mice of a wild stock were required to leave their thermally buffered burrows and run on a running wheel for various lengths of time for food pellets (Figure 8.6). A prolonged foraging requirement that allowed normal growth and reproductive development at 23°C (74°F) inhibited both at 10°C (50°F). Normal growth occurred at the latter temperature in the presence of excess food, however; indeed, these animals breed well even at minus 6°C if given excess food and bedding (Bronson and Pryor, 1983). Thus it is the length of time a small female must forage for food in relation to ambient temperature that is critical. Any degree of food scarcity when combined with even a mildly cool temperature presents a serious energetic challenge.

Related to this problem is the fact that small mammals have relatively

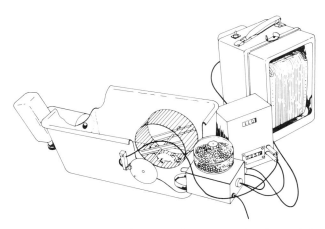

Figure 8.6. Special caging system designed by Glenn H. Perrigo for studying foraging and reproductive development in house mice. In this cage an animal can live in a thermally buffered burrow at the left, but to feed it must emerge into whatever conditions are imposed upon it by the investigator and run a predetermined number of revolutions on a running wheel. When that number of revolutions is achieved, an automatic pellet dispenser ejects a 45-mg pellet of food into a feeding cup. The electronic controls for programming the pellet dispenser are shown at the center right, and an automatic chart recorder at the upper right accumulates daily running patterns. (From Perrigo and Bronson, 1983)

little energy stored as fat to counter acute emergencies. A typical mammal weighing 25 grams carries only enough fat to survive two or three days without food at 27°C, and survival time drops to a matter of hours at 10°C. Because of this problem the energy-partitioning process of the small mammal probably always favors some fat storage over the demands of reproduction (Perrigo and Bronson, 1983).

Set against this background is the fact that the caloric costs of lactation are immense for the small female. As shown in Figure 8.7, even in the utopian conditions of the laboratory, a female mouse must more than double her food intake to nourish herself and her mass of offspring late in lactation. In a natural habitat the lactating female either must have hoarded a great amount of food ahead of time, or she must leave her nest many times each night to forage. This increases greatly her own thermoregulatory costs and those of her offspring which, in turn, necessitates still more foraging.

Thus during late lactation the small female rodent probably needs to find and consume as much as four or five times as much food as was required before she became pregnant. In a sense, then, late lactation comprises an enormous energetic bottleneck that is difficult to surmount under any conditions, but impossible if prolonged foraging is required in even mildly cool temperatures.

When one considers this energetic bottleneck, the small female's paucity of energy stores, and the regional, seasonal, and year-to-year variation in temperature and food availability that exists in the northern hemisphere, highly variable breeding patterns such as those seen in *Peromyscus* certainly are expected. One more factor must be considered here, however—life expectancy. The average life expectancy of most small mammals living in the

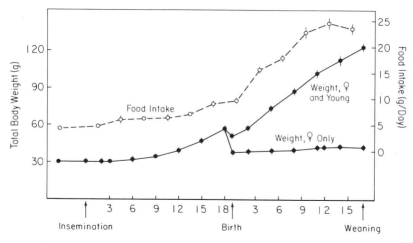

Figure 8.7. Changes in body weight of mother and young mice, in relation to food intake, throughout an entire reproductive cycle. (Bronson and Marsteller, 1985)

temperate zone is measured in weeks, or a few months at best. This means that small mammals must reproduce whenever there is any possibility of successfully meeting their lactational costs. Thus there usually is a high degree of flexibility associated with the breeding of most small mammals. In a sense they must push hard against their energetic constraints, both seasonally and regionally, because they live such a short time.

This undoubtedly is why one finds continuous breeding by these animals in some circumstances at unexpectedly high latitudes (e.g., Figure 8.2). One of the best examples of such opportunism was recorded by Linduska (1942), who found pregnant deermice in Michigan in January. These animals were exploiting the energetically good conditions of shocked corn standing in otherwise harshly open fields.

The Energetics of Reproduction in Males

What about the small male? Males and females differ fundamentally in the amount of energy they invest in their offspring. Stated differently, the two sexes differ greatly in the nature of the energetic costs of successful reproduction. Thus one expects the two sexes often to differ just as fundamentally in the way that their reproductive effort is regulated by existing energetic conditions (see Crook, 1977; Clutton-Brock et al., 1982).

The expected difference between the two sexes is best shown in relation to an experimental design whose many variations often have been used to study the relationship between body growth and reproductive development in laboratory rodents (Glass and Swerdloff, 1980). In one such variation often used in my laboratory and shown in Figure 8.8, animals are allowed to grow normally until a particular stage, at which time further growth is inhibited by restricting the amount of food available to them. Sometime later these animals are again

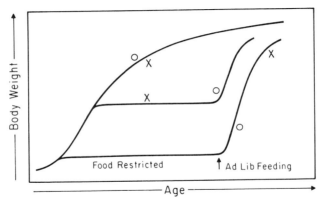

Figure 8.8. Relationship between age and body weight at which males (×) and females (○) achieve fertility when body growth is either allowed to proceed uninterrupted, or stopped at one of two body weights. In the latter case the animals are maintained at one of these two body weights by restricting their food intake until much later, when ad lib feeding is resumed and the animals experience "catch-up" growth. The generalized results shown here are modelled after studies done in the author's laboratory with wild house mice, domestic mice, and domestic rats. (Bronson and Rissman, 1986)

allowed unlimited access to food, at which time they experience rapid catch-up growth. We have used this design in studies with both wild and domestic stocks of house mice and with laboratory rats.

If growth is stopped early during somatic development, both sexes cease reproductive development. When ad lib feeding is resumed, females achieve their first ovulation in a few days, but males require much longer to achieve functional reproductive maturity. When maintained at a somewhat higher body weight, females again cease reproductive development, but they can ovulate more quickly when ad lib feeding is resumed. In contrast, males maintained at this weight become sexually mature despite their lack of further growth.

What is illustrated here are different adaptive strategies for balancing the length of the gametic cycle against two other factors: short life expectancy and the difference in energetic investment required for successful reproduction on the part of the two sexes. Most small mammals in the wild not only face short life expectancies, they also face decidedly uncertain energetic conditions after weaning. Usually at this time, either by choice or by force, they often leave their natal environs in search of a new home.

During these dispersal movements they must be prepared to abandon growth at any time. With their much shorter gametic cycle, females can proceed rapidly with the final stages of reproductive development after a new home with good energetic conditions has been found. The spermatogenic cycle of a male, however, is several weeks in length, and to initiate it only after dispersal is complete would be tantamount to genetic suicide. Thus natural selection has provided different strategies for the two sexes, with the final stages of reproductive development proceeding largely independently of growth in the small male, but not in the female. The female proceeds with her first ovulation only after a new home with a food supply adequate to support lactation has been secured.

A further strategy related to fertility onset in males is in evidence when one examines the timing of weaning in small mammals. Body size at weaning varies in mammals anywhere from 10% to 65% of adult body size (Millar, 1977). Wild house mice, domestic house mice, and laboratory rats are all weaned in the laboratory when they are about three weeks of age. This translates as 55%, 30%, and 15% of their adult body weight, respectively. Preventing further growth after weaning by restricting available food almost totally inhibits further reproductive development in the male rat while having only minor effects on wild house mice (Hamilton and Bronson, 1985). Reproductive development is totally inhibited by this procedure in the female of all these stocks, however. Time of weaning relative to body weight must have been an important focus of natural selection in the evolutionary history of these animals.

NUTRIENTS AND REPRODUCTION

While an argument can be made that a bioenergetic view of reproduction is a unifying force that can account for much of the variation seen in the annual patterns of breeding in small rodents, obviously it cannot account for all of it. Indeed, there can be no doubt that the availability of key nutrients can vary annually and seasonally in natural habitats, and when this occurs a partitioning process must decide among reproductive and nonreproductive needs. The most important nutrients here are the essential amino acids, certain polyunsaturated fatty acids, a variety of minerals, and some vitamins, all of which must be obtained from the mammal's food because none can be synthesized internally.

It is unfortunate that we know so little about the dietary requirements of rodents living in the wild. Considerable effort has been devoted to developing adequate breeding diets for our standard laboratory animals, and, as expected, diets that are deficient in a necessary nutrient deter growth, puberty, and adult reproductive success (Glass and Swerdloff, 1977).

Little more can be said here because of the paucity of available information, except that water balance, a subject seldom considered in relation to reproduction, could be a profound seasonal regulator in deserts and dry grasslands (e.g., Nelson et al., 1983). Specifically, it seems reasonable to expect that the extra water needed for milk production could be a potent limiting factor in these environments and could also have been a focus of concern for natural selection.

STRATEGIES INVOLVING SEASONAL PREDICTORS

Regardless of whether seasonal breeding is required because of energetic or nutritional variation, or both, it has long been recognized that a rodent may opt to use a predictor of this variation. This is the classic basis for distinguishing between the "ultimate" and "proximate" causes of seasonal breeding (Baker, 1938), and it distinguishes between the "obligatory" and "facultative" strategies proposed by Negus and Berger (1972).

Use of a predictor allows metabolic preparation for an oncoming period when food availability and climate will combine in such a way as to maximize the probability of reproductive success. Thus the use of a predictor can be an advantage in a seasonally changing environment, if these changes are predictable, but a disadvantage if they are not. It must be remembered, however, that the degree of predictability offered by an environment is in part a function of the life expectancy of the animal perceiving it. The simple fact that good and bad seasons alternate with each other on an annual basis may be an adequate level of predictability for a large animal that may live several years, but not for a small one with a life expectancy of only a few months at best.

Only three general strategies for using predictors are apparent at this time in muroid rodents. The first of these is wide-open opportunism, where no predictors of any kind are employed. In its extreme form this strategy would dictate that males remain sexually ready at all times of the year, and that females breed either seasonally or continually depending upon moment-to-moment energetic and nutritional considerations. The second strategy involves the use of photoperiod to time seasonal breeding, and the third involves the use of secondary plant compounds to predict an oncoming period of maximum food availability.

Opportunism

A reasonable argument can be made that the most common strategy employed by mammals involves opportunism in one form or another. The basis for this argument relates simply to the fact that the typical mammal on this planet is small in size and tropical in residence (see Eisenberg, 1980). Living in an area offering little thermoregulatory challenge suggests that these mammals will breed either seasonally or continuously depending upon rainfall pattern and hence variation in food availability. Figure 8.9 presents the patterns of reproduction of two muroid rodents living in a grassland in

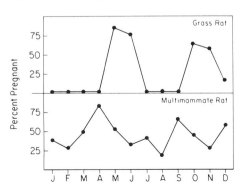

Figure 8.9. Percent of females pregnant each month in two muroid rodents living in an equatorial grassland in Uganda. (Redrawn from Delaney and Neal, 1969)

equatorial Uganda, as adapted from Delaney and Neal (1969). The two species of concern here are seed eaters, but they revert to herbacious food when necessary. Rainfall patterns are somewhat unpredictable in this part of Uganda and, as a consequence, so is the production of vegetation.

One of these animals, the multimammate rat (*Mastomys natalensis*), breeds throughout the year in Uganda. The other, the grass rat (*Arvicanthis abyssinicus*), breeds in relation to rainfall. In the year studied here by Delaney and Neal two rainy periods resulted in two distinct periods of breeding by this latter species. The difference in feeding strategies that allows one but not the other of these two mammals to breed year-around in Uganda is unknown. Males of both species apparently remain sexually active at all months of the year.

A purely opportunistic reproductive strategy also is found in global colonizers like the house mouse and the Norway rat, whose wild forms often live in man-made environments and whose domesticated forms serve as some of our most common laboratory mammals (e.g., Bronson, 1979). This strategy undoubtedly has been adopted also by many of the smaller mammals living in the southern part of the temperate zone.

Photoperiodic Prediction

Because photoperiodic prediction is used by many mammals to time their annual breeding efforts in the northern temperate zone, it has attracted the intense interest of biologists for decades. The question of who uses photoperiodic prediction is best approached in relation to the hemispheric breeding patterns presented earlier for *Peromyscus*.

Over millions of years the recent ancestral stocks of these mammals were forced southward repeatedly by advancing glaciers. The latest of these episodes occurred about 10,000 years ago, when few mammals lived above 35° of latitude. Since that time the climatic and dietary conditions of North America have changed immensely, and correlated with these changes has been a gradual northward spread of mammals into all possible habitats. Photoperiodic prediction obviously would provide an advantage in some of these habitats at one time or another, but not at other times or in other places.

Recent work in the laboratory of my colleague, Claude Desjardins, and in the laboratories of Robert Lynch and Irving Zucker, has shown that the use of photoperiodic prediction is still in a state of flux in *Peromyscus* populations. Desjardins and Lopez (1980), for example, reported a latitudinal gradient in which a few deermouse males collected in Alberta were insensitive to photoperiodic influence, more were insensitive in South Dakota, while none were photoperiodic in Texas.

The genetic basis for this heterogeneity has been documented now by selection experiments. Using a population of deermice in which about three-quarters of the animals normally are photoperiodic, Desjardins et al. reduced this proportion to one-quarter in just two generations of selection in the laboratory.

Except in the very northern part of their range deermice commonly produce two generations during a single breeding season. Thus the proportion of deermice that are photoperiodically sensitive probably is a highly labile statistic in the wild, shifting easily from year to year in the same population and, just as easily, from one locale to another.

Regarding the question of how photoperiod actually times an annual breeding cycle in small rodents, this question impinges upon a vast area of elegant research on the one hand, and a vast unknown on the other. How a light cycle is perceived, how it interacts with endogenous circadian rhythms of sensitivity, and how all of this is transduced in the brain to regulate gonadotropin secretion has been an intensely active area of research for two decades now (e.g., Reiter, 1980). Most of this research has involved only two or three domesticated species, however, and thus at this point in time we probably have only a shallow appreciation of how photoperiod actually acts to time seasonal breeding in the many populations of wild mammals living in their diverse habitats.

At least in theory, if a period of optimal climatic and food conditions is predictable, and if it is bracketed by the same critical daylength, then this cue could be used to trigger both the onset and the cessation of annual breeding. This may be the situation in some small mammals living in the temperate zone. On the other hand, the optimal period of breeding usually is not bracketed well by the same photoperiod. In this case, either the onset or the cessation of breeding can be cued by a critical daylength, but not both.

A common strategy here may be that which has been adopted by the male golden hamster. In this animal, cessation of breeding is cued by a critical short daylength, after which the animal becomes refractory to further short-day inhibition. Testicular recrudescence, and the onset of breeding, then occurs spontaneously after an endogenously programmed period of time (Elliott and Goldman, 1981).

There must be other continuously breeding mammals, probably many, in which the onset rather than the cessation of breeding is cued by a critical daylength, and in which the length of the breeding rather than the nonbreeding season is programmed endogenously. Indeed, a comparison of the way puberty is regulated by photoperiod in two distantly related hamsters illustrates the great importance of local selection here (Figure 8.10).

Testicular growth occurs spontaneously in the young golden hamster, even on short daylengths, but just as maturity is achieved the system collapses and the male becomes infertile. The Djungarian hamster shows a classical inhibition of reproductive development in response to short days, just as does the adult male of this species. The local factors that have yielded this difference in strategies are not known.

Prediction by Plant Cues

The use of plant predictors is a poorly researched area. It may or may not be a common strategy. Our best evidence for the existence of plant predictors

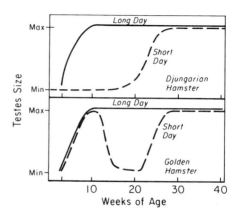

Figure 8.10. Change in testes weight in young Djungarian and golden hamsters maintained in the laboratory on long vs. short daylengths. (Bronson and Rissman, 1986, redrawn from Hoffman, 1978, and Darrow et al., 1980)

comes from work on the montane vole (*Microtus montanus*). This species lives at high altitude in the Rocky Mountains, where the season of food availability varies anywhere from 3 to 6 months each year. Daylength by itself is not a good predictor of the precise onset and cessation of plant growth at these high altitudes.

As shown convincingly by Negus, Berger and co-workers (e.g., Sanders et al., 1981), a secondary plant compound found in newly emerging grass, the phenol 6-methoxybenzoxalinone, is used by these voles to predict accurately the oncoming period of maximum availability of green grass. Indeed, reproduction can be stimulated in these voles in midwinter under a heavy snow cover by feeding them fresh green shoots (Negus and Berger, 1977).

The capacity to predict accurately an oncoming period of food availability is exceptionally important to montane voles, since their potential breeding season is short and unpredictable, their mortality rate is exceptionally high, and they must produce large numbers of rapidly maturing offspring, all on a calorically poor but seasonally abundant diet. Thus massive lactational costs must be supported under particularly trying conditions. The result is a strategy in which males but not females are regulated by photoperiod. Males come into breeding condition early and await the emergence of fresh grass which contains the melatoninlike phenol that, in turn, stimulates females to come into breeding condition.

MODULATION BY SOCIAL CUES

There can be no doubt that the social dimension of a rodent's environment can exert a profound influence on its reproduction, and that such cues can modulate efficiency during seasons when breeding is possible. A vast literature documents this fact. At the risk of oversimplification, three general categories will be proposed here to deal with all of the diverse ways in which social cues can modulate reproduction in rodents. The bases for distinguishing among these three categories include whether or not hormonal intervention is required for a reproductive event to be regulated by the social cues and, if so, the degree of specificity associated with both the cue and the hormonal response it invokes.

First, as is obvious, any social interaction, whether it involves animals of the same or different sex, requires organization by appropriate behavioral cues. Second, many mammals have evolved direct and specific neural and hormonal pathways via which reproductive events such as ovulation are regulated temporally by discrete social cues. Third, a variety of social situations can evoke nonspecific emotional states that secondarily influence reproduction. Only the last two categories will be considered further.

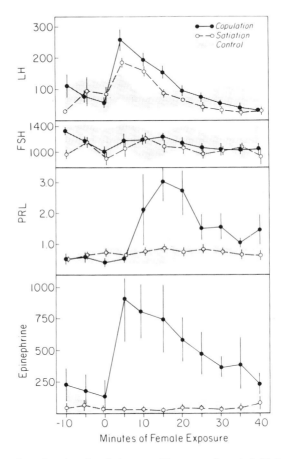

Figure 8.11. Reaction of male mice that were either sexually sated (Satiation) or sexually rested (Copulation) to a receptive female. Blood was collected via atrial cannulae, starting 10 minutes before the female was encountered and continuing for 40 minutes thereafter, and analyzed for epinephrine, prolactin (PRL), follicle-stimulating hormone (FSH), and luteinizing hormone (LH). All sexually rested males mated with their test females; no sexually sated male showed any interest in a female. Stippled area indicates the mean ± one standard error for a group of males not encountering a female. (Bronson and Rissman, 1986, redrawn from Bronson and Desjardins, 1982)

The distinction between these two categories are illustrated in Figure 8.11. Here, male mice bearing indwelling atrial cannulae were either sated sexually or not, and then exposed to receptive females. Both types of males experienced an immediate release of luteinizing hormone (LH) but not follicle-stimulating hormone (FSH) when a female was introduced into their cages. This is a specific response to a priming pheromone in the female's urine, and it initiates the release of only one of the two gonadotropins. The increase in prolactin (PRL) observed later in the test period was a specific response to ejaculation.

Sexually active but not sexually sated males showed an increase in circulating levels of epinephrine (and, not shown, also in norepinephrine and corticosterone) when they encountered a receptive female. This is a correlate of sexual arousal. Arousal undoubtedly involves multisensory input, and it is an emotional state that induces a nonspecific release of adrenal hormones. Thus in this figure one can discern both specific hormonal responses to discrete social cues and a generalized change in emotional state which, secondarily, influences hormonal activity.

Specific Priming

In regard to the highly specific pathways via which social cues can work, there are, of course, several classic examples of this type of cueing: the induction of ovulation in reflex ovulators by cervical stimulation, and the oxytocin/milk letdown response to suckling. The adaptive ways in which specific social cues can work in mammals, however, is best illustrated by the pheromonal/tactile regulation of puberty in house mice.

The first ovulation of these animals can occur at any time over a period of several weeks, depending upon the female's social environment (reviewed by Vandenbergh, 1983). In general, cues emanating from a sexually active male accelerate the final stages of sexual maturation in a young female, while cues from other females decelerate it. Furthermore, the relative dominance of male accelerating and female decelerating cues shifts dramatically during the development of a young female mouse (Figure 8.12). When newly weaned females are grouped with a male present, the female's decelerating cues totally override any acceleratory action of the male until the females reach about 20 g (for the CF-1 female), after which the male's cues assume dominance and the final stages of the female's sexual maturation ensue rapidly.

The cues, the sensory pathways, and the hormonal pathways underlying this cueing system all are relatively specific. That is, ovulation is regulated temporally by discrete social cues operating along direct neural pathways to change the secretion of only two tropic hormones. The cues include only specific urinary chemicals that act via vomeronasal input, i.e., priming pheromones, and less specific tactile cues. These cues combine synergistically to modulate only LH and prolactin secretion, thereby regulating the young female's peripubertal development (Bronson and Macmillan, 1983).

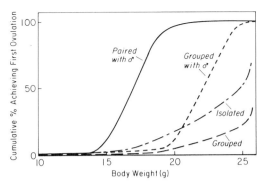

Figure 8.12. Cumulative percentages of CF-1 female mice achieving their pubertal ovulation depending upon whether or not they were housed alone or in groups, and whether or not a male was present. (Unpublished data)

Something akin to the house mouse's system of social modulation has been seen now in a wide variety of muroid rodents (Vandenbergh, 1983). A further richness is suggested by some of these studies where individuality is important (e.g., Rood, 1980).

The adaptive significance of the social priming of ovulation undoubtedly resides in the need to time this event in relation to existing familial and population conditions. As shown in Figure 8.13, for example, social priming can induce a marked blurring of the edge of the breeding season of deermice. In the absence of both a stimulatory daylength and social stimulation, male deermice of this particular population remain reproductively infantile until 6 or 7 months of age, the approximate length of the nonbreeding season in the area from which this population was collected (South Dakota). Obvious here, however, is the strong amelioratory effect of the presence of a female in short days. Any regulatory mechanism that allows flexibility in the onset or cessation of breeding is a decided advantage to short-lived mammals, who must breed maximally whenever socially and energetically possible.

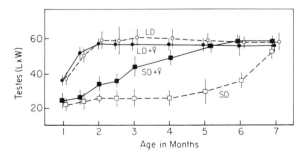

Figure 8.13. Mean testis size ($\pm$ SE) in photoperiodically sensitive deermice from one to seven months of age while being held on short days (SD) vs. long days (LD) (8 vs. 16 hours of light), with and without a female of the same age in their cage. Data collected by Desjardins and Bronson, and published in Bronson (1985).

Modulation via Emotional State

Regarding the second category of social regulation, that involving nonspecific responses to emotional states, it must be acknowledged immediately that we have few solid concepts with which to deal with this type of regulation. We know that a large number of experimental situations result in an enhancement of adrenal secretion. The release of epinephrine and corticosterone when a male mouse encounters a receptive female, for example, can be duplicated simply by placing the animal in a strange environment, by changing its cage, or even by exposing the male to a tennis ball (Craigen and Bronson, 1982).

There can be little doubt that these nonspecific responses are secondary reflections of complex emotional states which, in turn, reflect the animal's multisensory perception of its environment. Finally, we know that many of these nonspecific reactions also potentiate or interfere with some reproductive processes. If they promote reproductive success, we classify them under the rubric of "arousal"; if they act to the detriment of reproduction, we evoke the classic concept of "stress." In neither case do we have any real understanding of the emotional states involved.

Many common laboratory procedures can have aversive effects on the reproduction of rodents (see Ramaley, 1981). Perhaps the best examples of aversive reactions, however, are those found in mice living at high population density. The house mouse has been studied intensively in this regard (e.g., Christian and Davis, 1964). In a typical experiment, large and complex cages are seeded with a few pairs of mice and the population then is allowed to grow until it regulates itself. This dramatic regulation often involves a marked inhibition of sexual maturation among young animals, as well as a cessation of reproduction by adults. Dense populations are characterized by considerable intermale aggression. The losers of these fights, other social subordinates, and most of the onlookers are physiologically stressed in the classic sense.

Even more profound effects have been observed in crowded deermice. As shown in a long series of studies by Terman and colleagues, young deermice become fertile at 5 to 8 weeks of age when they are paired in small cages with adults of the opposite sex. When born and reared in dense, freely growing populations, however, as many as 95% of these deermice still are not fertile by 90 days of age; indeed, many die at well over a year of age without ever having achieved fertility (Terman, 1973). While it is debatable how often this type of regulation effectively limits population growth in the wild, the mechanisms do exist and they must often operate to at least some degree in wild populations to limit breeding during periods when it is energetically possible.

CONCLUSIONS

A physiological ecologist can work either in the laboratory or in the field, or both. However, the small nocturnal mammals of concern here are almost impossible to study in any physiological detail under field conditions. Thus my drive for some time now has been to study them in the laboratory, but to always view my experimental results within the context of what field ecologists have learned about natural populations of these animals.

The picture that has emerged from this effort is one in which the regulation of reproduction is dominated by a short life expectancy. Many of these animals do not survive long enough to achieve puberty, let alone reproduce. Furthermore, the environmental challenges facing mammals of this size in a natural habitat are both immense and complex. The numbers and distribution of these animals on this planet, nevertheless, documents the obvious fact that they have enjoyed unparalleled success in exploiting all kinds of habitats in all kinds of climates. The question is: how have they been able to do so?

The answer to this question is both simple and complicated. In a simplistic sense, one need only say that small mammals are supremely flexible, and that they are always opportunistic to some degree in tailoring their reproductive efforts to the environments in which they live. This generality, of course, hides a lot of complexity. This complexity probably is most easily seen in relation to the reproductive event that is so crucial to a short-lived animal—puberty. Here we can see an amazing number of forces at work, both in the evolutionary context and in relation to an animal's immediate reactions to its immediate environmental challenges.

One can see that the way that puberty is regulated energetically varies markedly between the two sexes. One can see where some individuals in some populations opt to use seasonal predictors, while other individuals in the same population do not. This seems a natural consequence of selection operating on short-lived individuals in unpredictable environments. One also can see adaptive regulation by pheromones to tailor the onset of fertility to existing social conditions, and one can see nonspecific inhibition of puberty as a consequence of adverse social conditions at the level of the population. All-in-all, one sees puberty as reflecting a summation of many responses to complex forces, but in all cases the result is flexibility and an overwhelming drive to somehow accomplish procreation before death intervenes.

Set against this background it is perhaps of interest now to consider what we really know and what we don't know about the environmental regulation of reproduction in small mammals. If we take as a final goal here the development of a reasonably large series of animal models, each of which encompasses a solid linkage between ecological and physiological concerns, and which in toto are representative of all small mammals, then several major gaps exist in our present body of knowledge. Each of these gaps offers a profitable avenue for future research.

First, at the most basic level, it is obvious that even though the muroid rodents are the best studied of all mammals, we still have not studied enough wild examples in sufficient detail both in the laboratory and in their natural habitats to provide a truly meaningful overview of the environmental control of their reproduction. Particularly obvious here is the lack of good information about tropical rodents. It is humbling indeed to realize that we have so much information about a few highly domesticated rodents, yet so little information about the annual breeding patterns and the factors responsible for these patterns in the most common mammals on this planet—the small- to average-sized muroid rodents living in the diverse parts of the tropics.

Most reproductive biologists live and work in the temperate zone, and almost all of the mammals we study have evolved here also. Had the science of reproductive biology developed in the tropics, where most mammals live, our current view of the environmental control of their reproduction might be quite different.

Still at a general level, conspicuously absent in this area are routine side-by-side comparisons of males and females, whether the concern is energetics, nutrients, predictors, or the neuroendocrine pathways through which these factors act to modulate reproduction. As discussed earlier, the reproductive efforts of the two sexes have been shaped by fundamentally different evolutionary forces, and there is every reason to suspect that the environmental control of their reproduction will often differ either quantitatively or qualitatively. A broad exploration of this possibility could add a great richness to our perception of the strategies employed by mammals generally when dealing with changing environments, as well as the neuroendocrine underpinnings of these strategies.

With regard to the specific environmental factors known to influence reproduction in these animals, each seems to present its own unique set of ignorances, and hence its own unique research opportunities. Our knowledge of the energetics of reproduction is limited in a major way. We have no broad theoretical understanding of the way the energy-partitioning process relates to the endocrine system in its entirety, and specifically to the neuroendocrine control of reproduction.

We have pieces of this puzzle derived from laboratory studies of isolated challenges and isolated responses. Unfortunately, animals did not evolve in small cages where they were subjected to one challenge at a time, and they did not evolve to respond in simple ways. Studying animals only in this way can yield artifactual constructs. In this regard, the development of a broad physiological overview of energy partitioning in relation to reproduction could provide a much-needed theoretical basis for the well-studied reactions to such diverse manipulations as food restriction, protein or fat restriction, enforced locomotion, and temperature variation. All of these manipulations are related energetically.

The simple bioenergetic relationship used here as a theoretical basis— namely one in which reproductive processes compete for available energy with all of the mammal's other demands, all within a framework of established hierarchical priorities—is an obvious oversimplification. Certainly these demands interact in much more complex ways than this (e.g., Wade and Gray, 1979). Developing a meaningful overview of this process, and how it varies between sexes and between populations, would seem to be one of the paramount challenges for physiologists interested in the environmental control of reproduction.

Nutrient partitioning could be another exciting area of research. We actually know very little about the physiological process whereby nutrients are partitioned between reproductive and nonreproductive needs, and we know little about the importance of specific nutrients for breeding. In the latter regard, particularly valuable might be attempts to induce winter breeding in strongly seasonal populations by using specific nutrient supplementation. Winter breeding has been induced in seasonally breeding populations of several rodents in British Columbia using food supplements, for example, but it is not known if all members of these populations reacted, nor is it known whether calories or nutrients were the important variables here (e.g., Fordham, 1971; Taitt and Krebs, 1981).

Regarding potential predictors of seasonal change, we may not have thought about this problem in sufficiently broad scope. There may be other potential predictors in addition to photoperiod and secondary plant compounds. Reasonable possibilities include a physical dimension of rainfall (Sadleir, 1969), the chemical composition of insects, which often are eaten when available by these animals, and some facet of the energetic cost/gain ratio of foraging.

The first could be important for animals living in deserts or dry grasslands; a chemical component of an insect could be an important trigger for the breeding of insectivores or omnivores, while a foraging parameter could be useful for small mammals generally. Could a small mammal use the energetic cost/gain ratio of the foraging conditions it encounters at the time of ovulation, for example, to predict whether or not it will be able later to support the much greater costs of lactation?

Despite a great amount of experimental interest, several gaps remain in our knowledge about photoperiodic control, many at a quite general level. The ways that critical daylength and short-term endogenous programming and circannual rhythms act and interact to regulate reproduction in different mammals living in different environments remain poorly understood. Do all photoperiodic rodents rely upon the critical-daylength model so well elucidated in the hamster? Can photoperiod be used to track rainfall patterns and vegetation cycles in the tropics, particularly near the equator? If so, is there an advantage for such prediction over pure opportunism? How does this choice relate to body size, life span, and social organization?

Particularly rewarding here might be the study of animals that are known to be extending their range latitudinally at this time, such as the neotropical cotton rat, *Sigmodon hispidus* (Johnston and Zucker, 1979). Also of interest would be studies directed toward understanding the physiological and genetic bases of the population heterogeneity noted in deermice, and a determination of the commonness of this phenomenon among rodents generally.

Documentation of the ability of one rodent to use a secondary plant compound to predict an oncoming period of high food availability certainly opens the door for further explorations that could be quite rewarding. There is indirect evidence now of the existence of other potential plant predictors—for example, the phytoestrogens (e.g., Labov, 1977). Critical in all such work, however, will be the experimental separation of the direct from the predictive effects of a cue. This is the problem that has proven so difficult in visualizing the use of ambient temperature as a predictor.

The biggest gap in our knowledge about the social priming systems of rodents concerns our inability to relate them in a meaningful way to the evolution of social organization and to visualize the adaptive advantage of these systems in natural populations. This field of interest began as a laboratory science and, unfortunately but not necessarily, it largely remains so today.

The emotional control of reproduction offers a host of research opportunities. This is one of the three factors that influence the reproduction of all mammals (Bronson, 1985). Our understanding of the relevant emotional states, the endocrine responses to them, and how all of this relates to specific reproductive processes is rudimentary. Particularly interesting here might be experiments involving subtle stimulation and fine-grained hormonal assessments.

Finally, from a purely physiological perspective, the drive here for some time now has been to study finer and finer dimensions of the neural and endocrine reactions of a few domesticated stocks to discrete environmental manipulations. This has been a rewarding approach, and one that will continue to be so in the future. As emphasized earlier, however, animals living in the wild are never subjected to one isolated factor at a time; they are barraged by many.

How are the brain and the endocrine system organized adaptively to accommodate multiple cueing? For example, in evolutionary, energetic, neural, and endocrine terms, why does the presence of a running wheel override inhibitory daylengths in female hamsters (Borer et al., 1983)? What happens to luteinizing hormone secretion if an animal is subjected to a permissive photoperiod while living in threshold energetic conditions? Can specific social cues override nutrient deficiencies, and can they potentiate the effect of plant predictors?

We rarely ask such questions, but real appreciation of the neuroendocrine organization of the rodent's reproductive effort probably awaits such efforts. These are the kinds of complexities that were faced by them during their evolution, and handling such complexities adaptively probably is what they are designed to do best.

REFERENCES

BAKER, J.R. (1938) The evolution of breeding season. In *Evolution: Essays on Aspects of Evolutionary Biology* (essays presented to E. Goodrich). G.R. de Beer, ed., pp. 161–177, Oxford University Press, Oxford, England.

BARNETT, S.A. (1973) Maternal processes in the cold adaptation of mice. Biol. Rev. *48*:477–508.

BERRY, R.J. (1982) The natural history of the house mouse. Field Stud. *3*:219–262.

BORER, K., C.S. CAMPBELL, J. TABOR, K. JORGENSON, S. KANDARIAN, and L. GORDON (1983) Exercise reverses photoperiodic anestrus in golden hamsters. Biol. Reprod. *29*:38–47.

BRONSON, F.H. (1979) The reproductive ecology of the house mouse. Quart. Rev. Biol. *54*:265–299.

BRONSON, F.H. (1985) Mammalian reproduction: An ecological perspective. Biol. Reprod. *32*:1–26. Reprinted by permission.

BRONSON, F.H., and E. RISSMAN (1986) The biology of puberty. Biol. Rev. *61*:157–195.

BRONSON, F.H., and C. DESJARDINS (1982) Endocrine responses to sexual arousal in male mice. Endocrinology *111*:1286–1291.

BRONSON, F.H., and B. MACMILLAN (1983) Hormonal responses to primer pheromones. In *Pheromones and Reproduction in Mammals.* J. Vandenbergh, ed., pp. 176–197, Academic Press, New York.

BRONSON, F.H., and F. MARSTELLER (1985) Effect of short term food deprivation on reproduction in female mice. Biol. Reprod. (in press). Reprinted by permission.

BRONSON, F.H., and S. PRYOR (1983) Ambient temperature and reproductive success in rodents. Biol. Reprod. *29*:72–80. Reprinted by permission.

CHRISTIAN, J.J., and D.E. DAVIS (1964) Endocrines, behavior and population. Science *145*:1550–1560.

CLUTTON-BROCK, T.H., F.E. GUINNESS, and S.D. ALBON (1982) *Red Deer: Behavior and Ecology of Two Sexes.* Wildlife Behavior and Ecology series. G.B. Schaller, ed. University of Chicago Press.

CRAIGEN, W., and F.H. BRONSON (1982) Deterioration of the capacity for sexual arousal in aged male mice. Biol. Reprod. *26*:869–874.

CROOK, J.J. (1977) On the integration of gender strategies in mammalian social systems. In *Reproductive Behavior and Evolution*, J.S. Rosenblatt and B.R. Komisaruk, eds., pp. 170–179, Plenum Publishing Corp., New York.

DARROW, J.M., F.C. DAVIS, J.A. ELLIOTT, M.H. STETSON, F.W. TUREK, and M. MENAKER (1980) Influence of photoperiod on reproductive development in the golden hamster. Biol. Reprod. *22*:443–450.

DELANEY, M.J., and B.R. NEAL (1969) Breeding seasons in rodents in Uganda. J. Reprod. Fert. Suppl. *6*:229–235.

DESJARDINS, C., and M.J. LOPEZ (1980) Sensory and nonsensory modulation of testis function. In *Testicular Development, Structure and Function.* A. Steinberger and E. Steinberger, eds., pp. 381–388, Raven Press, New York.

DESJARDINS, C., F.H. BRONSON, and J. BLANK (1986) Genetic selection for reproductive photoresponsiveness in deermice. Nature *322*:172–173.

EISENBERG, J.F. (1978) Evolution of arboreal herbivores in the class Mammalia. In *The Ecology of Arboreal Folivores*, G.G. Montgomery, ed., pp. 135–152, Smithsonian Institution Press, Washington, D.C.

EISENBERG, J.F. (1980) The density and biomass of tropical mammals. In *Conservation Biology*, M. Soule and B.A. Wilcox, eds., pp. 35–56, Sinauer Association, Sunderland, MA.

ELLIOTT, J.A., and B.D. GOLDMAN (1981) Seasonal reproduction: Photoperiodism and biological clocks. In *Neuroendocrinology of Reproduction*. N.T. Adler, ed., pp. 377–423, Plenum Publishing Corp., New York.

FORDHAM, R.A. (1971) Field populations of deermice with supplemental food. Ecology *52*:138–146.

GLASS, A.R., and R.S. SWERDLOFF (1977) Serum gonadotropins in rats fed a low-valine diet. Endocrinology *101*:702–707.

GLASS, A.R., and R.S. SWERDLOFF (1980) Nutritional influences on sexual maturation in the rat. Fed. Proc. *39*:2360–2364.

HAMILTON, G., and F.H. BRONSON (1985) Food restriction and reproductive development in wild house mice. Biol. Reprod. *32*:773–778.

HART, J.S. (1971) Rodents. In *Comparative Physiology of Thermoregulation*, Vol. 2. G.C. Whittow, ed., pp. 1–49, Academic Press, New York.

HOFFMANN, K. (1978) Effects of short photoperiods on puberty, growth and molt in the Djungarian hamster. J. Reprod. Fert. *54*:29–36.

JOHNSTON, P.G., and I. ZUCKER (1979) Photoperiodic influences on gonadal development and maintenance in the cotton rat, *Sigmodon hispidus*. Biol. Reprod. *21*:1–8.

LABOV, J.B. (1977) Phytoestrogens and mammalian reproduction. Comp. Biochem. Physiol. *57*:3–9.

LINDUSKA, J.P. (1942) Winter rodent populations in field shocked corn. J. Wildl. Manage. 6:353–363.

MILLAR, J.S. (1977) Adaptive features of mammalian reproduction. Evolution *31*:370–386.

MILLAR, J.S. (1984) Reproduction and survival of Peromyscus in seasonal environments. In *Bulletin of the Carnegie Museum: Proceedings of the Winter Ecology Symposium* (in press).

NEGUS, N.C., and P.J. BERGER (1972) Environmental factors and reproductive processes in mammalian populations. In *Biology of Reproduction: Basic and Clinical Studies*. J.T. Velardo and B.A. Kasprow, eds., pp. 89–98, Third Pan American Congress on Anatomy, New Orleans.

NEGUS, N.C., and P.J. BERGER (1977) Experimental triggering of reproduction in a natural population of *Microtus montanus*. Science *196*:1230–1231.

NELSON, R.J., J. DARK, and I. ZUCKER (1983) Influence of photoperiod, nutrition and water availability on reproduction of male California voles, *Microtus californicus*. J. Reprod. Fert. *69*:473–477.

PERRIGO, G., and F.H. BRONSON (1983) Foraging effort, food intake, fat deposition and puberty in female mice. Biol. Reprod. *29*:455–463. Reprinted by permission.

PERRIGO, G., and F.H. BRONSON (1985) Sex differences in energy allocation strategies in house mice. Behav. Ecol. Sociobiol. (in press).

RAMALEY, J.A. (1981) Stress and fertility. In *Environmental Factors in Mammal Reproduction*. D. Gilmore and B. Cook, eds., pp. 198–235, Macmillan Publ. Ltd., London.

REITER, R.J. (1980) Photoperiod: Its importance as an impeller of pineal and seasonal reproductive rhythms. Int. J. Biometeor. *24*:57–63.

ROOD, J.P. (1980) Mating relationships and breeding suppression in the dwarf mongoose, *Helogale-Parvula*. Anim. Behav. *28*:143–150.

SADLEIR, R.M.F.S. (1969) *The Ecology of Reproduction in Wild and Domestic Mammals*. Methuen and Co., London.

SADLEIR, R.M.F.S. (1974) The ecology of the deermouse *Peromyscus maniculatus* in a coastal coniferous forest. II. Reproduction. Can. J. Zool. *52*:119–131.

SANDERS, E.H., P.D. GARDNER, P.J. BERGER, and N.C. NEGUS (1981) 6-Methoxybenzoxazolinone: A plant derivative that stimulates reproduction in *Microtus montanus*. Science *214*:67.

TAITT, M.J., and C.J. KREBS (1981) The effect of extra food on small rodent populations: II. Voles *Microtus townsendii*. J. Anim. Ecol. *50*:125–137.

TERMAN, C.R. (1973) Recovery of reproductive function by prairie deermice *Peromyscus maniculatus bairdii* from asymptotic populations. Anim. Behav. *21*:443–448.

VANDENBERGH, J. (1983) Pheromonal regulation of puberty. In *Pheromones and Reproduction in Mammals*. J. Vandenbergh, ed., pp. 95–112, Academic Press, New York.

WADE, G.N., and J.M. GRAY (1979) Theoretical review: Gonadal effects on food intake and adiposity: A metabolic hypothesis. Physiol. Behav. *22*:583–593.

NINE
Hormonal Control of Sex Differences in the Brain and Behavior of Mammals

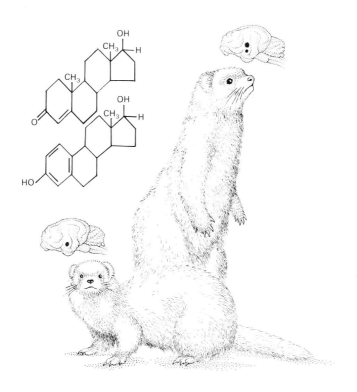

Michael J. Baum
Department of Biology
Boston University
Boston, Massachusetts

The casual observer notes differences between men and women (*Homo sapiens*) including body size, hair distribution, and, of course, the structure of the external genital organs. Upon closer inspection, one can also identify sex differences in the structure and function of the gonads and the internal genital ducts, in the ability of the liver and the kidney to metabolize drugs, and in the function of the brain. In humans differences in brain function have been studied only indirectly. Perceptual, cognitive, and overt behavioral differences between men and women have been identified under a variety of naturalistic and experimental situations, and the existence of sex differences in brain function has been inferred from these observations (see Chapter 12). More direct studies of the relationships among genetic sex, gonadal hormone secretions, brain structure and function, and the expression of behavior have, however, been carried out in a variety of nonhuman mammals. To date, reproductive behavior has been studied most widely in this context, and it is the aim of this chapter to identify some of the relevant issues currently under investigation. I will illustrate these topics by describing the action of sex steroid hormones in controlling the differentiation of masculine and feminine patterns of coital behavior in a carnivore, the ferret (*Mustela furo*). As will be seen, these experiments show that the relevant behavioral actions of sex steroid hormone exposure in the developing male ferret are closely correlated with the actions of these same hormones in creating a permanent, sexually dimorphic structure in the forebrain.

Research strategies for studying the mechanisms underlying the development of sexually dimorphic patterns of behavior in mammals have derived directly from earlier work of investigators such as Alfred Jost (1960) and Jean Wilson (Wilson et al., 1981), who described in detail the way in which testicular secretions in the male organize the masculine internal and external genital organs. They showed that in female mammals, which possess two X chromosomes (the homogametic sex), development of the genitalia occurs in the absence of any hormonal signal from the ovaries, whereas in males testicular secretions act during fetal life to program the embryogenesis of masculine internal and external genital structures. In male mammals (the heterogametic sex) possession of a Y chromosome (and a X chromosome) typically insures, via mechanisms which remain controversial, that testes will develop *in utero*. Note that in some other vertebrate classes (e.g., birds) the female is the heterogametic sex in which an active genetic signal is required for ovarian development.

In mammals, the fetal male, like the female, possesses both Mullerian and Wolffian ducts prior to the onset of the testicular secretion of hormones (see Figure 9.1). Working with rabbits, Jost (1960) showed that gonadectomy

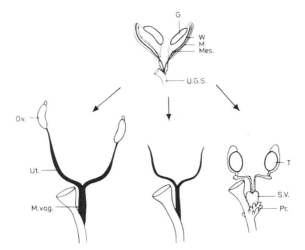

Figure 9.1. Schematic representation of the development of the internal genital ducts in fetal rabbits. The undifferentiated structures (top) differentiate into either the female (bottom left) or male (bottom right) organs. Castrated individuals of either sex develop the feminine structures (bottom middle). G = gonad; W = Wolffian duct; M = Mullerian duct; Mes = mesonephros; UGS = urogental sinus; Ov = ovary; Ut = uterine horns; M. vag. = Mullerian vagina; T = testis; S.V. = seminal vesicle; Pr = prostate. (Reproduced with permission from Jost, 1960)

of either male or female fetuses results in the differentiation of the Mullerian ducts into the uterus and the Mullerian portion of the vagina. The same events occur in females which possess ovaries. By contrast, possession of testes in the male causes the differentiation of the Wolffian ducts into the seminal vesicles and prostate, coupled with the inhibition of Mullerian duct development. Differentiation of the Wolffian ducts in males depends on the action of testosterone (T) during fetal life. By contrast, a second nonsteroidal secretion of the testes (Mullerian-inhibiting substance) actively inhibits the development of the internal Mullerian duct system. Although important details of the embryonic process controlling internal duct differentiation remain to be elucidated (e.g., the identity and mechanism of action of the Mullerian-inhibiting substance), the basic principles first proposed by Jost have been confirmed in a wide variety of mammalian species.

Prior to the age when the testes in males first produce T, male and female fetuses possess identical external genital structures (Figure 9.2). Feminine external genitalia develop in females without any contribution from ovarian secretions. In fetal males, however, T secreted by the testes reaches the external genital primordial structures where it is converted into 5-alpha-dihydrotestosterone (DHT). This metabolite of T promotes the differentiation of the penis and the closure of the scrotal folds, into which the testes later descend.

Given the widespread acceptance of these models for the normal regulation of internal and external genital development, respectively, it is perhaps not

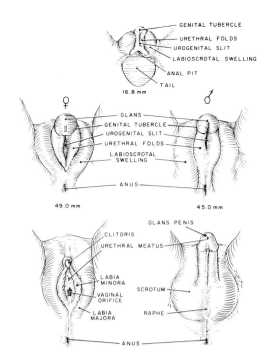

Figure 9.2. Schematic representation of the differentiation of the external genitalia in males (right side) and females (left side) from an indifferent primordium (top-middle), which is identical in the two sexes. (Reproduced with permission from Williams, 1981)

surprising that investigators attempted to extrapolate from them in studying the role of testicular hormones in controlling the development of sexually dimorphic patterns of behavior. Work to date strongly suggests that the differentiation of the neural mechanisms which enable the adult individual to display the sexually appropriate patterns of reproductive behavior parallels the differentiation of the *internal* genital duct systems. That is, during perinatal life male and female mammals possess the potential to develop neural control mechanisms for both masculine and feminine coital behaviors. Typically, in response to the neural action of testicular steroid hormones, males develop the capacity to express masculine sexual behavior whereas they lose the capacity to exhibit feminine coital behavior. However, it is not the case, as for the differentiation of the external genital structures, that these two facets of behavioral sexual differentiation are mutually exclusive. Thus in several mammalian species, males develop the neural mechanisms needed for the expression of masculine sexual behavior without losing the neural mechanisms needed for the adult expression of certain aspects of feminine coital behavior. These issues are discussed more extensively in the following sections.

COITAL MASCULINIZATION

The experiments of William Young and his co-workers (Phoenix et al., 1959; Young et al., 1964) first established that prenatal exposure of female guinea pigs (*Cavia porcellus*) to pharmacological amounts of T permanently enhanced their capacity to display masculine sexual behaviors as adults. That is, if individuals which receive T treatment early in life are gonadectomized as adults and treated with T, they will mount and copulate with an estrous female. This process is called *coital masculinization*. Subsequent work by numerous investigators confirmed this basic finding in several additional mammalian species, although the critical period for the organizational action of steroid hormones differs greatly among different orders. As used here, the term *critical period* refers to the ages during which exposure to steroid hormones affects the developing brain mechanisms which later control behavior. The existence of a critical period is inferred by the observation that perinatal exposure to hormones either prior to or after particular perinatal ages fails to affect behavioral development. In guinea pigs and rhesus monkeys (*Macacca mulatta*), with gestation periods of approximately 68 and 170 days, respectively, the process of coital masculinization seems to occur prenatally. In rat (*Rattus norvegicus*) and ferret, in which gestation lasts approximately 22 and 42 days, respectively, the process is initiated prenatally and completed after birth. In the discussion which follows, the process of coital masculinization will be described in detail for ferrets.

When confronted with an estrous female, a mature male ferret in breeding condition typically displays a combination of behaviors, including neck gripping, mounting, and pelvic thrusting behaviors (see Figure 9.3), which lead to the intromission of the penis into the female's swollen vulva, followed by ejaculation. Even after ovariectomy and treatment with T, adult females typically show little such behavior. In ferrets copulation by the male not only insures that sperm will be passed to the female, but it also initiates a neuroendocrine reflex in the female which causes the secretion of an

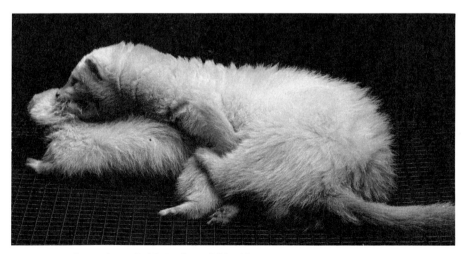

Figure 9.3. Receptive coital behavior exhibited by an estrous female ferret in response to a neck grip and mount by a male.

ovulatory surge in luteinizing hormone (LH) (Carroll et al., 1985). In an initial study groups of female ferrets were exposed to testosterone propionate (TP) either via subcutaneous (s.c.) injections to the pregnant mother during gestation (days 16–34 of a 42-day gestation) or via s.c. injections of the newborn offspring. Animals were then allowed to mature without further treatment, and in adulthood their masculine coital behavior was assessed in the presence of an estrous female. When adult, the ovaries of all females and the testes of control males were removed, whereupon all ferrets were tested for masculine sexual behavior while receiving first no steroid hormones and then daily s.c. injections of TP. As shown in Table 9.1, prenatal exposure to TP, combined with a single injection of TP on postnatal day 3, failed to masculinize females' sexual behavior appreciably, although it did promote the development of a male-like penile sheath. By contrast, other females exposed to TP over the first 10 days of life displayed levels of neck-gripping behavior which resembled that of control males. These females lacked penile structures, suggesting that the behavioral action of the neonatal steroid treatment could best be attributed to an action of the steroid on the developing nervous system.

TABLE 9.1. **Effect of perinatal treatment with testosterone propionate (TP) on neck-gripping behavior of female ferrets (*Mustela furo*) tested in adulthood with estrous females. All ferrets were gonadectomized in adulthood and tested with an estrous female after subcutaneous administration of TP (1 mg/kg) or no hormone. Data are expressed as total number of minutes of neck gripping over three 8-min. tests (mean ± SEM).**

Sex and perinatal treatment	N	Endocrine condition when tested	
		No hormone	TP
Females			
Control	7	0.2 ± 0.1	5.2 ± 1.9
TP days E16–34; day 3	6	0.3 ± 0.1	7.4 ± 2.0
TP day 3	5	0.1 ± 0.1	7.9 ± 3.0
TP days 0–10	4	1.0 ± 0.7	$18.6 \pm 2.9^*$
Males			
Control	6	1.0 ± 0.3	$13.9 \pm 2.9^*$

SOURCE: Adapted from Baum, 1976.

$^*p < .05$, compared with the first three groups of females.

In another study, female ferrets were exposed to either a low or a high dosage of T during different perinatal periods. In addition, males were deprived of their testicular secretions by castration at different postnatal ages. After concurrent T treatment in adulthood, very little neck-grip behavior was displayed by female ferrets which received either high or low dosages of T over the last 11 days of gestation (Figure 9.4). By contrast, females exposed to a high dosage of T (administered via s.c. implantation of

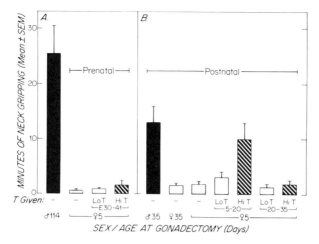

Figure 9.4. Effect of prenatal (A) versus neonatal (B) exposure of female ferrets to testosterone (T) on their expression of neck-grip behavior after T treatment in adulthood. Lo and Hi T refer to low versus high dosages of testosterone given over the perinatal ages indicated. E30–41 refers to postconception days in utero. (Data are adapted from Baum and Erskine, 1984, and from Tobet and Baum, 1986)

a Silastic capsule containing the steroid) over postnatal days 5–20 showed a high degree of coital masculinization. No such effect was obtained in females given T over days 20–35. Males castrated on postnatal days 20 and 35 displayed equivalent levels of neck gripping after treatment with T in adulthood, whereas males castrated on day 5, like control females, displayed very low levels of this behavior (Figure 9.5). Taken together, these behavioral data suggest that in the male ferret the critical period for coital

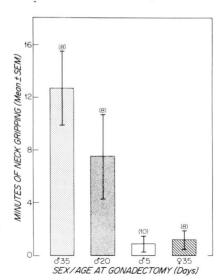

Figure 9.5. Effect of neonatal castration of male ferrets on the expression of neck-grip behavior after testosterone treatment in adulthood. (Adapted from Baum and Erskine, 1984)

masculinization begins shortly after birth and is completed by postnatal day 20.

In light of these results, it was of interest to know whether circulating concentrations of T differ in male and female ferrets during perinatal development. The results of such a study are shown in Figure 9.6. Significant sex differences in plasma T occurred at several perinatal ages, the first being 5 days prior to birth (earlier ages were not studied) followed by postnatal days 10 and 15. Clearly, there is a correspondence between the existence of greater plasma T levels in males at postnatal days 10 and 15 and the suggestion from the behavioral studies already described that coital masculinization normally occurs in male ferrets between birth and postnatal day 20.

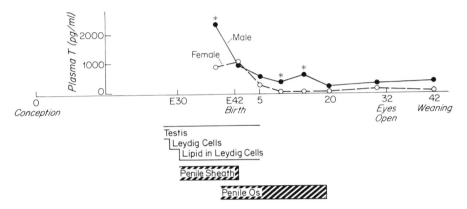

Figure 9.6. Plasma testosterone in male and female ferrets during perinatal development. The timing of critical events in testicular and external genital development in males is also indicated. *$p < .05$, male values greater than female values. E30 and E42 refer to postconceptional days. (Adapted from Erskine and Baum, 1982)

When taken together, these data suggest that in the male ferret, as in males of all other mammalian species which have been studied to date, T acts during a specific perinatal period to cause coital masculinization. By themselves, the behavioral results presented above suggest that in male ferrets this period extends between postnatal days 5 and 20. However, additional data call into question such a simplistic explanation of the neuroendocrine events which lead to coital masculinization. To examine this, groups of male and female ferrets were exposed to the same dosages of T (either delivered to fetuses via T administration to the pregnant mother or directly to the newly born offspring) as had been used in the behavioral study whose results are shown in Figure 9.4. Interestingly, when killed on gestational day 41, fetuses whose mothers were exposed to a low dosage of T had circulating concentrations of T that were slightly higher than those measured in males at this age. Fetuses derived from mothers which received the high dosage of T had considerably higher plasma levels of T (Figure 9.7).

Hormonal Control of Sex Differences in Mammals   Chap. 9

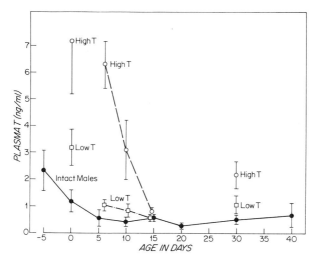

Figure 9.7. Plasma concentrations of testosterone (T) resulting from exogenous perinatal treatment of ferrets with T. High or low dosages of T were given via subcutaneous implantation of Silastic capsules containing this steroid: (a) to pregnant mothers over days 30–42 of gestation, (b) on postnatal day 5 to males and females which were gonadectomized at the same time, and subsequently killed on days 6, 10, or 15, or (c) on postnatal day 20 to males and females which were gonadectomized at the same time and killed on day 30. Data for gonadally intact male ferrets for the ages indicated are given for sake of comparison. (Adapted from Baum and Erskine, 1984; Erskine and Baum, 1982; and Tobet et al., 1985)

Neither group of females was coitally masculinized, a finding which strengthens the argument that an important aspect of this process normally occurs neonatally in the male ferret. The fact that females exposed to both low and high dosages of T between postnatal days 20 and 30 were not coitally masculinized, even though they had plasma T levels which were elevated over that previously measured over this age range in gonadally intact males, further points to the period between birth and day 20 as a critical one for coital masculinization in males. It is important to note, however, that females exposed to the low dosage of T between postnatal days 5 and 20 had plasma levels of T which were slightly higher than those measured in gonadally intact males at the same ages, yet these females were only slightly masculinized (see Figure 9.4). Females exposed over days 5–20 to a high dosage of T later exhibited a high level of masculine coital behavior; however, during the neonatal period of exposure to T it seems likely that plasma T levels were six times higher than those which are typically present in gonadally intact males at this age.

These data suggest that considerably less circulating T is required neonatally in the gonadally intact male ferret to cause coital masculinization than is required in females when they receive their steroid from an exogenous source. Stated differently, during neonatal life the male brain is more sensitive than the female brain to the masculinizing action of T. This observation in ferrets provides empirical support for a similar hypothesis first made by Judith Weisz and Ingeborg Ward in 1980. They suggested that prenatal elevations in circulating T, which normally occur in male rats, sensitize the developing nervous system to the postnatal action of testicular steroids, thereby promoting the organization of masculine behavioral capacities. As shown in Figure 9.6, plasma T concentrations are elevated prenatally in male ferrets, just as they are in male rats. The question is whether prenatal exposure of the brain to steroid hormones contributes to the process of coital masculinization in males. Data already presented show that prenatal elevation of plasma T levels in females, by itself, fails to cause coital masculinization. This observation does not, however, rule out the possibility that prenatal exposure to T, or a neural metabolite of T, enhances the ability of postnatal hormone exposure to cause masculinization in normal males. This question will be dealt with in the following section, insofar as the answer is closely linked to the issue of which steroid molecule acts in the developing male brain to cause coital masculinization.

NEURAL METABOLISM OF TESTOSTERONE: CONTRIBUTION TO COITAL MASCULINIZATION

As stated at the outset, research on the neuroendocrine regulation of behavioral sexual differentiation has evolved directly from work on genital differentiation. An important aspect of this work is the demonstration that differentiation of the external genitalia in the male depends on the conversion of T into its 5-alpha-reduced metabolite, DHT, in the undifferentiated external genital tissues. Metabolism of T by 5-alpha reduction occurs in the brains of fetal and adult individuals in a wide variety of vertebrate species. In addition to 5-alpha reduction of T, certain subcortical brain structures contain an enzyme complex, aromatase, which catalyzes the conversion of T into estrogenic metabolites. Studies have been conducted using the ferret to determine whether neural aromatization of T occurs during the period of sexual differentiation, and whether any aspect of behavioral sexual differentiation depends on the action of estrogenic metabolites of T formed in the developing male nervous system.

In an initial study the brains of male and female ferrets were collected at various pre- and postnatal ages and dissected as shown in Figure 9.8. Brain areas were then homogenized in phosphate buffer and incubated for one hour with the androgen [3H]19-hydroxyandrostendione, an immediate precursor of the estrogen, estrone. The cofactor, NADPH, was also added as a source of electrons in the formation of estrone. High levels of aromatase activity were present in several subcortical regions, including the preoptic area (POA), mediobasal hypothalamus (MBH), and temporal lobe (amygdala) during the late gestational and early postnatal periods (Figure 9.9). Very low aromatase activity was detected in cerebral cortex at these perinatal ages; in adulthood aromatase activity was also greatly reduced in subcortical sites. Aromatase activity in the POA + MBH was significantly

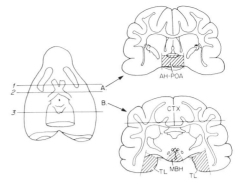

Figure 9.8. Schematic diagram of the dissection used to obtain neural tissues from the anterior hypothalamus-preoptic area (AH-POA), temporal lobe, including amygdala (TL), mediobasal hypothalamus (MBH), and cerebral cortex (CTX) of male and female ferrets. Two slabs of brain tissue (A and B) were formed by making three coronal cuts (1, 2, and 3). (Reproduced with permission from Vito et al., 1985)

higher in males than in females at both prenatal ages studied, whereas there were no significant sex differences during postnatal life.

It is well established that steroid hormones exert their action on target cells by interacting with subcellular protein receptors. These receptors

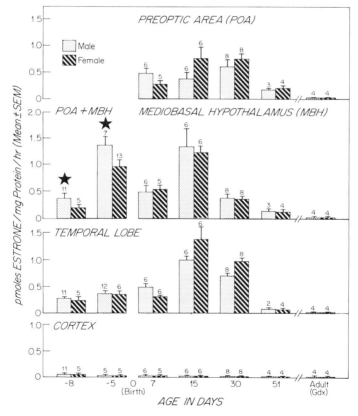

Figure 9.9. Aromatase activity in different brain regions of male and female ferrets killed at different perinatal ages or in adulthood after gonadectomy (Gdx). At star, $p < .05$ sex comparison. (Reproduced with permission from Tobet et al., 1985)

facilitate the interaction of the steroid with DNA in the cell nucleus, leading to the synthesis of messenger RNA and eventually to changes in the intracellular synthesis of protein. Much research suggests that the developing CNS, like nonneural target tissues, responds to androgen and estrogen only if the respective receptors for these hormones are present. As shown in Figure 9.10, receptors for androgen (e.g., either T or DHT) as well as estrogen (e.g., estradiol or estrone) are present in the brains of male and

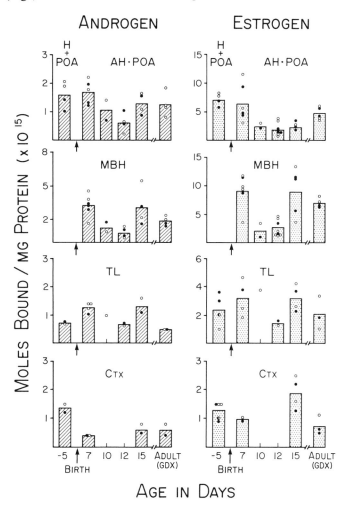

Figure 9.10. Concentration of androgen and estrogen receptors in cytosol extracts of pooled male (black dots) and pooled female (open dots) regions of brains taken from ferrets at different perinatal ages and in adulthood after gonadectomy (Gdx). See caption to Figure 9.8 for abbreviations. Quantitation of receptor concentrations was carried out using DNA-cellulose affinity chromatography. Cytosols were incubated with saturating concentrations of 3H-dihydrotestosterone (to measure androgen receptor) or 3H-estradiol (to measure estrogen receptor). (Reproduced with permission from Vito et al., 1985)

female ferrets as early as 5 days prior to birth (the earliest age sampled) and extending into adulthood. Thus the potential for androgenic as well as estrogenic effects on neural and behavioral differentiation exists throughout the neonatal period (e.g., postnatal days 5–20) when testicular secretions seem to promote coital masculinization. Moreover, the potential for both androgen and estrogen action is also present prenatally, when the developing male brain is probably being "sensitized" to the later postnatal masculinizing action of sex steroids.

Several studies have been conducted with ferrets to assess the relative roles of prenatal and neonatal estrogen versus androgen receptor activation in controlling the process of coital masculinization. In an initial study high dosages of T, DHT, or estradiol (E2) were administered over postnatal days 0–15 to gonadally intact female ferrets and their masculine coital behavior was studied in adulthood (Figure 9.11). Females exposed neonatally to this dosage of T displayed as much neck-gripping behavior in adulthood as control males, provided T was given at the time of testing. Females given DHT neonatally were no more active than control females which received empty capsules over postnatal days 0–15. A slight stimulation of masculine coital behavior occurred in females exposed neonatally to E2; however, the level of behavior exhibited by these females was significantly lower than that displayed by T-treated females and control males.

In another study male ferrets were implanted s.c. over postnatal days 0–15 with androst-1,4,6-triene-3,17-dione (ATD), a steroid which inhibits aromatase activity by competing with T for the enzyme. Although hypotha-

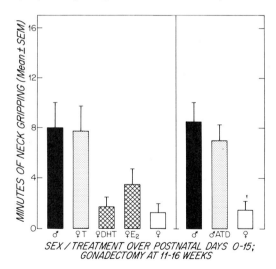

Figure 9.11. Effect of neonatal administration of testosterone (T), dihydrotestosterone (DHT), or estradiol (E2) to female ferrets (left panel) or the aromatase inhibitor, ATD, to male ferrets (right panel) on the expression of neck-grip behavior after testosterone treatment in adulthood. Hormones or drugs were given between postnatal days 0–15 via Silastic capsules which were implanted subcutaneously. (Adapted from Baum et al., 1982, and Baum et al., 1983)

lamic aromatase activity was strongly inhibited, males given this neonatal treatment and later tested for masculine sexual behavior in adulthood displayed levels of neck-gripping which were equivalent to those of control males (Figure 9.11). These findings strongly suggest that aromatization of T during neonatal life contributes little, if anything, to the process of coital masculinization. Likewise, the inability of DHT to mimic the masculinizing action of T in females suggests that this 5-alpha-reduced metabolite of T is not involved in the control of coital masculinization. As in the case of the internal Wolffian duct system, T itself appears to act neonatally in the male ferret brain to promote coital masculinization.

The results of another study strongly suggest that prenatal exposure of the male brain to estrogenic metabolites of circulating T sensitizes it to the subsequent masculinizing action of T during early postnatal life. Pregnant ferrets were given different treatments over gestational days 30–41, whereupon the litters were delivered by caesarian section, cross-fostered to other lactating females, gonadectomized on postnatal day 5, and then tested for masculine coital behavior in adulthood while receiving daily injections of a high dosage of TP. Under these testing conditions control males gonadectomized on day 5 still showed a measurable level of neck-gripping behavior, although it was significantly lower than the level displayed by other males which were castrated on postnatal day 114 (Figure 9.12A, B, and C). Administration of Silastic capsules containing the aromatase inhibitor, ATD, to pregnant mothers strongly inhibited the activity of aromatase in the hypothalami of male and female offspring. Other male offspring, whose mothers received ATD in addition to being ovariectomized and given progesterone to maintain pregnancy, displayed significantly lower levels of neck gripping in adulthood than control males. Administering a low dosage of E2 to mothers failed to counteract the suppressive effect of maternal ovariectomy and ATD treatment on neck gripping. Administration of a high

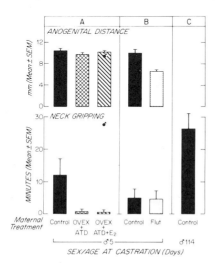

Figure 9.12. Effect of prenatal reductions in estrogenic (A) versus androgenic (B) stimulation of male ferret fetuses on the expression of neck-grip behavior after testosterone treatment in adulthood and on anogenital distance measured at the time of caesarian delivery on day 42 of gestation. Ovex = maternal ovariectomy; ATD = subcutaneous implantation into pregnant ferrets of Silastic capsules containing the aromatase inhibitor, ATD; E$_2$ = estradiol given in a dilute dosage; flut = 2× daily subcutaneous injections of the antiandrogen, flutamide, to pregnant ferrets; ♂ = data from 1 surviving male whose mother was ovariectomized and received progesterone, ATD, and a high dosage of E$_2$. (Adapted from Tobet and Baum, 1986)

dosage of E2 to other ovariectomized, ATD-treated mothers caused a high incidence of mortality in newborn offspring; however, one male whose mother had received this treatment survived into adulthood, and when given TP and tested with an estrous female it displayed as high a level of neck-gripping as the control males which had been castrated on day 114. Surprisingly, this occurred even though this estrogen-exposed male had been castrated on day 5.

Prenatal exposure of male ferrets to the androgen receptor antagonist, flutamide, caused significant reductions in anogenital distance, a sensitive index of androgenic action in the developing genital tubercle (Figure 9.12B, top). This proves that flutamide passes across the placenta and reaches the fetuses. Yet prenatal exposure to this antiandrogen failed to attenuate the coital responsiveness of males, assessed in adulthood after further treatment with TP. As already described, plasma concentrations of T are significantly higher in male than in female ferrets prenatally, and the activity of aromatase in the hypothalamus + POA is also higher in males than in females. Both of these factors likely result in a significantly higher production of estrogen in specific brain regions of developing male ferrets. The behavioral results suggest that this estrogen contributes to the process of coital masculinization. Studies by Pierre Corbier (Corbier et al., 1978) and Koos Slob (Slob et al., 1980) show that plasma levels of T rise dramatically in male, but not female, rats within a few hours after birth. Plasma T then drops precipitously within a few hours. Mary Erskine, Stuart Tobet, and I have recently observed a similar phenomenon in male ferrets within 2 hours after caesarian delivery. The behavioral data shown in Figure 9.12 suggest that prenatal exposure of the male ferret to estrogen, produced locally in the brain, contributes to coital masculinization. It is possible that in the control males castrated on postnatal day 5 this estrogenic stimulation sensitized the developing brain to the masculinizing action of an acute, postdelivery surge in circulating T. In males castrated at later postnatal ages this immediate postnatal surge in T, plus the more sustained elevation in circulating T previously observed in male ferrets between days 5 and 20 (Figure 9.6), may further facilitate coital masculinization.

Although the research of others using rats and hamsters (*Mesocricetus auratus*) has implicated estrogenic metabolites of androgen in the control of coital masculinization, these results in the ferret are the first to suggest a sequential action of estrogen and androgen in controlling this aspect of behavioral sexual differentiation. They also raise the possibility that these two steroids act synergistically to cause coital masculinization in diverse orders of mammals. To date, no experimental studies on the role of estrogen in controlling any aspect of brain or behavioral sexual differentiation have been conducted using nonhuman primates. However, Anke Erhardt and co-workers (Erhardt et al., 1985) reported that the incidence of bisexual or homosexual orientation is significantly higher in women whose mothers received a potent synthetic estrogen, diethylstilbestrol, during pregnancy. This estrogen was widely prescribed during the 1950s and 1960s to pregnant women thought to be at risk for spontaneous abortion. Attention was subsequently drawn to their female offspring, who frequently contracted vagino-cervical cancer. The recent observation of a higher incidence of homo/bisexual orientation in these women raises the question of whether in man, as in ferrets and other nonprimate mammals, estrogen formed in the developing male brain normally contributes to the process of masculine psychosexual differentiation (see Chapter 12).

COITAL DEFEMINIZATION

As explained above, the differentiation of the Mullerian ducts in fetal males is actively inhibited by the action of the Mullerian-inhibiting substance produced by the testes. To date there is no evidence that this protein hormone is secreted into the peripheral circulation of the male during fetal life, nor is it known whether this hormone affects the development of the male's central nervous system (CNS) in any way. It is clear, however, that the ability to exhibit certain feminine coital behaviors, which normally develops in females, is in some instances actively blocked in the male by the action of testicular steroid hormones. For example, exposing fetal female guinea pigs to T permanently reduces their ability as adults to express the receptive posture of lordosis, following ovariectomy and injection of ovarian hormones in adulthood (Phoenix et al., 1959).

Males of numerous rodent species will exhibit low levels of feminine reproductive behavior, if castrated and treated with estrogen and progesterone in adulthood. By contrast, males which are castrated at birth, or which are given ATD neonatally to block the neural synthesis of estrogen from circulating androgen, display high levels of receptive behavior in adulthood, if given exogenous ovarian hormones. These findings suggest that in rodents estrogenic metabolites of circulating androgen act perinatally to *defeminize* the receptive capacity of males. It seems likely that a similar process occurs in males of several additional nonrodent mammalian species, including dog (*Canis familiaris*), pig (*Sus scrofa*), and sheep (*Capra ammotragus*).

Given the ubiquity of these findings, it was very surprising to discover that perinatal administration of TP to female ferrets fails to attenuate their capacity to display the receptive coital posture illustrated in Figure 9.3. As shown in Table 9.2, neither pre- nor early postnatal treatment with TP reduced females' later acceptance of male neck-grips, regardless of whether they were tested while gonadally intact and in estrus or after ovariectomy and daily injections of estrogen. Also notable is the finding that male ferrets, castrated as adults and treated with estrogen, are as receptive to the courtship behavior of other males as the various groups of females which have been tested. The work of several investigators, including Jan Thorton, Steve Pomerantz, and Robert Goy (Pomerantz et al., 1986; Thornton and Goy, 1986) as well as Kathleen Chambers and Charles Phoenix (Phoenix et al., 1983), has revealed a similar persistence of feminine receptive behavior

TABLE 9.2. Effect of perinatal treatment with testosterone propionate (TP) on receptive behavior of female ferrets (*Mustela furo*) tested in adulthood with a sexually active male. Ferrets were tested in adulthood while in estrus (females) and after gonadectomy and subcutaneous administration of no hormone or estradiol benzoate (EB; 10 µg/kg) (all animals). Data are expressed as the percentage of time that animals tested displayed a limp, receptive posture in response to a neck grip by the stimulus male (mean ± SEM).

Sex and perinatal treatment	N	Endocrine condition when tested		
			Gonadectomized	
		Intact estrus	No hormone	EB
Females				
Control	7	96 ± 2	2 ± 1	97 ± 1
TP days E16–34; day 3	6	97 ± 1	1 ± 1	95 ± 2
TP day 3	5	98 ± 1	0	96 ± 1
TP days 0–10	4	98 ± 1	5 ± 3	98 ± 1
Males				
Control	6	–	–	97 ± 1

SOURCE: Adapted from Baum, 1976.

in female rhesus monkeys exposed prenatally to T. Rhesus males castrated soon after birth (at a time well after the prenatal period of brain sexual differentiation) also show receptive feminine sexual behavior after adult treatment with ovarian hormones.

It is not understood why perinatal exposure to testicular hormones defeminizes receptive behavior in some mammalian species but not in others. It is the case, however, that male ferrets and rhesus monkeys can both be induced to express the posture normally associated with feminine receptivity in the context of social interactions which are not explicitly sexual. For example, rhesus monkeys of both sexes frequently signal subordinance to a more dominant animal by displaying a behavior which is indistinguishable from a receptive response. Unlike lordotic responses, this receptive behavior is not reflexive, and in males the neural mechanisms which control its expression are not defeminized during perinatal life.

Until fairly recently, investigators interested in the hormonal regulation of feminine sexual behavior and in the process of behavioral defeminization, as it occurs in males undergoing sexual differentiation, concentrated exclusively on the regulation of receptive behavior. This behavior could only be studied in the presence of a specific somatosensory stimulus (e.g., a neck-grip from a male ferret, or a mount with flank palpation from a male rat or rhesus monkey). Primatologists such as Barry Keverne (Keverne, 1976) and Ronald Nadler (Nadler, 1981) had described seasonal and monthly fluctuations in the degree to which females of several nonhuman primate species will seek out and initiate sexual interaction with males. Based on an analysis of this primate work, and as a result of some of his own observations on rats, dogs, and hamsters, Frank Beach (Beach, 1976) proposed that the term *proceptive behavior* be applied to aspects of feminine sexual behavior which initiate or maintain sexual interaction with a male partner. This conceptual distinction between receptive and proceptive feminine sexual behavior has had important consequences for research on behavioral sexual differentiation.

Several investigators, including Paula Davis, Bruce McEwen, Barbara Fadem, and Ronald Barfield (Davis et al., 1979; Fadem and Barfield, 1981) have shown that proceptive behavior in male rats, like receptive responsiveness to ovarian hormones, is greatly attenuated as a consequence of the action of testicular hormones during perinatal life. Similar data have been obtained in dogs by Frank Beach (Beach et al., 1977). In light of the nonoccurrence of receptive defeminization in male ferrets, it became of interest to assess the development of proceptive responsiveness in males of this species. Tests of sexual behavior typically occur in a confined observation box, and under these circumstances estrous female ferrets display very little proceptive behavior. Primatologists had found, however, that requiring a female to perform an operant response (e.g., pressing a lever to gain access to the male) enabled the investigator to assess more precisely the proceptive capacity of the animal. In my experiments, ferrets are required to perform an operant response (running over a distance of nearly 2 meters) in order to gain access to a stud male. As shown in Figure 9.13, control females ovariectomized on postnatal day 35 display a progressive reduction in their latency to approach a stud male in response to daily administration of increasing

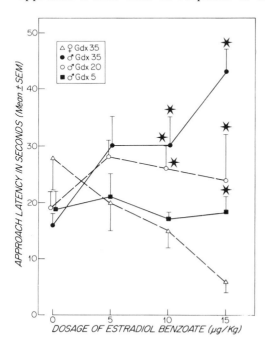

Figure 9.13. Proceptive behavior of male and female ferrets which were gonadectomized (Gdx) at different early postnatal ages and which in adulthood received daily injections of increasing dosages of estradiol benzoate (EB) while being allowed to approach a stud male in an L-shaped runway. Stars indicate significantly greater than female control value for each indicated EB dosage. (Reproduced with permission from Baum et al., 1985)

dosages of estradiol benzoate (EB). Males castrated on day 35 ran progressively slower to a stud male in response to EB, and males castrated on days 20 and 5 were intermediate between the extremes of the male and female control groups. These findings suggest that postnatal exposure of the male ferret to testicular secretions (or neural metabolites thereof) promotes the defeminization of the mechanism controlling proceptive behavior. It was interesting to discover, however, that castration on postnatal day 5 did not cause males to display approach latencies which were similar to those of control females. This suggests that testicular hormones also act in the male prior to this age to cause proceptive defeminization.

The results of another study (Figure 9.14) indicate that the estrogenic metabolites of T formed prenatally in the male ferret brain exert such an action. The males used in this study were the same ferrets used in the study of coital masculinization (Figure 9.12). All males were castrated on postnatal day 5, thereby reducing the defeminizing action of any testicular hormone which would otherwise have occurred after this age. Control males were derived of mothers which were simply given s.c. implants containing progesterone on gestational day 30 and were subjected to caesarian section on gestational day 42. These males displayed approach latency profiles which were very similar to those of the day-5 castrates shown in Figure 9.13; approach latencies were short, but constant irrespective of the dosage of EB received at the time of testing. By contrast, males in which the availability of estrogenic stimulation was reduced over the last part of gestation displayed significant reductions in approach latencies as a consequence of EB treatment which very much resemble those of normal females (compare Figures 9.13 and 9.14). Administration of a low dosage of E2 to pregnant females failed to reverse the effects of maternal ovariectomy + ATD treatment on the approach latencies of male offspring. Significantly, however, one surviving male whose mother received a high dosage of E2, in addition to being ovariectomized and given ATD, showed approach latencies similar to those of control males.

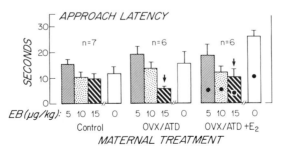

Figure 9.14. Effect of prenatal deprivation of estrogenic stimulation on proceptive responsiveness of male ferrets which were castrated on postnatal day 5 and subsequently in adulthood were treated with estradiol benzoate (EB) and allowed to approach a stud male in an L-shaped runway. Arrows point to a significant dose-dependent reduction in approach latency. See caption to Figure 9.12 for more information. (Adapted from Baum and Tobet, 1986)

These results show that male ferrets, like males of the other nonprimate mammalian orders studied to date, are defeminized proceptively as a consequence of the perinatal action of testicular steroids. Again, this process depends at least in part on the neural conversion of androgen into estrogen. Studies already referred to (Thornton and Goy, 1986; Pomerantz et al., 1986) have shown that proceptive defeminization also typically occurs in rhesus monkeys as a consequence of prenatal exposure to T. When tested with a sexually active stud male tethered in one corner of a large observation cage, female rhesus monkeys which had been exposed prenatally to T or DHT displayed lower levels of proceptive behavior (i.e., solicitational responses) than did control females while receiving estrogen. The same was true of males castrated shortly after birth and tested in this situation. As stated earlier, no experiments have been conducted to assess the contribution in male primates of estrogenic metabolites of T to any aspect of behavioral sexual differentiation. Until such studies are attempted, we can only speculate, based on results obtained in studies of rats, hamsters, and ferrets, that a similar estrogen-dependent process occurs in primates.

SEXUAL DIFFERENTIATION OF THE BRAIN

In the discussion of their paper describing the long-term behavioral consequences of prenatal exposure of female guinea pigs to T, Phoenix, Goy, Gerall, and Young (1959) speculated that the prenatal steroid treatment had somehow "organized" brain mechanisms which later control the expression of reproductive behavior. Their use of the term *organizational* represented a direct extrapolation from a by then well-established dogma in embryology. As discussed earlier, it was and continues to be thought that androgens secreted by the fetal testes organize the transformation of primordial internal and external genitalia into the genital structures characteristic of the newborn male. Phoenix et al. (1959) distinguished this developmental effect of hormones from the "activational" effect of sex steroids in adult individuals. In the case of genital tissues, such activational effects of adult hormone exposure are reflected either in the occurrence of cell proliferation or a stimulation of secretory activity in existent organs. By analogy, in the case of the brain it has been proposed (Young et al., 1964) that sex steroid hormones activate existent hormonal circuits, thereby contributing to the expression of patterns of sexually dimorphic behavior.

Despite the publication of numerous behavioral studies representing several different mammalian species, as well as the publication of data showing that in nonprimate mammals the neuroendocrine regulation of luteinizing hormone and prolactin secretion is different in the two sexes, scientists remained skeptical that such functional sex dimorphisms could be explained in terms of visible, morphological differences between the brains of males and females. Such evidence was eventually forthcoming in 1973, however, when Geoffrey Raisman and Pauline Field used electron microscopy to analyze the synaptic connectivity of the rat preoptic area (POA). They discovered that the dendrites of the POA receive a higher proportion of afferent inputs onto dendritic spines in females than in males. Furthermore, neonatal castration of male rats created the female phenotype of dendritic organization, whereas neonatal administration of TP to females created the male phenotype. This work was the first to suggest that sex steroid hormones act directly on the developing male brain literally to "organize" neural circuits which in later life control behavior and other aspects of neuroendocrine function.

After this discovery, progress linking sex steroid hormone-induced changes in neural morphology with functional changes was, however, very limited. In 1976, Fernando Nottebohm and Arthur Arnold working with zebra finches (*Poephila guttata*) and canaries (*Serinus canarius*) reported that the volume of forebrain nuclei which control singing is significantly greater in males than in females. This sex difference, which was subsequently shown to depend in part on post-hatching exposure of the male to estrogen (Gurney, 1981), correlated beautifully with the dimorphic control of song production in these species (typically only the male sings). Since this early work, numerous studies representing several different vertebrate classes have established unambiguously that sex differences in neural morphology exist, and that sex steroid hormones acting perinatally in the male brain are responsible for these differences.

Following the work of Nottebohm and Arnold, other investigators including Roger Gorski and co-workers (Gorski et al., 1980; Hines et al., 1985) and Pauline Yahr and Deborah Commins (Commins and Yahr, 1984a) found that nuclei exist in the POA of the rat, guinea pig, and gerbil which are significantly larger and contain more neurons in males than in females. Working with ferrets, Stuart Tobet, David Zahniser, and I (Tobet et al., 1986) found that males possess a nucleus in the dorsal portion of the anterior hypothalamus-POA (AH-POA) which is not present in females. As shown diagrammatically in Figure 9.15, this sexually dimorphic dorsal nucleus of the AH-POA is visible in the same coronal plane as another ventral nucleus, which is present in both sexes. The dorsal nucleus in males consists primarily of neurons with large cell bodies.

Additional experiments showed that neither neonatal nor adult administration of sex steroids to female ferrets succeeded in organizing dorsal POA nuclei. Also, neonatal castration of males failed to block the development of a dorsal nucleus, suggesting that the organization of this nucleus in males occurs prenatally. Tobet confirmed this prediction by showing that prenatal exposure of female ferrets to T (administered to their mothers over gestational days 30–41) promoted the formation of dorsal nuclei of the AH-POA (Figure 9.16A); female offspring of these T-treated mothers possessed dorsal nuclei whose estimated volumes were similar to those of untreated control males.

Additional evidence suggests that the organization of dorsal nuclei in males depends on the action of estrogenic metabolites of circulating T, as

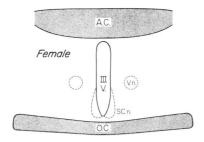

Female

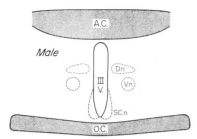

Male

Figure 9.15. Sexual dimorphism in ferrets at the border of the preoptic-anterior hypothalamic area. Bilateral ventral nuclei (V.n.) are present in both sexes, whereas only males possess dorsal nuclei (D.n.). A.C. = anterior commissure; III V. = third ventricle; SC.n. = suprachiasmatic nuclei; O.C. = optic chiasm. (Adapted from results presented in Tobet et al., 1986)

opposed to the action of androgen. Thus, prenatal exposure to the androgen receptor antagonist, flutamide, failed to block the development of dorsal nuclei in males. By contrast, prenatal reduction of estrogenic stimulation, achieved via ovariectomy + ATD treatment of the mother, completely inhibited the development of dorsal AH-POA nuclei in males (Figure 9.16B and 9.16C). Administration of a low dosage of E2 to females, in addition to

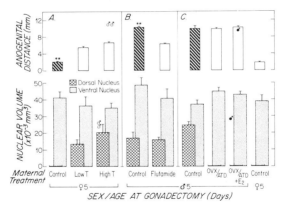

Figure 9.16. Effect of prenatal exposure to (A) different dosages of testosterone (T), (B) the antiandrogen, flutamide, or (C) treatments which reduce estrogen availability on the estimated volume of the dorsal and ventral nuclei of the preoptic-anterior hypothalamic area and on anogenital distance at birth in male and female ferrets. Data are expressed as mean ± SEM. ♂ = data for two male ferrets whose mother received the high dosage of testosterone. ♂̇ = data from one male whose mother was ovariectomized and received progesterone, ATD, and a high dosage of E_2. See the caption to Figure 9.12 for further details. (Reproduced with permission from Tobet et al., 1986a)

ovariectomy and ATD treatment, failed to restore dorsal nuclei in males; however, the one surviving male whose mother received a high dosage of E2 in addition to ovariectomy and ATD possessed dorsal nuclei of the AH-POA which were indistinguishable from those of control males. As shown in Figure 9.16, the volumes of the ventral nuclei of POA/AH were equivalent in all groups of ferrets.

These results show that in a carnivore, the ferret, the development of a gross structural dimorphism of the AH-POA depends on the action of estrogen in the male. Data supporting the same conclusion have been obtained by Klaus Dohler in the rat (Dohler et al., 1984) and by Mark Gurney (Gurney, 1981) in the zebra finch. Although more data are needed from additional species representing other vertebrate classes, the available evidence consistently suggests that estrogens act in the developing male forebrain to organize its nuclear structure. In songbirds this estrogen may be derived directly from the circulation, insofar as John Hutchison, Rose Hutchison, and John Wingfield (Hutchison et al., 1984) have reported that circulating concentrations of estradiol are actually higher immediately after hatching in male than in female zebra finches. In mammals, however, consistent sex differences in circulating levels of estradiol during perinatal life have not been detected. By contrast, in the few mammalian species which have been studied (e.g., rat, rabbit, ferret) significant sex differences in circulating T and/or in brain aromatase activity have been found, both of which could result in greater neural production of estrogen from androgenic precursor in males than in females.

Beginning early in development, large numbers of neurons throughout the brain are predestined to die. It has been suggested, though not proven, that exposure to E2 during the perinatal period somehow protects forebrain neurons from degeneration and death (Arnold and Gorski, 1984). Some evidence suggests that the source of this estrogen to the developing male brain may have changed in the course of evolution. As discussed earlier, in birds the primary source seemingly resides outside the brain, insofar as in at least one species circulating levels of estradiol are higher in males than in females shortly after hatching. By contrast, in several mammalian species (Erskine and Baum, 1984) plasma concentrations of estradiol are equivalent in males and females during the period of brain sexual differentiation. It seems likely that male mammals attain higher degrees of estrogenic stimulation than females in particular brain regions via local aromatization of greater amounts of androgenic substrate. The fact remains, however, that in ferrets, as well as in other mammalian and nonmammalian vertebrate species, the female is also exposed perinatally to considerable estrogenic stimulation. This raises the question of whether, in addition to its selective action in the male forebrain, estrogen also promotes neuronal longevity in the female. Clearly, much more information concerning the effects of estrogen on neuronal survival is needed to answer this question.

As stated earlier, a strong relationship has been demonstrated in songbirds between the existence of larger song-control nuclei in males than in females and the ability of the male to learn song and to sing after adult exposure to T. In male rats no correlation has been found between the existence of a large nucleus of the medial AH-POA and any sexually dimorphic, functional attribute (Arendash and Gorski, 1983). By contrast, in gerbils the presence in males of a dense group of cells in the dorsal portion of the AH-POA (which resembles the sexually dimorphic nucleus present in male ferrets) has been correlated with the males' ability to exhibit masculine sexual behavior after androgen exposure in adulthood (Commins and Yahr, 1984b). Additional examples of similar relationships between sexually dimorphic neuronal structure and function are awaited in other mammalian species.

In the ferret a correlation clearly exists between the ability of prenatal inhibition of estrogen biosynthesis to inhibit dorsal nucleus formation in males and the severe disruption of their later ability to exhibit masculine coital behavior (i.e., coital masculinization is presumably inhibited). The possible relationship between this morphological effect of prenatal estrogenic deprivation on POA neurons and the deficit in masculine coital capacity is particularly obvious in light of the extensive work of Benjamin Hart and co-workers (Hart et al., 1973), who showed that damage to the medial POA disrupts masculine coital performance in males of diverse mammalian orders, as well as in other vertebrate classes. It is clear, however, that in ferrets the mere possession of dorsal nuclei of the AH-POA does not guarantee that an individual will be able to exhibit masculine behavior in response to T exposure in adulthood: females exposed prenatally to T possess dorsal nuclei, yet display low (female-like) levels of neck-gripping, mounting, and pelvic thrusting (see Figure 9.4). Estrogenic metabolites of T may act prenatally in male ferrets to preserve the dorsal nuclei, whereas T itself may act neonatally to insure that appropriate connections are established between cells in these nuclei and other brain sites (Tobet et al., 1986). Both events may be needed to insure that an individual is maximally responsive to the later activational effect of T in controlling the expression of masculine coital behavior.

Evidence already summarized shows that sex steroid hormones, acting in the male mammal, independently affect the processes of coital masculinization and defeminization. The occurrence of coital masculinization and of proceptive defeminization has been documented in every mammal species studied to date, whereas the defeminization of receptive behavior occurs in some mammals but not in others. In males at least some of the behavioral actions of testicular hormone during development depend upon the neural aromatization of androgen to estrogen. An emerging body of literature has clearly shown that permanent sex differences in neuronal organization exist at different levels of the CNS. The central challenge for future research is to identify the mechanisms whereby androgen and estrogen promote the development of these dimorphisms and to establish in mammals unambiguous links between sex differences in neural morphology and the ability of members of each sex to exhibit particular patterns of overt behavior and neuroendocrine function.

ACKNOWLEDGMENT

Research in the author's laboratory is supported by U.S. Public Health Service grant HD21094. The author is recipient of Research Scientist Development Award MH000392 from the National Institute of Mental Health. I gratefully acknowledge the contributions of my colleagues, Mary Erskine, Stuart Tobet, Jacob Canick, Christine Vito, and Tom Fox to the research findings and ideas presented in this chapter.

REFERENCES

ARENDASH, G.W., and R.A. GORSKI (1983) Effects of discrete lesions of the sexually dimorphic nucleus of the preoptic area or other medial preoptic regions on the sexual behavior of male rats. Brain Res. Bull. *10*:147–154.

ARNOLD, A.P., and R.A. GORSKI (1984) Gonadal steroid induction of structural sex differences in the central nervous system. Ann. Rev. Neurosci. *7*:413–442.

BAUM, M.J. (1976) Effects of testosterone propionate administered perinatally on sexual behavior of female ferrets. J. Comp. Physiol. Psychol. *90*:399–410.

BAUM, M.J., and M.S. ERSKINE (1984) Effect of neonatal gonadectomy and administration of testosterone on coital masculinization in the ferret. Endocrinology *115*:2440–2444.

BAUM, M.J., C.A. GALLAGHER, J.T. MARTIN, and D.A. DAMASSA (1982) Effect of testosterone, dihydrotestosterone, or estradiol administered neonatally on sexual behavior of female ferrets. Endocrinology *111*:773–780.

BAUM, M.J., C.A. GALLAGHER, J.H. SHIM, and J.A. CANICK (1983) Normal differentiation of masculine sexual behavior in male ferrets despite neonatal inhibition of brain aromatase or 5-alpha-reductase activity. Neuroendocrinology *36*:277–284.

BAUM, M.J., E.R. STOCKMAN, and L.A. LUNDELL (1985) Evidence of proceptive without receptive defeminization in male ferrets. Behavioral Neuroscience *99*:742–750.

BAUM, M.J., and S.A. TOBET (1986) Effect of prenatal exposure to aromatase inhibitor, testosterone, or antiandrogen on the development of feminine sexual behavior in ferrets of both sexes. Physiol. Behav. *37*:111–118.

BEACH, F.A. (1976) Sexual attractivity, preceptivity, and receptivity in female mammals. Horm. Behav. *7*:105–138.

BEACH, F.A., A.I. JOHNSON, J.J. ANISKO, and I.F. DUNBAR (1977) Hormonal control of sexual attraction in pseudohermaphroditic female dogs. J. Comp. Physiol. Psychol. *91*:711–715.

COMMINS, D., and P. YAHR (1984a) Adult testosterone levels influence the morphology of a sexually dimorphic area in the mongolian gerbil brain. J. Comp. Neurol. *224*:132–140.

COMMINS, D., and P. YAHR (1984b) Lesions of the sexually dimorphic area disrupt mating and marking in male gerbils. Brain Res. Bull. *13*:185–193.

CORBIER, P., B. KERDELHUE, R. PICON, and J. ROFFI (1978) Changes in testicular weight and serum gonadotropin and testosterone levels before, during, and after birth in the perinatal rat. Endocrinology *103*:1985–1991.

CARROLL, R.S., M.S. ERSKINE, P.C. DOHERTY, L.A. LUNDELL, and M.J. BAUM (1985) Coital stimuli controlling luteinizing hormone secretion and ovulation in the female ferret. Biol. Reprod. *32*:925–933.

DAVIS, P.G., C.V. CHAPTAL, and B.C. MCEWEN (1979) Independence of the differentiation of masculine and feminine sexual behavior in rats. Horm. Behav. *12*:12–19.

DOHLER, K.-D., S.S. SRIVASAVA, J.E. SHRYNE, B. JARZAB, A. SIPOS, and R.A. GORSKI (1984) Differentiation of the sexually dimorphic nucleus in the preoptic area of the rat brain is inhibited by postnatal treatment with an estrogen antagonist. Neuroendocrinol. *38*:297–301.

EHRHARDT, A.A., H.F.L. MEYER-BAHLBURG, L.R. ROSEN, J.F. FELDMAN, N.P. VERIDIANO, I. ZIMMERMAN, and B.S. MCEWEN (1985) Sexual orientation after prenatal exposure to exogenous estrogen. Arch. Sex. Behav. *14*:57–75.

ERSKINE, M.S., and M.J. BAUM (1982) Plasma concentrations of testosterone and dihydrotestosterone during perinatal development in male and female ferrets. Endocrinology *111*:767–772.

ERSKINE, M.S., and M.J. BAUM (1984) Plasma concentrations of oestradiol and oestrone during perinatal development in male and female ferrets. J. Endocrinol. *100*:161–166.

FADEM, B.H., and R.J. BARFIELD (1981) Neonatal hormonal influences on the development of proceptive and receptive sexual behavior in rats. Horm. Behav. *15*:282–288.

GORSKI, R.A., R.E. HARLAN, C.D. JACOBSEN, J.E. SHRYNE, and A.M. SOUTHAM (1980) Evidence for the existence of a sexually dimorphic nucleus in the preoptic area of the rat. J. Comp. Neurol. *193*:529–539.

GURNEY, M.E. (1981) Hormonal control of cell form and number in the zebra finch song system. J. Neurosci. *1*:658–673.

HART, B.L., C.M. HAUGEN, and D.M. PETERSEN (1973) Effects of medial preoptic-anterior hypothalamic lesions on mating behavior of male cats. Brain Res. *54*:177–191.

HINES, M., F. DAVIS, A. COQUELIN, R.W. GOY, and R.A. GORSKI (1985) Sexually dimorphic regions in the medial preoptic area and the bed nucleus of the stria terminalis of the guinea pig brain: A description and an investigation of their relationship to gonadal steroids in adulthood. J. Neurosci. *5*:40–47.

HUTCHISON, J.B., J.C. WINGFIELD, and R.E. HUTCHISON (1984) Sex difference in plasma concentrations of steroids during the sensitive period for brain differentiation in the zebra finch. J. Endocrinol. *103*:363–369.

JOST, A. (1960) Hormonal influences in the sex development of the bird and mammalian embryo. Mem. Soc. Endocrinol. *7*:49–62. Reprinted with permission of Cambridge University Press.

KEVERNE, E.G. (1976) Sexual receptivity and attractiveness in the female rhesus monkey. In *Advances in the Study of Behavior*, Vol. 7. J.S. Rosenblatt, R.A. Hinde, E. Shaw, and C. Beer, eds., pp. 155–200, Academic Press, New York.

NADLER, R.D. (1981) Laboratory research on sexual behavior of the great apes. In *Reproductive Biology of the Great Apes.* C.E. Graham, ed., pp. 191–238, Academic Press, New York.

NOTTEBOHM, F., and A.P. ARNOLD (1976) Sexual dimorphism in vocal control areas of the songbird brain. Science *194*:211–213.

PHOENIX, C.H., R.W. GOY, A.A. GERALL, and W.C. YOUNG (1959) Organizing action of prenatally administered testosterone propionate on the tissue mediating mating behavior in the female guinea pig. Endocrinology *65*:369–382.

PHOENIX, C.H., J.N. JENSEN, and K.C. CHAMBERS (1983) Female sexual behavior displayed by androgenized female rhesus macaques. Horm. Behav. *17*:146–151.

POMERANTZ, S.M., M.M. ROY, J.E. THORNTON, and R.W. GOY (1985) Expression of adult female patterns of sexual behavior by male, female and pseudohermaphroditic female rhesus monkeys. Biol. Reprod. *33*:878–889.

RAISMAN, G., and P.M. FIELD (1973) Sexual dimorphism in the neuropil of the preoptic area of the rat and its dependence on neonatal androgen. Brain Res. *54*:1–29.

SLOB, A.K., M.P. OOMS, and J.T.M. VREEBURG (1980) Prenatal and early postnatal sex differences in plasma and gonadal testosterone and plasma luteinizing hormone in female and male rats. J. Endocrinol. *87*:81–87.

THORNTON, J., and R.W. GOY (1986) Behavior of rhesus and defeminization by androgen given prenatally. Horm. Behav. (in press).

TOBET, S.A., and M.J. BAUM (1986) Estrogen and androgen act sequentially to cause coital masculinization in the male ferret (submitted).

TOBET, S.A., J.A. SHIM, S.T. OSIECKI, M.J. BAUM, and J.A. CANICK (1985) Androgen aromatization and 5-alpha-reduction in ferret brain during perinatal development: Effects of sex and testosterone manipulation. Endocrinology *116*:1869–1877.

TOBET, S.A., D.J. ZAHNISER, and M.J. BAUM (1986) Sexual dimorphism in the preoptic/anterior hypothalamic area of ferrets: Effects of adult exposure to sex steroids. Brain Res. *364*:249–257.

TOBET, S.A., D.J. ZAHNISER, and M.J. BAUM (1986a) Differentiation in male ferrets of a sexually dimorphic nucleus of the preoptic/anterior hypothalamic area depends upon prenatal exposure to estrogen. Neuroendocrinol. (in press). Reprinted by permission of S. Karger AG, Basel.

VITO, C.C., M.J. BAUM, C. BLOOM, and T.O. FOX (1985) Androgen and estrogen receptors in perinatal ferret brain. J. Neurosci. *5*:268–274.

WEISZ, J., and I.L. WARD (1980) Plasma testosterone and progesterone titers of pregnant rats, their male and female fetuses and neonatal offspring. Endocrinology *106*:309–316.

WILLIAMS, R.H., ed. (1981) *Textbook of Endocrinology*, 6th ed., p. 444. W.B. Saunders, Philadelphia.

WILSON, J.D., F.W. GEORGE, and J.E. GRIFFIN (1981) The hormonal control of sexual development. Science *211*:1278–1284.

YOUNG, W.C., R.W. GOY, and C.H. PHOENIX (1964) Hormones and sexual behavior. Broad relationships exist between the gonadal hormones and behavior. Science *143*:212–218.

TEN
Reproduction in Carnivores and Ungulates

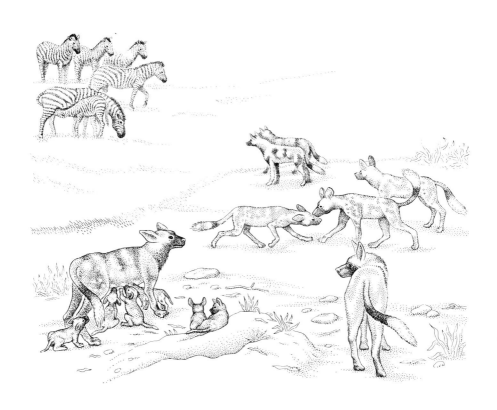

Cheryl S. Asa
New York Zoological Society
Bronx, New York
and
The Population Council
Center for Biomedical Research
New York, New York

There are no a priori reasons for a discussion of carnivore and ungulate reproduction to occur in the same chapter. However, considering them together does present an opportunity to compare and contrast their respective reproductive strategies and how they are influenced by their interactions as predator and prey while at the same time coping with the same environmental pressures. The fact that one group serves as a food source for the other has affected sexual interactions by shaping social organization. Both the threat of predation on ungulates and the hunting strategies of carnivores are reflected in their social systems and sexual behavior.

THE CARNIVORES

The order Carnivora is composed of mammals that evolved as predators. Care must be taken, however, to distinguish between the use of the term carnivore, the ecological designation referring to a meat-eating animal, and the taxonomic category which includes not only meat-eaters, but species which are omnivorous, and in the extreme case of the pandas, completely herbivorous. This chapter will deal with members of the Carnivora, whether or not they are exclusively meat-eaters. The fact that some families of this order have come to rely on food sources other than meat presents an opportunity to assess the potential impact of differing modes of food acquisition on sociosexual relationships.

There are seven families in the order Carnivora (Table 10.1), which are divided into 238 species (Nowak and Paradiso, 1983), although larger numbers are sometimes reported as a result of subspecies' being accorded

TABLE 10.1.   Families of the order Carnivora with common representatives.

Order Carnivora
Families: Viverridae (36/70)*—civets, genets, mongooses
Mustelidae (23/64)—weasels, mink, ferrets, skunks, badgers, wolverine, otters
Ursidae (3/8)—bears, pandas
Procyonidae (7/19)—raccoons, coatis
Felidae (4/37)—cats
Canidae (16/36)—foxes, wolf, coyote, jackals, dog
Hyenidae (3/4)—hyenas, aardwolf

SOURCE: Adapted from Nowak and Paradiso, 1983.
*(number of genera/number of species).

the status of species. Two superfamilies are usually recognized: the Canoidea (or Arctoidea), including the canids, ursids, procyonids, and mustelids; and the Feloidea (or Aeluroidea), composed of felids, hyenids, and viverrids.

The majority of carnivores are solitary, or associate in pairs or small groups, although the complex, highly evolved social systems of some of the canids are comparable to those described for primates. Among the smaller members of the order, e.g., the viverrids, females may reproduce two to three times per year, whereas among the bears and large cats several years may pass between births. Most, however, produce one litter annually.

Partly because of the reduced threat of predation on the offspring of carnivores, in contrast to herbivores, the young are altricial. They are usually born blind and helpless, requiring much maternal attention. Most notably in canids, males, and sometimes other family members, contribute to the care of the young. A long period of dependence is necessary in species which rely heavily on freshly killed meat, to learn hunting techniques.

Several unusual adaptations of reproductive physiology are found among carnivores. Examples are induced ovulation (some felids and mustelids); delayed implantation (some mustelids and ursids); a lengthy proestrus accompanied by a bloody uterine discharge (some canids); and a copulatory tie (some canids). Most remarkable is the hypertrophied clitoris and pseudoscrotum of the female spotted hyena (*Crocuta crocuta*).

Much of the following discussion of carnivore social organization and reproduction is based on information contained in the excellent, comprehensive review by Ewer (1973). The variety of social systems found in viverrids, the most primitive family of the carnivores, is probably due to the variety of strategies used in food procurement. The most detailed information comes from African mongooses and has shown that the more predacious species are solitary, which prevents interference when hunting small vertebrates. Those species whose diets include invertebrates and fruit, who are more diurnal, or live in more open habitat are more likely to be gregarious. They also may share a burrow system which affords better protection from predators. The basic social group is the male/female/young-family group. Even among the more solitary species, male/female pairs are often seen foraging together and may have stable bonds.

The mustelids, many of which are comparable in size to the viverrids, are considerably less social, perhaps related to their heavy reliance on predation of small vertebrates. The characteristic living arrangement is that of mutually intolerant males holding permanent territories, each of which encompasses the smaller territories of one or more females. The relatively larger male may be aggressively dominant to the females within his territory and is likely to have mating rights to all of them. Badgers (*Taxidea taxus*) may be the most social of this family, using communal burrow systems.

Little is known of the procyonids, despite the common occurrence of their best-known member, the raccoon (*Procyon lotor*). Young littermates may be found together, but adults den singly, although they may scavenge in proximity to each other. Bears are basically solitary, and some may be territorial. However, as with raccoons, they will congregate in places where food is concentrated, such as brown bears (*Ursus arctos*) at a river where salmon are running or polar bears (*U. maritimus*) at a whale carcass.

The social structure of most felids, including the domestic cat (*Felis catus*), lynx (*F. lynx*), puma (*F. concolor*), leopard (*Panthera pardus*), and tiger (*P. tigris*), seems to be similar to the model proposed for mustelids. Female territories are contained within a larger, male territory, but the degree of intrasexual tolerance may vary. Cheetahs (*Acinonyx jubatus*) are probably not territorial and are basically solitary, although pairs are sometimes seen together. Adult groups are likely littermates that have yet to disperse.

The lion (*P. leo*) is by far the most gregarious of the felids. The social group is composed of a family of females and cubs, with one or two adult males. The cohort of adult females is stable, whereas the young may emigrate and the position of the adult male(s) may be usurped by challenging male(s). This is in contrast to the solitary nature of the closely related and similar-sized tiger and is probably due to the difference in habitat and the concentration of prey. The prey of lions are often found in large herds on the open plains, a situation which facilitates cooperative hunting even in a species which stalks. The size of a lion pride appears positively correlated with the density of prey and negatively correlated with the density of cover.

Some canids, such as the red fox (*Vulpes vulpes*), have a social system like what seems to be the prototypical carnivore form, one or more female territories within one male territory. In cases where there is only one female, the association is thought to be monogamous, with the same pair mating again in subsequent years. However, when the male controls multiple female territories, he likely mates with all. Defense of the territory is related to seasonal gonadal activity and decreases after mating in January. However, males remain during the period of offspring dependence, then range from the territory in autumn when the young disperse.

Jackals (*Canis aureus, C. mesomelas*) are monogamous, remaining together year-round, year after year. They may hunt small vertebrates alone, but can cooperate in the capture of the young of small gazelles. Depending on local conditions, offspring may not disperse before the arrival of the next litter. Those which stay contribute to the care of the new pups and probably enhance their chances of survival. The additional time for maturation and practice at tending young may also increase the chances of survival for their own future offspring (Moehlman, 1980).

Cape hunting dogs (also called African wild dogs, *Lycaon pictus*), which inhabit the African plains, are found in large groups of about ten individuals, although numbers of up to 50 have been counted. There are separate male and female hierarchies, but all members share in the care of young and even of injured and sick adults. In contrast to the lion pride, related adult males make up the stable unit of the group. Young females are more likely than males to disperse from their natal packs and enter an established pack of males (Nowak and Paradiso, 1983). Typically, only the dominant male and female reproduce, and they actively inhibit breeding by subordinates.

The size of the average wolf pack (*Canis lupus*) with five to eight animals is somewhat smaller than that of Cape hunting dogs. The pack is a family group consisting of an adult pair and their offspring of successive years. There are separate male and female hierarchies, with the parents at the top of their respective hierarchies and younger animals subordinate to their older siblings. As with Cape hunting dogs, the dominant pair are usually the only ones to breed, behaviorally suppressing sexual activity of subordinates (Packard et al., 1985).

The social relationships of the coyote (*Canis latrans*) appear to be flexible, adapting to local conditions. It may be solitary, live in pairs, or in packs, but long-term monogamous pairs may be the modal social unit (Nowak and Paradiso, 1983). Like wolves, they are seasonally territorial.

The wolf's territorial behavior is most notable during the breeding season, with male urine-marking increasing in autumn and continuing at a relatively higher rate through spring. Unlike most other species, the dominant female also begins to urine-mark at this time, using a modified leg-lift posture. At the time of pair formation between a previously lone male and female, urine-marking behavior is most intense and often entails tandem-marking by both members of the pair in succession (Rothman and Mech, 1979). Established pairs also tandem-mark during the breeding season, but frequencies are lower than for new pairs.

In experiments on the relative importance of olfactory communication in a wolf pack, two of three males and two of three females were made anosmic by transection of the olfactory peduncle. The subsequent failure of the operated wolves to detect biologically relevant substances such as food, urine, and anal-gland secretions confirmed their inability to smell. One anosmic female succeeded in securing the dominant position among the females but failed to bond normally to the dominant male, who was intact. Her concomitant very low level of urine-marking, despite her status, suggests that either performance of the behavior in concert with the male, or transmission of urine-borne chemical messages between the pair, may be an integral part of the bonding process (Asa et al., 1986).

The striped hyena (*Hyaena hyaena*) is solitary or paired, depending on the relative distribution of food. When the sexes are together, the female is dominant over the male. Brown hyenas (*H. brunnea*) are organized into clans in which males are dominant. They den communally but often scavenge alone.

Spotted hyenas (*Crocuta crocuta*) also live in clans, but females are not only larger and dominant, they possess genitalia that are superficially indistinguishable from those of males. The clitoris is hypertrophied, and a pair of swellings composed of fibrous tissue resembles a scrotum. Plasma levels of testosterone in adult females are similar to those of adult males, in contrast to striped and brown hyenas whose females have lower testosterone than males. Testosterone was also high in female spotted hyenas in utero, suggesting fetal as well as adult testosterone influence on male-type genitalia and behavior (Racey and Skinner, 1979).

Mutual genital sniffing is the focal point of spotted hyena social greetings within the clan, preceded by a display of erect penis or clitoris. The female's hypertrophied clitoris and pseudoscrotum may be necessary for her to maintain a dominant position. This hypothesis is strengthened by the observation that in the closely related viverrids, binturong and especially fossa females possess enlarged clitorides and scrotum-like swellings. Although information is not available on their social relations, it is common among other viverrid females to be slightly larger than and dominant to males.

Most carnivores, even equatorial species, produce young only once a year. Exceptions are found among the small, often tropical species. Although most of these have two litters annually, up to four have been reported for the dwarf mongoose (*Helogale parvula*). In temperate and arctic zones, the reproductive cycle of carnivores is constrained by environmental factors. The birth of young must coincide with conditions favorable for optimum growth, so mating must be properly timed to allow for gestational development.

Changes in photoperiod are the most reliable predictor of seasonal change and are believed to mediate sexual cyclicity in many mammals (see Chapter 8). Photic information impinges on retinal receptor cells and is relayed by neural connections via the retino-hypothalamic tract and suprachiasmatic nucleus to the superior cervial ganglia (part of the sympathetic nervous system) and then to the pineal gland. Here the message is transduced into endocrine form, mainly melatonin, which is carried by the blood to the hypothalamus and pituitary, centers which control gonadotropin production and secretion (Legan and Winans, 1981).

The effect of changing daylength on parameters of reproduction have been studied extensively in the golden hamster (*Mesocricetus auratus*), domestic sheep (*Ovis aries*), and the white-tailed deer (*Odocoileus virginianus*) (Turek et al., 1984; Plotka et al., 1979; see Chapter 8). Pinealectomy or superior cervical ganglionectomy in these photoperiod-sensitive species results in either abolition or disruption of their annual rhythm of gonadal activity.

Among the carnivores, changes in photoperiod have been shown to influence seasonality in many species, especially the mustelids. However, involvement of the pineal has been evaluated in only the ferret (*Mustela putorius*) and the wolf. The sensitivity of the ferret to experimentally manipulated daylength was an early model of photoperiod sensitivity, since exposure to extended daylengths during the fall anestrous period when females typically were reproductively inactive reliably stimulated ovarian activity (Rowlands and Weir, 1984). Subsequent studies of ferrets pinealectomized or blinded by transection of the optic tract resulted in disruption of the annual cycle after the first reproductive season (Herbert et al., 1978).

Thus it was quite unexpected when pinealectomy failed to disrupt the seasonal reproductive cycles of both male and female wolves (Asa et al., submitted). Measures of testosterone and luteinizing hormone for males and progesterone and estradiol for females revealed no differences from intact pack members. To control for possible synchronization with intact wolves by pheromonal communication, some pinealectomized wolves were also made anosmic; these animals continued to cycle regularly. Likewise, removal of the superior-cervical ganglia did not alter the annual rhythm (Asa et al., submitted).

The reason for the discrepancy between the wolf and other photoperiod-sensitive species is unclear. It is likely that the timing of reproductive events in the wolf and other canids is influenced by photoperiod, since (1) breeding is seasonal at higher latitudes, (2) mating occurs later at higher latitudes, and (3) translocation of the maned wolf (*Chrysocyon brachyurus*) and the red fox (the species for which data exist) resulted in a 6-month phase-shift in their breeding cycles. However, as is often the case in research, as additional species are studied, exceptions to earlier models are likely to be discovered.

Mediation of seasonal peaks in mating and birth of young for equatorial species is uncertain but probably is related to rainfall. Phytochemicals present in the new plant growth which follows a rainy period may account for such a phenomenon in herbivorous animals. Whether carnivores respond to changes in environmental cues such as humidity or barometric pressure, or to the higher plane of nutrition or other factor(s) supplied by the increasing abundance of prey, has not been determined.

Major seasonal changes in climate, such as equatorial dry periods or temperate and arctic zone winters, are often accompanied by reductions in prey density. Births must occur as early as possible in milder seasons, when food is also more plentiful, to give the young adequate time to develop before conditions again become unfavorable. With gestation periods of one to three months for the majority of carnivores, breeding would have to take place during harsh conditions, e.g., winter. Yet, courtship and mating activity require a considerable energy expenditure.

Some species such as bears have solved the problem of cold and inadequate food supply by denning during the winter, but this period of isolation and inactivity makes mating even more problematic. For many mustelids, procyonids, and bears, delayed implantation has alleviated this problem by making the times of mating and birth independent of gestation length. Thus, for brown (*Ursus arctos*) and black bears (*U. americanus*), mating can take place during the summer and not interfere with the period of heavy feeding in fall when fat has to be accumulated before denning. For the polar bear, spring mating is preferable because animals are widely dispersed during the summer. For small temperate or arctic zone mustelids there are obvious advantages to mating in spring or summer when conditions are favorable, while delaying the time of parturition to the following spring.

The range of delay duration is considerable, from as little as 2 weeks in spotted skunks (*Spilogale putorius*) and mink (*Mustela vison*) up to 11 months in ermine (*M. erminea*). That a delay as brief as two weeks can confer an advantage seems improbable. An effect of domestication may account for the phenomenon in mink, but too little is known at this time of the natural history of the spotted skunk to provide an explanation.

The Canoidea are most commonly monestrus, i.e., an infertile cycle is followed by an interval of ovarian quiescence, or anestrus. In contrast, many Feloidea, particularly felids, are polyestrus with an infertile cycle soon followed by another cycle. In northern latitudes, felids are likely to be seasonally polyestrous, with multiple cycles interrupted by periods of anestrus during harsher environmental conditions.

Very few studies have been conducted on the physiological parameters of the estrous cycles in carnivores. Notable exceptions have been the domestic dog and cat, plus a few other canids and felids. The female domestic dog (*Canis familiaris*) has approximately two monestrous cycles per year, although there may be breed and individual differences. The cycle may be divided into several phases: proestrus, estrus, pregnancy or pseudopregnancy, and anestrus. Proestrus and estrus each last approximately one to two weeks (Concannon et al., 1977), followed by two months of increased progesterone levels. Ovulation is spontaneous and unless the female conceives, an obligate pseudopregnancy ensues. Although this nonpregnant, progestational phase is often termed metestrus, pseudopregnancy seems more apt, since hormonal profiles are similar in amplitude and duration to those of the pregnant female. There is individual variation in the expression of maternal behavior and in the degree of abdominal and mammary swelling which accompanies the condition. Some females are affected to the extent of lactation and/or mothering phantom pups at the termination of pseudopregnancy (Smith and McDonald, 1974). A short anestrus precedes the next cycle.

The wolf, a probable ancestor of the domestic dog, is also monestrous, but has only one cycle per year. The durations of estrus and pregnancy or pseudopregnancy are similar to those of the dog, but the proestrous phase is often longer (Figure 10.1; Seal et al., 1979). Anestrus is, of course, much longer, lasting six to eight months.

The social system of the wolf suggests an explanation for obligate pseudopregnancy in the absence of pregnancy. The dominant female is usually the only one of a pack to breed, and yet subordinate females contribute to the care of her pups, their own younger siblings (Mech, 1970). Observations of the behavior of female domestic dogs confirm that the hormones of pseudopregnancy can stimulate maternal behavior. Thus in a wolf pack, subordinate females are primed by the same endocrine milieu as the mother herself, ensuring not only that they will not be hostile toward the pups, but will help provision and protect them. Pseudopregnancy has been

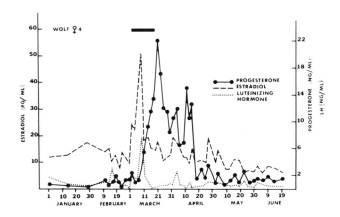

Figure 10.1. Serum concentrations of progesterone, estradiol, and LH from January through June in a female wolf (*Canis lupus*) paired with a male (the black bar indicates the observed duration of proestrus and the clear bar the observed duration of estrus). (By permission of Seal et al., 1979)

shown to be hormonally similar to pregnancy in the ferret, mink, and arctic fox (*Alopex lagopus*) as well, but less is known about the possible adaptive significance of this physiological state in these species (Rowlands and Weir, 1984).

An interesting feature of proestrus in the dog and wolf is the bloody discharge from the uterus, superficially similar to the menstrual flow of primate females. However, the endocrine milieu during proestrus is quite different from that of the primate menstrual phase. Proestrual bleeding in the dog and wolf is correlated with elevated levels of estrogen (Seal et al., 1979; Concannon et al., 1977), whereas primate menstrual bleeding follows the decline of estradiol and progesterone at the end of the luteal phase. Apparently not all canids have proestrual bleeding, e.g., the red fox, despite a cycle similar to that of the wolf in many other respects. However, slight vaginal hemorrhage during proestrus has been reported for the raccoon (Rowlands and Weir, 1984).

In contrast to the dog and wolf, the domestic cat is seasonally polyestrous and an induced ovulator. Two peaks of sexual activity have been described, January to March and May to June (Verhage et al., 1976). If ovulation is not induced, estrus recurs every two to three weeks. Sterile mating causes pseudopregnancy, during which progesterone and estradiol may attain amplitudes similar to pregnancy, but with shorter duration (Figure 10.2).

Hormonal profiles of the cycling Siberian tiger (*Panthera tigris altaica*) (Figure 10.3) are similar to those of the domestic cat. The tiger is seasonally polyestrous, with cycles extending from late January to early June (Seal et al., 1985). Unfortunately, endocrine measures of pregnancy and pseudopregnancy are not available, despite efforts to induce ovulation by administration

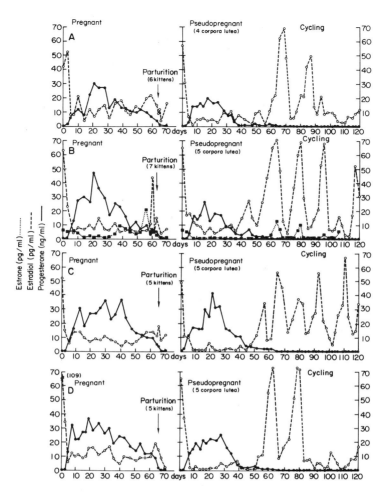

Figure 10.2. Profiles of circulating concentrations of estradiol and progesterone in four individual cats (*Felis catus*) and estrone in one (B) during pregnancy, pseudopregnancy, and polyestrus. (By permission of Verhage et al., 1976)

of PMSG (pregnant mares serum gonadotropin). Peaks in serum testosterone were found to accompany most estradiol peaks.

Because they are widely considered to be male hormones, testosterone and other androgens are not commonly measured in females. Although testosterone may be converted to estradiol in brain target tissues, it or its androgen metabolites may be involved in the support of female sexual behavior (Beach, 1976). In fact, the relative rates of conversion of testosterone to estradiol versus the androgen dihydrotestosterone may be important in the induction of female sexual initiative (Wallen and Goy, 1978).

In most female mammals, ovulation occurs spontaneously at a specific point in the estrous cycle, whether or not copulation occurs. However, in

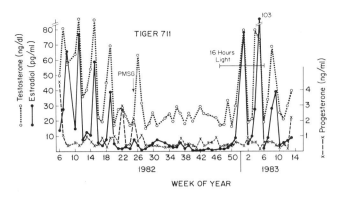

Figure 10.3. Serum concentrations of estradiol, testosterone, and progesterone in the tiger (*Panthera tigris*). Blood samples were taken each week. On June 25 pregnant mares' serum gonadotropin (PMSG) was given IM as a single dose of 1200 IU by blow dart. Twenty weeks later the photoperiod was extended to 16 hours by 240-watt floodlight. (By permission of Seal et al., 1985)

some species ovulation must be induced by vaginal and/or cervical stimulation such as that provided by coitus. In still others, ovulation may occur spontaneously, but its timing can be influenced by copulatory stimulation. It appears that all cats are polyestrous, and that most are induced ovulators. However, in the lion, ovulation may sometimes be induced, but increases in progesterone following estradiol surges which occur even in the absence of copulation are indicative of ovulation and corpus luteum (CL) formation (Schmidt et al., 1979).

The mink and brown bear are unusual among the carnivores studied, in that an additional wave of follicular growth follows the first estrus and ovulation, even if mating during the first was fertile (Rowlands and Weir, 1984). Because the second cycle occurs during the period of gestational delay, the follicles may be necessary for formation of additional CL to support implantation and gestation.

For the mink, mating during the second estrus causes expulsion of the blastocysts from the first; consequently the male which copulates during the second estrus sires the young of that year (Short, 1984). Although these data are from domestic mink, the physiology of the wild mink may be similar. It would be interesting to know the social dynamics surrounding this phenomenon, e.g., whether the pair remains together for the second mating and if the male faces competition at that time.

The duration of estrus is relatively long in most carnivores (Table 10.2). In contrast, most female ungulates and rodents are receptive for only a matter of hours. The comparative vulnerability of prey species during courtship and copulation must be at least partly responsible for the difference. Estrus in the small, black-footed cat (*Felis nigripes*) lasts only 5 to 10 hours, perhaps as a protective adaptation to predatory pressure in relatively open habitat.

TABLE 10.2. **Duration of estrus and of copulation and type of ovulation for selected carnivores.**

Species	Duration of estrus	Duration of copulation	Type of ovulation
Ferret	3–5 d	0.5–2 hr	induced
Raccoon	2–3 d		induced
Brown bear	≤10 d	20–30 min	spontaneous?
Domestic cat	9–10 d (w/o mating) 4d (with mating)	several seconds	induced
Lion	4–16 d	6–68 sec	can be spontaneous
Domestic dog	7–10 d	15–30 min	spontaneous
Wolf	~9 d	15–30 min	spontaneous
Fox	2–4 d		spontaneous
Spotted hyena		12 min	spontaneous

SOURCES: Rowlands and Weir, 1984; Nowak and Paradiso, 1983; Ewer, 1973; Schaller, 1972.

Many predators are solitary and do not interact socially and may even be hostile toward each other outside the breeding season. Even where territories or home ranges overlap and a male and female are familiar, associations during most of the year are not close. A period of time is required for partners to locate one another and become sufficiently acquainted to allow contact. The latter has special significance for carnivores, which are well armed for killing.

Induced ovulation, which is common among felids and mustelids, is also thought to be related to the time needed for partner location and acclimation. If ovulation is spontaneous and estrus duration brief, proper coordination of partners is critical. Such timing may not be possible for species where males and females are not in regular, close contact. If ovulation occurs only by copulatory stimulation and the period of receptivity is long, timing of social relations can be more flexible.

Prolonged courtship can be important for the social carnivores also. Except perhaps for the lion and spotted hyena, males of the more social species contribute to the care of young and sometimes of the mother. Extended association prior to copulation may help formulate or strengthen the bond necessary to insure male allegiance to the female and offspring.

The period of proestrus in the wolf (and probably other canids) prolongs the period of precopulatory association. The length of proestrus for the wolf (Young, 1944) and coyote (Kennelly and Johns, 1976) has been reported to extend for one to four months, although that of the dog is much shorter (seven to ten days, Concannon et al., 1977).

Even before the appearance of the proestrous bloody discharge, male and female wolves begin to tandem urine-mark their territory (Asa et al., 1985) and to travel and rest in close proximity (Mech and Knick, 1978).

Although the urine-marking ritual involves sniffing each other's urine, when the female enters proestrus male interest seems to intensify. He sniffs and licks the urine spot and performs what is probably the canid version of *flehmen*. This behavior entails the rapid opening and closing of the mouth with the tongue slightly extruded. Such contact of the tongue with the roof of the mouth, the site of the paired openings to the nasopalatine ducts, may deliver urinary compounds to the vomeronasal organ (VNO) in a somewhat similar manner to that shown in guinea pigs (Wysocki et al., 1980). The analogous behavior in cats is called a grimace because of the accompanying facial expression.

The function of flehmen is apparently to introduce nonvolatile material, most commonly from urine, into the VNO. This organ is composed of paired, tubular structures lying on the floor of the nasal cavity. The VNO is the peripheral sensory organ of the accessory olfactory system, which has projections to the medial preoptic area and medial hypothalamus, brain areas identified with stimulation of sexual behavior and gonadotropic-hormone production. This tract remains distinct from that of the main olfactory system, which receives input from the nasal epithelium (Scalia and Winans, 1981).

Thus, the flehmen/VNO/accessory olfactory system appears to transduce an olfactory message (or messages) contained in urine or other fluids to brain sex centers, presumably to provide the male with information regarding the estrous status of the female. A metabolite or product of estradiol, which is elevated during proestrus, may mediate the male response.

The attractive component(s) may originate in the urine itself or be washed from the vaginal canal during urination. At the inception of estrus, the period of sexual receptivity, the focus of the male's olfactory attention shifts from the female's urine to the vulval area (Asa, unpublished personal observation). The hormone change which induces receptivity may also mediate the changes in components of urine or vaginal secretions.

As with urine, the male sniffs and licks the vulval area and performs the mouthing behavior. The importance of such interactions was suggested by experiments with anosmic male wolves (Asa et al., 1986). Over a period of three breeding seasons, two sexually naive, anosmic males failed to respond in the customary way to urine or vaginal secretions of their female partners. In spite of sexual solicitation by the females, neither male was observed to mate and neither female conceived.

In the first year after surgery, the behavior of a sexually experienced, anosmic male was similar to that of the naive males. However, in the subsequent season, he responded to the sexual invitations of his kennel-mate, copulated successfully, and sired pups. He was not seen responding to her urine, but did lick the genital area when she presented and deflected her tail.

The levels of circulating testosterone, seasonal testicular growth, and sperm concentrations of the anosmic males were not different from those of controls. These results indicate that olfactory signals from proestrous and perhaps estrous urine are not required for activation of the endocrine system or for spermatogenesis, but are important cues for behavioral stimulation of sexually naive males. Behavioral cues from estrous females are apparently adequate for experienced males. Because these animals were housed in relatively close contact in kennels, other undoubtedly important roles of urinary signals such as the location of a mate or the attractivity sufficient to maintain proximity for bond formation could not be evaluated.

The primary stages of pairing in the red fox resemble those of the wolf during the proestrous phase. Presumably, a bond is formed, because the male remains after mating to assist in the care of the young and is likely to be the same male to pair with the female in subsequent years. In newly forming pairs, the female initially exhibits hostility toward the male, but he is apparently sufficiently attracted by glandular or urinary compounds to persist. She eventually becomes tolerant and a period of close contact, grooming, and play follows.

The endocrine events of the estrous cycle of the wolf are like those of the domestic dog. The relationship of ovulation to the onset of estrus and concomitant hormone changes have been summarized for the dog by Concannon et al. (1977): (1) ovulation (38 to 44 hours post-LH surge) may occur from one day before to five days after the onset of estrus; (2) progesterone secretion may precede or coincide with the onset of the LH surge (60 to 70 hour before ovulation); and (3) progesterone synergizes with the estrogen peak that terminates proestrus, initiating estrus. Estrogen alone makes the female attractive, but progesterone is required to synergize with the estrogen to induce sexual receptivity. These observations concur with what is known for the wolf.

The timing of sexual receptivity in the wolf and the dog is unusual in that estrus can continue for up to a week post-ovulation, and in the presence of steadily increasing progesterone. In other species in which progesterone has been found to synergize with estradiol [guinea pig (*Cavia porcellus*) and rat (*Rattus rattus*): Morali and Beyer, 1979; horse (*Equus caballus*): Asa et al., 1984], progesterone administration beyond the first day was inhibitory to sexual behavior. No neuroendocrine explanation is apparent for the absence of inhibition in the face of sustained levels of progesterone in the wolf and dog.

Interestingly, the ovum of the dog is relatively immature at ovulation, being a primary rather than secondary oocyte, as in most mammals. Yet this cannot be responsible for the tendency for later mating, because fertilization can take place at an earlier stage of oocyte development in the dog (Short, 1984).

Progesterone is not involved in the estrous behavior of cats and increases only when genital stimulation is sufficient to induce ovulation, a process associated with premature demise of estrus. Estradiol is the major steroid hormone circulating at the time of estrus (Figure 10.2; Verhage et al., 1976) and is sufficient to induce sexual behavior in the domestic cat (Michael & Scott, 1957).

Elements of aggression are often obvious components of sexual interaction in carnivores. In canids it takes the form of play-fighting, but in mustelids and felids the potential for injury is present. In these latter families, males and females typically do not associate and may not be tolerant of proximity outside the breeding season. Among mustelids, precopulatory behavior of pine martens (*Martes americana*), weasels (*Mustela rixosa, M. nivalis*), and striped skunks (*Mephitis mephitis*) includes, besides a dramatic increase in scent-marking, play and chases which may end in fighting. Just prior to mating the male grasps the neck of the female with his teeth. If she does not immediately assume the mating posture, with hindquarters elevated and tail deflected, he drags her about until she does so. The male maintains the neck-bite throughout copulation, which may last an hour or more, as the animals lie on their sides. Pairs usually mate several time in succession, with copulatory bouts alternating with periods of fighting. In spite of the integral role of fighting in the mating sequence, injuries seldom occur, probably due to a strong bite inhibition and the ritualized nature of the aggression.

Copulation in felids is much like that described for mustelids, with the addition of characteristic male and female vocalizations. Mating sequences throughout the felids are similar to those of the domestic cat, which has been studied in the most detail.

Although a proestrous phase has not been reported for the cat, the female apparently becomes attractive to the male several days prior to becoming receptive. During this time she is likely to be pursued by more than one male, resulting in intermale competition and possible fighting. The victorious male must then be accepted by the female, a process during which his approaches are at first repulsed by spitting, hissing, and striking with extended claws. Despite the often much larger size of the male, he does not retaliate but persistently reapproaches, giving the "entreaty" call. The female's resistance gradually subsides till she tolerates his presence. Ultimately she becomes proceptive, i.e., she solicits copulation. After a sequence of rolling, purring, and patting at him playfully, she assumes the mating posture with hindquarters elevated and tail deflected, a stance which can be induced by the male neck-bite which often precedes mating.

Copulation is brief, only a few seconds, but may be repeated several times. An indication of how many times is given by Schaller (1972) in which a male lion copulated 157 times in 55 hours with two females. As coitus ends, the female rolls away, strikes out at the male and gives a loud cry. Whether this sudden aggressiveness is coincident with ejaculation or withdrawal is uncertain. The penis is covered with backwardly directed, horny spines whose development is androgen-dependent. Because of the correlation in species studied between the presence of penile spines and induced ovulation, it is thought the stimulation provided by the spines may be requisite for ovulation.

Mating in viverrids is similar to that in the felids, except for the postejaculatory cry and aggression. Viverrids are not induced ovulators and most have no penile spines. An exception is the fossa (*Cryptoprocta ferox*), a species in which the female gives a low cry upon intromission, not withdrawal. Male brown and striped hyenas, but not spotted hyenas, also have penile spines, but the mechanism of ovulation is unknown. Obviously, further investigation is required before conclusions about adaptive significance can be drawn, but the observation that all species of carnivora in which spines occur are members of the superfamily Feloidea suggests a common origin.

Of the hyenids, mating behavior has been reported only for the spotted hyena. The absence of an extended period of courtship has been attributed to their social structure, the clan, which keeps males and females in contact throughout the year. Although this eliminates the need for the preliminary stages of acquaintance, the wolf with its highly evolved social system has one of the longest periods of close precopulatory association. Yet, the lion, another social species, engages in little courtship activity. It is true that while year-round sociality reduces the time needed to acquire a mate, potential paternal involvement also influences a female's selection. In the lion and hyena, males offer protection to females and cubs of their social group, but do not contribute food. In lion prides, females are the primary hunters, regardless of the presence of young. In spotted hyena clans, food is not carried to the young. Instead, the mother suckles her cubs for 12 to 16 months, until they are nearly full grown (Nowak and Paradiso, 1983). Most other carnivore mothers nurse for about two months. This complete dependence on the hyena mother for sustenance obviates participation by the male. All clan members share food, so there is no advantage to a particular male's provisioning his mate.

In contrast, in a wolf pack a female cannot depend on subordinate adults to bring food to the den. During the first year, a newly formed pair has no other pack members on which to rely, and even in the subsequent year, if the first litter survives, they will be only yearlings and still relatively inexperienced hunters (Mech, 1970).

In view of these comparisons, the brief precopulatory interactions of the spotted hyenas is not surprising. There is, however, a period of rivalry among males for access to an estrous female, much as is seen in the cats. Here again, the female need select only for prowess, because the male has primarily protection to offer. Mating itself is preceded by mutual sniffing of anal pouches and genitals, as occurs during nonsexual greeting rituals. During this time the male's penis and the female's hypertrophied clitoris partially erect and are directed backward. Then, as the penis erects further, it curves forward, while the female's erection subsides. The male mounts with his hindquarters almost in a sitting position.

In the spotted hyena, the urogenital canal traverses the clitoris of the juvenile female, as it does the male penis. Then at puberty the opening elongates, forming a slit beneath the clitoris to accommodate copulation and parturition. Thus the female's male-type genitalia appear to be important principally in the context of social signaling and play only a small role in sexual interactions.

Coitus is remarkable in canids primarily for the copulatory tie or lock that occurs upon intromission, due to the swelling of the bulbus glandis near the proximal end of the penis (Figure 10.4). The male dismounts after ejaculation, but withdrawal is precluded for several minutes to an hour, depending on species and individual differences. A copulatory tie has been reported for all canids and may be an extreme form of postcoital mate-guarding. Work with laboratory rats, which leave a gelatinous plug in the vagina of the female at ejaculation, has shown that prevention of further mating during an approximately 15-minute period ensures fertilization by the sperm of the first male (Adler and Zoloth, 1970). Because canids are predators with few enemies, the danger resulting from such a vulnerable position is reduced. Still, the tie lasts only a few minutes in the Cape hunting dog, a species which inhabits open terrain, whereas in the wolf 15 to 30 minutes is more typical. An additional advantage for social canids is a reduction in intermale competition during the critical postcopulatory period.

Little is known about mating in ursids. The 20- to 30-minute duration of copulation, recurring on successive days, is surprising in animals that are believed to be spontaneous ovulators with no male contribution to care of young. Lengthy copulation is generally associated with induction of ovula-

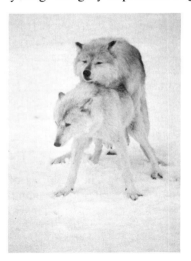
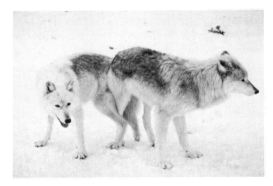
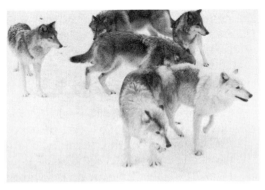

Figure 10.4. (A) Copulation by a dominant pair of wolves, (B) followed by an approximately 20-minute postcopulatory tie, (C) during which time subordinate pack members mill excitedly around the pair.

tion or is believed to help form or maintain pair bonds. Further investigation of these species may reveal other contributing factors.

THE UNGULATES

The term *ungulate* refers to all hoofed mammals, but taxonomically they are divided into two orders, the Perissodactyla, meaning odd-toed, and the Artiodactyla, or even-toed. The order Perissodactyla is considerably smaller, having only 16 species, which include the equids or horselike animals, tapirs, and rhinoceros (Table 10.3). The success of the much more numerous artiodactyls, 192 species, is attributed primarily to the ruminants, which comprise about 90% of the order.

Some species have been well studied as a result of domestication. In fact, most domestic mammals are ungulates—for example, the horse (*Equus caballus*), donkey (*E. asinus*), sheep (*Ovis aries*), goat (*Capra hircus*), cow (*Bos taurus*), pig (*Sus scrofa*), camels (*Camelus bactrianus, C. dromedarius*), llama (*Lama glama*), alpaca (*L. pacos*), and yak (*Bos grunniens*). For most of the others, field work has contributed valuable information on behavior and ecology, but data are still lacking for most on parameters of reproductive physiology. A conspicuous exception is the white-tailed deer, which has been studied largely because of its economic value as a North American game species.

The most primitive ungulates are believed to be the Tragulids, represented by the chevrotain or mouse deer (*Tragulus meminna, T. napu, T. javanicus*), small forest-dwelling ruminants that are primarily solitary. The

TABLE 10.3.   Families of the two orders of Ungulata with common representatives noted.

Order Perissodactyla
Families: Equidae (1/8)*—horses, zebras, asses
Tapiridae (1/4)—tapirs
Rhinocerotidae (4/5)—rhino
Order Artiodactyla
Families: Suidae (5/8)—pigs, warthog
Tayassuidae (2/3)—peccaries
Hippopotamidae (2/2)—hippos
Camelidae (3/6)—camels, llama, guanaco, alpaca, vicuna
Tragulidae (2/4)—chevrotains, mouse deer
Cervidae (17/38)—deer, moose, elk
Giraffidae (2/3)—giraffe, okapi
Antilocapridae (1/1)—pronghorn antelope
Bovidae (45/128)—antelopes, cattle, bison, gazelles, goats, sheep

SOURCE: Adapted from Nowak and Paradiso, 1983.
*(number of genera/number of species).

relatively primitive swine and tapirs also typically inhabit forests, although swine are more gregarious and often are found in groups. However, the ecology of these early forms is not representative of the majority of extant ungulate species. Most now inhabit open grasslands, primarily the plains of Africa and southern and central Asia. Here they may be found in large herds, although the advanced social systems seen in some carnivores are conspicuously absent. Social structure beyond the basic mother/young unit is seldom observed outside the breeding season.

Leuthold (1977) has summarized the types of social organization for the African ungulates, but his rankings are based more heavily on spatial arrangements (e.g., territoriality) than on social units. Although territoriality may influence sexual interaction, the degree of male/female association afforded by the social unit of a species is undoubtedly more important. Viewed from the perspective of the basic social unit, the chevrotains and duikers (*Cephalophus*) represent the most solitary forms. The most complex structure is found in the plains (*Equus burchelli*) and mountain zebras (*E. zebra*), where a stable group of females and young is permanently attended by one adult male.

Intermediate forms appear to be based on the mother/young unit, either singly or in aggregations. Seldom are adult males permanently attached to the female group. Exceptions are found in the two zebra species mentioned, in African buffalo (*Syncerus caffer*), horses, and the lamoids of South America [llama, alpaca, guanaco (*L. guanicoe*), and vicuna (*Vicugna vicugna*): Walther, 1984]. African buffalo live in large, relatively cohesive herds consisting of females and young plus some adult males. The number of males increases during the breeding season, but the highest-ranking males associate most closely with the herd and achieve most of the matings.

The social system of the feral domestic horse is like that of the plains and mountain zebras, consisting of a stable band of females, their young, and a male (Feist and McCullough, 1975). The same pattern is seen in lamoids, except that the latter are usually territorial (Raedeke, 1979). Males of the other equid species, Grevy's zebra (*Equus grevyi*), the feral domestic donkey, and the African wild ass (*E. asinus*, progenitor of the domestic donkey), have mating territories during the breeding season but do not associate with females at other times.

Interestingly, considerable social flexibility exists among the equids in response to different habitats. In some areas a group of females may be tended by more than one adult male (Miller, 1981). Males of feral ponies become territorial when living where adequate resources can be defended without difficulty (Rubenstein, 1981), and feral donkeys are more social where vegetation is lush than in arid habitat and may even form harems (Moehlman, 1970).

Such plasticity may be common to other species and just more apparent in feral animals that may have access to a wider variety of conditions than their wild relatives. Evidence from a naturally occurring population of guanacos supports this contention. Where animal density is low and forage relatively poor, guanaco bands more closely resemble horses and are not territorial (Raedeke, 1979).

Most ungulates reproduce seasonally, even in equatorial regions where rainfall, not temperature, affects food availability. Their social systems, as well as physiology, are often profoundly changed by the advent of breeding season, since for many species males and females do not associate other than at the time of mating.

With the approach of the reproductive season, males which had previously lived singly or coexisted in bachelor herds begin to compete for access to females and perhaps for territories. During the rut, aggression increases and males may fight fiercely. Because most species are polygynous, males which do not succeed in the competition do not mate at all. Such high stakes have resulted in the evolution in many ungulate males of impressive horns or antlers for both display and combat. Although the horns of some bovids are remarkable for their size and their curved or spiral shapes, the most elaborate forms are found in the antlers of some of the cervids.

Except for the musk deer (*Moschus moschiferus*) and water deer (*Hydropotes inermis*), which instead have tusklike upper canines, all deer have antlers which go through a yearly cycle of growth and shedding in response to cyclic changes in testosterone (Figure 10.5). Initial stages of antler growth in the white-tailed deer, the species for which the most complete data exist, appear to be independent of gonadal hormones. Continued growth and maturation, including shedding of the velvet, require increasing levels of circulating testosterone. Antler shedding results from testosterone withdrawal at the close of the breeding season (McMillan et al., 1974).

In species where males hold territories during the few weeks or months of the breeding season, females visit for a few hours or days, but are not held within the territory. In nonterritorial species, intermale competition results in a dominance hierarchy which determines access to females. An individual, high-ranking male will typically tend a female only during her period of estrus, then move to another.

Species living in open habitat have developed a reliance on vision, which is obvious in the relative importance of postural displays in precopulatory rituals. Many with large horns or antlers seem not to use them in displays to females, but adopt postures with heads lowered or tipped to minimize the visual impact of their weapons (Leuthold, 1977).

Perhaps the most curious male display is that of the camel, in which he extrudes a portion of his soft palate, called the dulaa, by filling it with air. This structure appears to be under the control of testosterone also, because it is largest in breeding males and much reduced in females and castrated males (Gauthier-Pilters and Dagg, 1981).

In most bovids and cervids, contact between adult males and females is rare outside the breeding season, so not only are the potential mates probably unfamiliar with each other, they are not accustomed to proximity. Endocrine changes appear to stimulate both male approach to females and

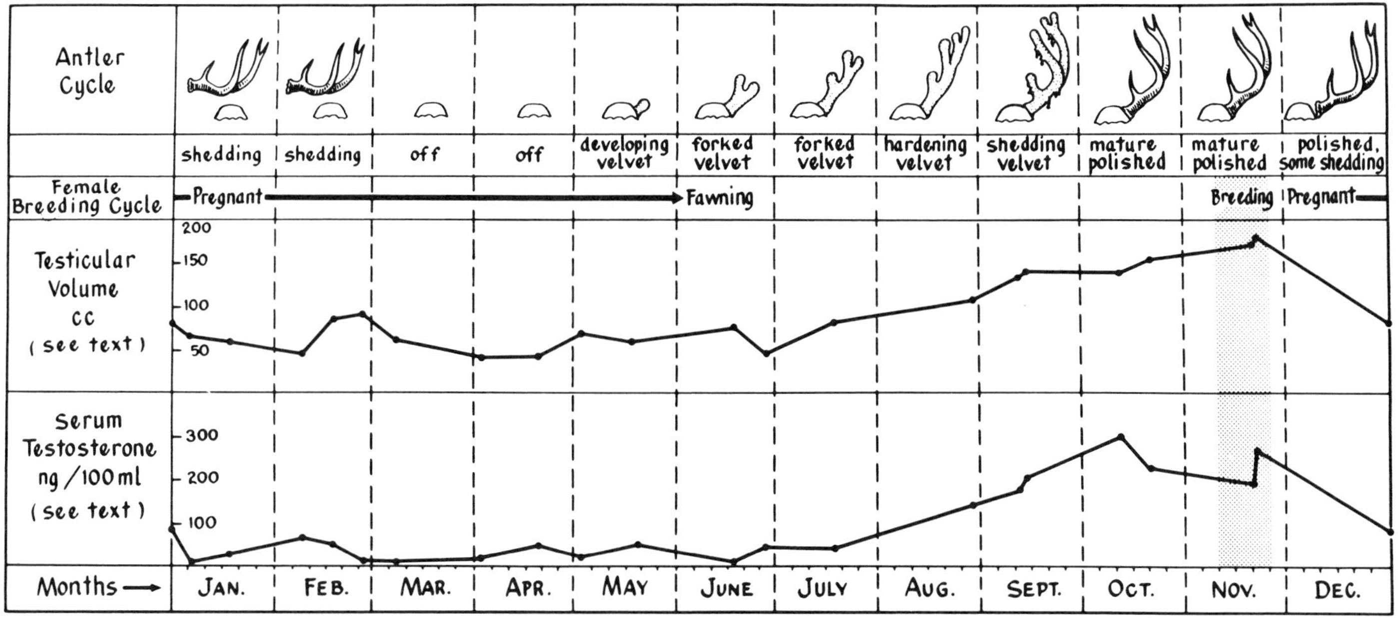

Antler Cycle	shedding	shedding	off	off	developing velvet	forked velvet	forked velvet	hardening velvet	shedding velvet	mature polished	mature polished	polished, some shedding
Female Breeding Cycle	Pregnant					Fawning					Breeding	Pregnant
Testicular Volume cc (see text)	200 150 100 50											
Serum Testosterone ng/100ml (see text)	300 200 100											
Months →	JAN.	FEB.	MAR.	APR.	MAY	JUNE	JULY	AUG.	SEPT.	OCT.	NOV.	DEC.

Figure 10.5. Relationship of the antler and breeding cycle to testicular size and circulating concentrations of testosterone in male white-tailed deer (*Odocoileus virginianus*). (By permission of McMillan et al., 1974)

278

female approach or tolerance of male proximity. Still, approach and acceptance seem to proceed in delicately balanced stages.

Driving is a component of courtship common to many ungulate species. At one extreme it entails high-speed chases, while at the other it diminishes to tandem circling with partners head-to-tail. For larger bovids such as the aurochs (*Bos taurus*), males do not drive at all, but the pair stands in the reverse parallel position seen in circling (Walther, 1984). Here again, a continuum is apparent. There are many behavioral similarities among species with differences only a matter of intensity or degree.

The much poorer eyesight of the more primitive ungulates, such as tapirs, rhinos, hippos, and pigs, has resulted in a stronger dependence on sensory modalities other than vision. Although little is known about their significance, vocalizations are a notable part of courtship, particularly by males. Some calls likely serve to soothe the female and thus allow approach, whereas others seem to excite her in preparation for copulation. The intensity of these vocalizations is greatest in the tapirs and rhinos (Walther, 1984).

The most dramatic incorporation of olfaction into courtship rituals also is found in tapirs and rhinos. Females splash great quantities of urine, often while being chased by the male. The frequency of male urination is also higher at this time.

Olfactory communication probably plays a major role in mediating the attractiveness of the estrous female. Flehmen, the behavior which serves to introduce urinary compounds into the vomeronasal organ (Wysocki et al., 1980), is seen in males of most ungulate species, although females and young occasionally flehm. Its increased occurrence during the breeding season and decreased frequency following castration suggest at least some androgen influence (Ladewig et al., 1980).

Males are especially interested in female urine, and urinary behavior is an integral part of courtship behavior of most ungulate species. The frequency of female urination increases during estrus, but if she does not do so spontaneously in response to a male approach, he may stimulate urination by sniffing, licking, or nudging the perineal area, or in more extreme cases by chasing her. After sniffing and/or licking the anogenital area or the urine of the female, the male performs flehmen, or lip-curl, which consists of lifting the head so that the nose is tilted upward (Estes, 1972). There is disagreement, perhaps as a result of species differences, as to whether the nares are closed and whether air is transpired during the behavior.

In species where more careful investigations have been performed, males have shown more interest in urine from females in late diestrus or proestrus, periods that might signal impending estrus to the male (Ladewig et al., 1980). Because of competition for females, a male may better choose which female to defend or follow if he can detect early signs of estrus.

Involvement of urine in courtship rituals is not restricted to transmission from female to male. In domestic goats, in particular, male displays include spraying themselves with urine, especially the beards under their chins, or even into their own mouths (Ladewig et al., 1980). Wetting the hair with urine may conceivably provide an olfactory message to estrous females which could be attractive or stimulating. However, a function for urine drinking is more obscure. The male Nile lechwe (*Kob megaceros*), an African antelope, also urinates onto the long hair of his lower neck, but then rubs his wet neck-mane on the female, marking her (Leuthold, 1977).

Male odor also plays a prominent role in the courtship behavior of pigs, but in this case, the sources are the preputial glands of the penile sheath and saliva (Sink, 1967; Patterson, 1968). This odor induces the immobilization reflex, the porcine equivalent of lordosis, in estrous females. Tactile stimulation and vocalizations by the boar can also cause this response, but a combination of these sensory modalities plus vision has the strongest effect (Signoret and Du Mesnil Du Buisson, 1961). The domestic pig-breeding industry has capitalized on this phenomenon by isolating the androgen metabolites of the boar's preputial gland and saliva. These are marketed as an aerosol to be sprayed on the snouts of females for estrus detection.

In addition, males communicate with a variety of skin glands, many of which seem to be androgen sensitive. These are used during courtship but also for territorial demarcation (Walther, 1984). For example, secretions from the occipital gland of the male camel increase during the breeding season and are thought to influence the occurrence of estrus in females (Ayorinde et al., 1982).

A typical copulatory sequence begins with the male placing his chin on the female's rump, perhaps as a final test of her readiness to mate. If she is receptive, he then mounts, achieves intromission and ejaculates. There is a remarkable range in copulatory duration among ungulates, from a few seconds in most species (Leuthold, 1977) to the 30–60 minutes with multiple ejaculations indulged in by rhinos (Owen-Smith, 1974).

Although it is common for a female to mate with many males during estrus, she may be tended, or guarded, after copulation. In those with lengthy periods of intromission, guarding may be unnecessary. An alternative method of preventing sperm competition by another male is to leave a copulatory plug. Among ungulates, the collared peccary (*Tayassu tajacu*) is the only species known to deposit such a gelatinous plug in the vagina upon ejaculation (Sowls, 1966). The plug may remain in place for up to an hour. The males does not guard the female during this time, and she may mate with other males before estrus ends. However, no information exists on whether she accepts, or is able to achieve copulation with, another male during the time the plug remains in place. Neither is it known if deposition of a vaginal plug increases the chances of paternity. The suids and tayassuids are the only ungulates which commonly have at least 3–5 fetuses per pregnancy. The others have 1 or 2, very rarely 3. Multiple paternity is documented in other orders (rabbits: Fischer and Adams, 1981; rats: Gartner et al., 1981) and could well occur in pigs.

Small equatorial species with shorter gestations, such as the dik-dik (*Madoqua saltiana*) and duiker, can breed twice a year, providing conditions are favorable. Larger ungulates breed once a year or less. In areas where conditions vary little throughout the year, there is still a trend for mating, and thus births, to occur seasonally. Where rainfall patterns are biannual, there may be two peaks.

As detailed for carnivores, environmental constraints on reproduction are focused primarily on the time of parturition, not mating. An exception is the roe deer (*Capreolus capreolus*), the only ungulate to show delayed implantation, and in fact, the first species in which the phenomenon was described (Nowak and Paradiso, 1983). The reason for the delay to occur only in this species is unclear but is perhaps related in some way to another unique feature. It is also the only territorial cervid. More interestingly, females as well as males are territorial, and mating occurs on female territories. Perhaps parameters of territorial defense require that mating be earlier in the year than it is for other deer. Of further interest is the observation that some roe deer females mate in fall and implant without undergoing delay.

In higher latitudes, births are timed to occur in spring or summer when temperatures are warmer and food more plentiful. Thus, depending on gestation length, breeding seasons tend to occur during the previous fall or early winter (white-tailed deer, sheep, goat) or spring and early summer (horse, donkey). Obviously, environmental cues are not the same for animals that breed in spring as for those breeding in fall, yet all respond to the perceived changes in daylength that occur at those times. The lengthening days of spring stimulate gonadal recrudescence in horses and donkeys, whereas the progressively shorter days of autumn are stimulatory to deer, sheep, and goats.

The mechanisms for transduction of photoperiodic information have been studied extensively in the domestic sheep and white-tailed deer. As described in the section on carnivores, light impinging on the retina is transduced into a hormonal message via the pineal gland (Legan and Winans, 1981).

The mechanism for transduction of information regarding the rainy season has not been established for ungulates. Estrus in the white rhino (*Ceratotherium simum*) has been noted to occur shortly after a flush of green grass following a dry period (Owen-Smith, 1974) and has been documented to coincide with the rains in dry plains areas for other species as well (Rowlands and Weir, 1984). Although changes in humidity and barometric pressure have not been eliminated, reproductive stimulation is more likely to come from the resultant vegetation. Increased nutritional level may be the trigger, or, as in rodents, specific compounds found in the new growth may stimulate gonadal activity (Sanders et al., 1981).

Tighter synchronization of estrus and parturition in species such as the wildebeest (*Connochaetes gnou*; Sinclair, 1977) and impala (*Aepyceros melampus*; Murray, 1982) is believed to be mediated by the lunar cycle. Because predators take more young of the early and late breeders (Estes, 1976), a concentration of births is thought to result in predator swamping— i.e., providing more than predators can eat during a shorter period of time and resulting in a lower total number of calves lost.

Another form of estrous synchronization which occurs in sheep, and probably other species, is mediated by pheromones. Feral ewes from the same social group tend to enter estrus together (Grubb, 1974), which implies interfemale olfactory communication. However, because rams were present and rams have been shown to cause advancement of first ovulation and of first estrus in ewes at the inception of the breeding season (Fraser, 1968), females are likely to be responding to male odor. The phenomenon is similar to that described in detail for laboratory mice, in which introduction of a male to a group of females results in rapid onset of synchronous estrus (Whitten, 1956).

The length of the estrous, or ovulatory, cycle varies by species. The modal value is about 3 weeks (Table 10.3), but most reported values are based only on behavioral observations and not on endocrine or ovarian measures. The most detailed information on physiological aspects of the ovulatory cycle come, of course, from domestic species such as the horse, cow, pig, and sheep (Cole and Cupps, 1977). Although seasonal constraints on reproduction have been eliminated in many domestic species—resulting for some, such as the cow and pig, in year-round cycles—it is unlikely that domestication has appreciably changed the dynamics of the ovulatory cycle itself. Unfortunately, endocrine data for wild counterparts of domestic stock have not been published.

For domestic ungulates, the estrous cycle is divided into the estrous (follicular) and diestrous (luteal) phases. Proestrus is not usually distinguished. A peak in estradiol, the primary estrogen produced by ripening ovarian follicles, stimulates a release of pituitary luteinizing hormone (LH), the timing of which typically coincides with behavioral estrus. Progesterone from the corpora lutea dominates the subsequent diestrous phase.

The white-tailed deer is the nondomestic species for which the most detailed hormone measurements are available (Figure 10.6; Plotka et al., 1980). Except that the preovulatory estradiol peak is less defined, the pattern is like that of the domestics. Hormone profiles for the ovulatory horse (Figure 10.7, Ginther, 1979) are basically similar, but the LH elevation is a curve rather than a peak and is in closer phase with estradiol.

Behavioral estrus in ungulates is often of less than 24 hours duration (Table 10.2). Estrus of more than 2 days is uncommon. Equids have the longest estrus of the spontaneous ovulators (Table 10.4). The camelids have extremely variable estrous periods because ovulation, which results in cessation of estrus, must be induced (Novoa, 1970).

Female camels, being induced ovulators, have less regular cycles, but are not monestrous and will come into heat again if not pregnant. Because reported cycle lengths vary from 2 to several weeks and pseudopregnancy following sterile mating is only 3 to 4 weeks, these states cannot be readily distinguished.

Experiments in which the ovaries are removed and sex hormones are injected have shown that estradiol alone is sufficient to induce estrous behavior in the cow, pig, and horse. However, in the horse, addition of progesterone on

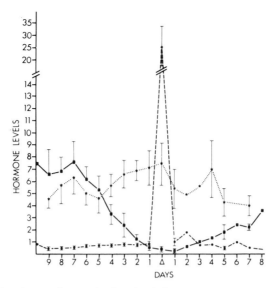

Figure 10.6. Periovulatory changes in the circulating concentrations of LH, estradiol, and progesterone from 10 days before estrus (△) through 8 days after estrus in the white-tailed deer (*Odocoileus virginianus*). LH (– – –) levels (N = 53) are expressed as ng NIH-LH-S7/ml serum. Estradiol (····) levels (N = 53) and progesterone (——) levels (N = 53) are pg/ml and ng/ml, respectively. (By permission of Plotka et al., 1980)

the first day of treatment only, results in an enhancement of the effect of estradiol on female proceptive behavior (Asa et al., 1984). Administration of progesterone with estradiol on subsequent days inhibits all aspects of sexual behavior, whereas treatment with estradiol alone continues to be moderately stimulatory. These results are similar to those reported for the guinea pig in regard to the synergy of progesterone and estradiol. However, the female guinea pig requires prior exposure to subthreshold levels of estradiol for progesterone facilitation to occur (Morali and Beyer, 1979).

An explanation for this discrepancy may lie in another anomaly of the horse, the failure of ovariectomy to abolish sexual behavior (Asa et al., 1980a). The phenomenon, described previously only in primates, is probably due in the horse and rhesus monkey (*Macaca mulatta*) to adrenal sex steroids (Asa et al., 1980b; Everitt et al., 1972). More extensive investigation revealed that mares exhibit sexual behavior (proceptivity, receptivity, and attractiveness) during seasonal anestrus as well as during the preovulatory period and following ovariectomy, but not during diestrus or pregnancy (Asa et al., 1983). These results suggest that the mare has the capacity to engage in sexual behavior except when under the influence of progesterone. However, an increase in progesterone or one of its metabolites just prior to ovulation may be the cause of the more intense estrus often seen at that time.

Progesterone has yet another effect on the expression of estrous behavior in the ewe and, to a lesser extent, the cow (Clemens and Christensen, 1975). Exogenous estrogen will induce estrus in the

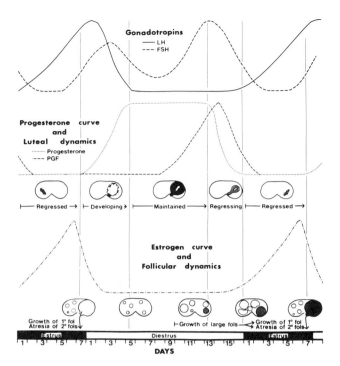

Figure 10.7. Temporal relationships among hormones and ovarian events during the estrous cycle of the horse (*Equus caballus*). (By permission of Ginther, 1979)

ovariectomized sheep and cow, but much smaller doses of estrogen are required if progesterone is added. However, progesterone administration must precede, not follow that of estradiol if facilitation is to occur.

The necessity for this can be better understood when the natural cycle of the intact ewe is examined. In early autumn, at the inception of the breeding season, the first ovulatory cycle is not accompanied by estrous behavior. This is called a "silent" estrus. Only after exposure to circulating progesterone from the corpus luteum of that previous cycle does the ewe show interest in the ram. Although ovariectomy and hormone-replacement studies have not been performed in other fall-breeding ungulates, the first ovulation of the season is not accompanied by estrous behavior in those for which data are available (Rowlands and Weir, 1984).

The absence of a proestrous phase in ungulates is somewhat surprising, considering the often complete segregation of the sexes outside the breeding season. Well before a female's first behavioral estrus, male testosterone increases stimulate species-specific aggression and dominance or territorial interactions. Rowlands and Weir (1984) suggest that males and females may respond to different cues or at different times to the same cues because of the longer period required to initiate and complete spermatogenesis.

There remains, however, the need for locating a partner, and perhaps early courtship or tending prior to the onset of estrus. Changes in female

Species	Breeding season	Duration of estrus	Estrous cycle length	Length of gestation
Asiatic tapir	Apr.–May			390–395 d
S. Amer. tapir	All year			390–400 d
Black rhino	Nov.–Dec.		17–60 d	419–476 d
White rhino	All year			
Domestic donkey	Mar.–Aug.	6 d	21–28 d	365 d
Domestic horse	Mar.–Aug. (some all year)	5–7 d	21 d	11 mo
Zebra	Jun.–Aug.	2–9 d	21 d	11–12 mo
Wild pig	All year, tropics; fall, temperate	2–3 d	21 d	100–140 d
Domestic pig	All year	2–3 d	21 d	112–115 d
Hippopotamus	Feb. & Aug. peaks	3 d		227–240 d
Dromedary camel	Dec.–Mar.			12–13 mo
Vicuna	Mar.–Apr.			11 mo
Giraffe	All year		12–15 d	457 d
White-tailed deer	Oct.–Jan.	24 hr	28 d	195–212 d
Moose	Sept.–Oct.	24 hr	20–22 d	226–264 d
Roe deer	Jul.–Aug.			285 d
Afr. buffalo	Feb.–Jul. peaks	5–6 d	23 d	340 d
Domestic cow	All year	< 24 hr	21 d	277–290 d
Amer. bison	Jul.–Sept. (all year in captivity)	2 d	21 d	285 d
Domestic goat	Sept.–Jan.	1–4 d	21 d	150 d
Domestic sheep	Sept.–Jan. (some breeds year-round)	1–2 d	16.5 d	150 d

SOURCES: Asdell, 1964; Rowlands and Weir, 1984; Nowak and Paradiso, 1983.

behavior do occur before the time of sexual receptivity. Most commonly these include hyperreactivity, restlessness, and an increase in urination (Fraser, 1968). Females and/or their urine have been reported to be attractive to males before sexual receptivity. The increase in estradiol which precedes both the LH surge and receptivity may influence these "pre-estrous" signs.

Several lines of evidence, albeit from disparate species, support this hypothesis. Administration of estradiol to ovariectomized mares increases the frequency of urination and approaches to the male (Asa et al., 1984). Increased estradiol during proestrus in female wolves correlates with both increased urination and attractiveness of the urine to male wolves (Seal et al., 1979; Asa et al., 1985; unpublished personal observations). Exogenous estradiol is necessary and sufficient to make ovariectomized rhesus monkeys attractive to males (Everitt et al., 1972). Male goats were shown to be more interested in late diestrous than estrous urine (Ladewig et al., 1980). Although ovariectomized domestic ungulates have been treated with estradiol to induce estrus, aspects of female response other than acceptance of the male for mating have not been carefully evaluated.

Among seasonally breeding cervids and bovids, the apparent widespread occurrence of behavioral estrus reliably accompanying the second but not first ovulation may be involved also. In this case, hormonal changes do occur in advance of the first period of receptivity and may affect female behavior or attractiveness.

Perhaps not coincidentally, most seasonally reproducing ungulates fall into the category of autumn, or short-day, breeders. Long-day breeders such as the horse may have silent ovulations, but the percentage is so low as to suggest social or clinical causes. Additionally, mate location is seldom required for female horses and lamoids which have males permanently in attendance. Mediation of social bonding in these species may be related to their relatively long estrous phases and, in the horse, by their ability to respond sexually outside the regular breeding season.

SUMMARY

The social systems of both ungulates and carnivores are correlated with their roles as prey and predator, respectively. Small ungulates (chevrotain, mouse deer) can escape detection by living more or less solitary lives in wooded habitat. In contrast, larger ungulate species more commonly rely on flight from predators in open terrain, often coupled with a tendency to associate with large groups (most bovids). Among carnivores, those which hunt small prey such as insects and rodents are typically solitary (bears, weasels) or live in pairs (foxes, jackals). Those which specialize in large prey often hunt cooperatively and thus form larger social groups (wolves, lions).

With the exception of some of the equids and South American lamoids, male and female ungulates seem not to develop bonds which endure beyond the period of female sexual receptivity, whether the species is solitary or gregarious. However, gregarious species are more likely to be polygynous; that is, although not all males succeed in mating, those that do are likely to mate with more than one female. Despite male attempts to maintain exclusive mating rights, females will breed promiscuously as well. Less gregarious species are more likely to form consort pairs during the period of sexual interaction.

Among the canids, monogamy is not uncommon, whether the association endures throughout the year (wolves, jackals) or reforms during the breeding season (foxes). In contrast to the large assemblages of ungulates, carnivore social groups are typically extended families (wolves, lions, Cape hunting dogs). Whereas the gregariousness of ungulates serves primarily as a predatory defense strategy, i.e., "safety in numbers," carnivore groups appear more cohesive. The long-term familial bonds may enable development of more complex communicative and cooperative hunting skills.

Smaller carnivores may themselves be vulnerable to predation. It may be no coincidence that these species are more likely to be solitary or to form pairs, in contrast to the larger species with larger social groups. In contrast to the lion, most felid species hunt relatively large game but lead primarily solitary lives, because their hunting technique entails stalking or springing at close range from cover, a strategy which would not benefit from assistance.

Vulnerability to predation is also reflected in such aspects of breeding activity as duration of copulation. Ungulates and smaller carnivores typically have very brief copulatory interactions. The longest durations are found among the larger canids and the large, relatively nonvulnerable ungulates such as rhinoceroses.

Generalizations regarding the reproductive strategies of carnivores and, especially, ungulates are constrained most severely by a dearth of information on their comparative reproductive physiologies. This interesting area of research awaits further investigation.

REFERENCES

ADLER, N.T., and S.R. ZOLOTH (1970) Copulatory behavior can inhibit pregnancy in female rats. Science *168*:1480–1482.

ASA, C.S., D.A. GOLDFOOT, M.C. GARCIA, and O.J. GINTHER (1980a) Sexual behavior in ovariectomized and seasonally anovulatory mares. Horm. Behav. *14*:46–54.

ASA, C.S., D.A. GOLDFOOT, M.C. GARCIA, and O.J. GINTHER (1980b) Dexamethasone suppression of sexual behavior in ovariectomized mares. Horm. Behav. *14*:55–64.

ASA, C.S., D.A. GOLDFOOT, and O.J. GINTHER (1983) Assessment of the sexual behavior of pregnant mares. Horm. Behav. *17*:405–413.

ASA, C.S., D.A. GOLDFOOT, M.C. GARCIA, and O.J. GINTHER (1984) The effect of estradiol and progesterone on the sexual behavior of ovariectomized mares. Physiol. Behav. *33*:681–686.

ASA, C.S., L.D. MECH, and U.S. SEAL (1985) The use of urine, faeces, and anal-gland secretions in scent-marking by a captive wolf (*Canis lupus*) pack. Anim. Behav. *33*:1034–1036.

ADA, C.S., U.S. SEAL, M.A. LETELLIER, and E.D. PLOTKA (submitted) Lack of effect of pinealectomy and superior-cervical-ganglionectomy on reproduction in the wolf (*Canis lupus*).

ASA, C.S., U.S. SEAL, E.D. PLOTKA, M.A. LETELLIER, and L.D. MECH (1986) Effect of anosmia on reproduction in male and female wolves (*Canis lupus*). Behav. Neural. Biol.

ASDELL, S.A. (1964) *Patterns of Mammalian Reproduction*, 2nd ed. Cornell University Press, Ithaca.

AYORINDE, F., J.W. WHEELER, C. WEMMER, and J. MURTAUGH (1982) Volatile components of the occipital gland secretion of the bactrian camel (*Camelus bactrianus*). J. Chem. Ecol. *8*:177–183.

BEACH, F.A. (1976) Sexual attractivity, proceptivity and receptivity in female mammals. Horm. Behav. 7:105–138.

CLEMENS, L.G., and L.W. CHRISTENSEN (1975) Sexual behavior. In *The Behaviour of Domestic Animals*. E.S.E. Hafez, ed., Williams and Wilkins, Baltimore.

COLE, H.H., and P.T. CUPPS (1977) *Reproduction in Domestic Animals*, 3d ed. Academic Press, New York.

CONCANNON, P., W. HANSEL, and K. McENTREE (1977) Changes in LH, progesterone and sexual behavior associated with preovulatory luteinization in the bitch. Biol. Reprod. 17:604–613.

ESTES, R.D. (1976) The significance of breeding synchrony in the wildebeest. E. Afr. Wildl. J. 14:135–152.

EVERITT, B.J., J. HERBERT, and J.D. HAMER (1972) Sexual receptivity of bilaterally adrenalectomized female rhesus monkeys. Physiol. Behav. 8:409–415.

EWER, R.F. (1973) *The Carnivores*. Cornell University Press, Ithaca.

FEIST, J.D., and D.R. McCULLOUGH (1975) Reproduction in feral horses. J. Reprod. Fert., Suppl. 23:13–18.

FISCHER, B., and C.E. ADAMS (1981) Fertilization following mixed insemination with "cervix-selected" and "unselected" spermatozoa in the rabbit. J. Reprod. Fert. 62:337–343.

FRASER, A.F. (1968) *Reproductive Behavior in Ungulates*. Academic Press, London.

GARTNER, K., B. WANKEL, and D. GAUDSZUHN (1981) The hierarchy in copulatory competition and its correlation with paternity in grouped male laboratory rats. Z. Tierpsychol. 56:243–254.

GAUTHIER-PILTERS, H., and A.I. DAGG (1981) *The Camel: Its Evolution, Ecology, Behavior and Relationship to Man*. University of Chicago Press, Chicago.

GINTHER, O.J. (1979) *Reproductive Biology of the Mare: Basic and Applied Aspects*. Published by the author, Dept. Veterinary Science, University of Wisconsin, Madison.

GRUBB, P. (1974) Mating activity and the social significance of rams in a feral sheep community. In *The Behaviour of Ungulates and Its Relation to Management*, Vol. I. V. Geist and F.R. Walther, eds. IUCN Publ. no. 24:457–476.

HERBERT, J., P.M. STACEY, and D.H. THORPE (1978) Recurrent breeding seasons in pinealectomized or optic-nerve-sectioned ferrets. J. Endocrinol. 78:389–397.

KENNELLY, J. J., and B.E. JOHNS (1976) The estrous cycle of coyotes. J. Wildl. Mgmt. 40:272–277.

LADEWIG, J., E.O. PRICE, and B.L. HART (1980) Flehmen in male goats: Role in sexual behavior. Behav. Neural Biol. 30:312–322.

LEUTHOLD, W. (1977) *African Ungulates*. Springer-Verlag, Berlin.

McMILLAN, J.M., U.S. SEAL, K.D. KEENLYNE, A.W. ERICKSON, and J.E. JONES (1974) Annual testosterone rhythm in the adult white-tailed deer (*Odocoileus virginianus borealis*). Endocrinology 94:1034–1040.

MECH, L.D. (1970) *The Wolf*. Natural History Press, New York.

MECH, L.D., and S.T. KNICK (1978) Sleeping distances in wolf pairs in relation to the breeding season. Behav. Biol. 23:521–525.

MICHAEL, R.P., and P.P. SCOTT (1957) Quantitative studies on mating behaviour of spayed female cats stimulated by treatment with oestrogens. J. Physiol. *138*:46–47.

MILLER, R.K. (1981) Male aggression, dominance and breeding behavior in Red Desert feral horses. Z. Tierpsychol. *57*:340–351.

MOEHLMAN, P.D. (1970) Behavior and ecology of feral asses (*Equus asinus*). Nat. Geog. Res. Reports: 1970 papers. pp. 405–411.

MOEHLMAN, P.D. (1980) Jackals of the Serengeti. Nat. Geog. *158*:840–850.

MORALI, G., and C. BEYER (1979) Neuroendocrine control of mammalian estrous behavior. In *Endocrine Control of Sexual Behavior*. C. Beyer, ed., Raven Press, New York.

MURRAY, M.G. (1982) The rut of the impala: Aspects of seasonal mating under tropical conditions. Z. Tierpsychol. *59*:319–337.

NOVOA, C. (1970) Review: Reproduction in Camelidae. J. Reprod. Fert. *22*:3–20.

NOWAK, R.M., and J.L. PARADISO (1983) *Walker's Mammals of the World*, 4th ed., Vol. II. Johns Hopkins University Press, Baltimore.

OWEN-SMITH, R.N. (1974) The social system of the white rhinoceros. In *The Behaviour of Ungulates and Its Relation to Management*. V. Geist and F.R. Walther, eds. IUCN Publ. no. *24*:341–351.

PACKARD, J.M., U.S. SEAL, L.D. MECH, and E.D. PLOTKA (1985) Causes of reproductive failure in two family groups of wolves (*Canis lupus*). Z. Tierpsychol. *68*:24–40.

PATTERSON, R.L.S. (1968) Identification of 3α-OH-5α-androst-16-ene as the musk odour component of boar submaxillary salivary gland and its relationship to the sex odour taint in pork meat. J. Sci. Food Agric. *19*:434–438.

PLOTKA, E.D., U.S. SEAL, M.A. LETELLIER, L.J. VERME, and J.J. OZOGA (1979) Endocrine and morphologic effects of pinealectomy in white-tailed deer. In *Animal Models for Research on Contraception and Fertility*. M.J. Alexander, ed., Harper and Row, Hagerstown, Md.

PLOTKA, E.D., U.S. SEAL, L.J. VERME, and J.J. OZOGA (1980) Reproductive steroids in deer. III. Luteinizing hormone, estradiol and progesterone around estrus. Biol. Reprod. *22*:576–581.

RACEY, P.A., and J.D. SKINNER (1979) Endocrine aspects of sexual mimicry in spotted hyenas *Crocuta crocuta*. J. Zool., Lond. *187*:315–326.

RAEDEKE, K.J. (1979) Population dynamics and socioecology of the guanaco (*Lama guanicoe*) of Magellanes Chile. Ph.D. Thesis, University of Washington.

ROTHMAN, R.J., and L.D. MECH (1979) Scent-marking in lone wolves and newly-formed pairs. Anim. Behav. *27*:750–760.

ROWLANDS, I.W., and B.J. WEIR (1984) Mammals; Non-primate eutherians. In *Marshall's Physiology of Reproduction*, 4th ed., Vol. 1, *Reproductive Cycles of Vertebrates*. G.E. Lamming, ed., Churchill Livingstone, Edinburgh.

RUBENSTEIN, D.I. (1981) Behavioural ecology of island feral horses. Equine Vet. J. *13*:27–34.

SANDERS, E.H., P.D. GARDNER, P.J. BERGER, and N.D. NEGUS (1981) 6-methoxy-benzoxazolinone: A plant derivative that stimulates reproduction in *Microtus montanus*. Science *214*:67–69.

SCALIA, F., and S.S. WINANS (1981) The differential projection of the olfactory bulb and accessory olfactory bulb in mammals. J. Comp. Neur. *161*:31–56.

SCHALLER, G.B. (1972) *The Serengeti Lion.* University of Chicago Press, Chicago.

SCHMIDT, A.M., L.A. NADAL, M.J. SCHMIDT, and N.B. BEAMER (1979) Serum concentrations of oestradiol and progesterone during the normal oestrous cycle and early pregnancy in the lion (*Panthera leo*). J. Reprod. Fert. *57*:267–272.

SEAL, U.S., E.D. PLOTKA, J.M. PACKARD, and L.D. MECH (1979) Endocrine correlates of reproduction in the wolf: I. Serum progesterone, estradiol, and LH during the estrous cycle. Biol. Reprod. *21*:1057–1066.

SEAL, U.S., E.D. PLOTKA, J.D. SMITH, F.H. WRIGHT, N.J. REINDL, R.S. TAYLOR, and M.F. SEAL (1985) Immunoreactive luteinizing hormone, estradiol, progesterone, testosterone, and androstenedione levels during the breeding season and anestrus in Siberian tigers. Biol. Reprod. *32*:361–368.

SHORT, R.V. (1984) Oestrous and menstrual cycles. In *Reproduction in Mammals*, 2d ed., Book 3. C.R. Austin and R.V. Short, eds., Cambridge University Press, Cambridge.

SIGNORET, J.P., and F. DUMESNIL DUBUISSON (1961) Etude du comportement de la truie en oestrus. IVth Cong. Int. Reprod. Anim., La Haye: 171–175.

SINCLAIR, A.R.E. (1977) Lunar cycle and timing of mating season in Serengeti wildebeest. Nature *267*:832–833.

SINK, J.D. (1967) Theoretical aspects of sex odor in swine. J. Thero. Biol *17*:174–180.

SMITH, M.S., and L.E. MCDONALD (1974) Serum levels of luteinizing hormone and progesterone during the estrous cycle, pseudopregnancy and pregnancy in the dog. Endocrinol. *94*:404–412.

SOWLS, L.K. (1966) Reproduction in the collared peccary (*Tayassu tajacu*). In *Comparative Biology of Reproduction in Mammals.* I.W. Rowlands, ed. Symp. Zool. Soc. Lond. *15*:155–172.

TUREK, F.W., J. SWANN, and D.J. EARNEST (1984) Role of the circadian system in reproductive phenomena. Rec. Prog. Horm. Res. *40*:143–184.

VERHAGE, H.G., N.B. BEAMER, and R.M. BRENNER (1976) Plasma levels of estradiol and progesterone in the cat during polyestrus, pregnancy, and pseudopregnancy. Biol. Reprod. *14*:579–585.

WALLEN, K., and R.W. GOY (1977) Effects of estradiol benzoate, estrone, and propionates of testosterone or dihydrotestosterone on sexual and related behaviors of ovariectomized rhesus monkeys. Horm. Behav. *9*:228–248.

WALTHER, F.R. (1984) *Communication and Expression in Hoofed Mammals.* Indiana University Press, Bloomington.

WHITTEN, W.K. (1956) Modification of the oestrous cycle of the mouse by external stimuli associated with the male. J. Endocrinol. *13*:399–404.

WYSOCKI, C.J., J.L. WELLINGTON, and G.K. BEAUCHAMP (1980) Access of urinary nonvolatiles to the mammalian vomeronasal organ. Science *207*:781–783.

YOUNG, S.P. (1944) *The Wolves of North America.* Part I. American Wildlife Institute, Washington, D.C.

ELEVEN
Stress, Social Status, and Reproductive Physiology in Free-Living Baboons

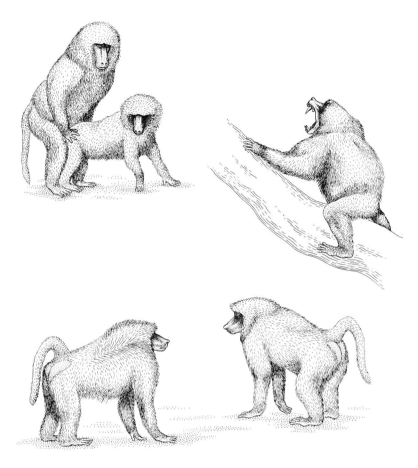

Robert M. Sapolsky
Department of Biological Sciences
Stanford University
Stanford, California
and
Institute of Primate Research
National Museums of Kenya
Nairobi, Kenya

During the Second World War, in the Nazi concentration camp of Theresienstadt, a German doctor examined the 800 women interned and found that 54% had ceased menstruating. Few of us are likely to be surprised by this statistic; the horrors of the camps included hard labor and malnutrition, and as calories and energy available to the body plummet under such conditions, unessentials like reproduction are typically curtailed. However, what was striking was that the amenorrhea in the majority of the women began during the first month of internment, long before the malnutrition had become pronounced (discussed in Reichlin, 1974). Research in behavioral biology and psychosomatic medicine helps explain this pattern in the women of Theresienstadt: emotional stress can disrupt reproductive physiology as profoundly as can malnutrition, physical abuse, or a wide variety of diseases. The endocrine literature is filled with similar examples of reproductive failure predominantly attributable to stress, such as in English populations during the bombings of London or in Northern Irish populations during civil strife. But the stressors that wreak havoc with reproductive function need not be as extreme as the horror of the Blitzkrieg or of entering a death camp. A change in living condition, in occupation, or in level of exercise are among the most frequently cited correlates of psychogenic amenorrhea, the failure of ovulation which cannot be attributed to organic pathology (Ross et al., 1981). Clearly, reproductive physiology is exquisitely sensitive to our emotional state.

A major advance in medical thought has been the recognition that this relationship of mental health and physical well-being extends far beyond the confines of reproduction. Emotional status, level of stress, and means of coping can influence veritably all aspects of health and disease. Most laypeople and health professionals have accepted this notion to the point where some maladies are now principally thought of as being "stress-related"—among them, peptic ulcers, colitis, and certain forms of impotency or hypertension. Physiologists continue to provide mechanisms by which stress can influence disease processes which are less readily viewed as being sensitive to emotions—cholesterol metabolism and the formation of sclerotic plaques in blood vessels, the establishment and growth of tumors, or the survival of neurons following a stroke (Kaplan et al., 1983; Sapolsky and Donnelly, 1985; Sapolsky and Pulsinelli, 1985).

Medical professionals have not always accepted a role for stress in disease processes. Only relatively recently have they seriously considered the vagaries of feelings, thoughts, and experiences when wrestling with questions of pancreatic enzymes, blood gases, and cardiac cycles. While the idea of a role for stress has often occurred in medical thought, it typically has been only in an anecdotal fashion. However, the concept of stress affecting physiology has gained credibility in recent decades through rigorous experiments. As a consequence, there is now substantial information known about the psychologic components of experience which are "stressful," the consistent manner in which the endocrine and nervous systems respond to such stress, and the mechanisms by which this stress-response is in the short term adaptive but in the long run pathogenic.

STRESS AND THE STRESS-RESPONSE

A *stressor* can be viewed as any environmental perturbation which disrupts homeostasis—the optimum of pH, oxygenation, and so on at which physiological systems function. The *stress-response* is the set of physiological adaptations which the body consistently musters in reestablishing homeostasis. Hans Selye, the scientist, physician, and indisputable father of modern stress physiology, was the first to note the consistency of the body's responses to varied insults. From his earliest days of medical training, Selye was interested in the general features similar to all diseases and the body's responses to them—as he called it in his memoirs, the "syndrome of just being sick" (Selye, 1979). In a landmark 1936 paper and in subsequent work, Selye showed that there are consistent patterns to how the body responded to a wide range of diseases as well as to varied emotional challenges (Selye, 1936, 1971). What he first noted is that cold stress, forced exercise, exposure to toxins, and numerous other insults all caused the same responses in rats: the adrenal glands enlarge, the thymus gland atrophies, and peptic ulcers develop. The first pathology is due to the sustained secretion by the adrenals of the principal stress hormones, epinephrine (also known as adrenaline), and glucocorticoids. The demand for their secretion during the sustained stress in these rats leads to hypertrophy of the adrenals. The atrophy of the thymus and development of peptic ulcers are two (and the most dramatically visible) of the many consequences of the elevated glucocorticoid concentrations in the blood. Selye's intellectual descendants have since shown that in addition to the secretion of epinephrine and glucocorticoids, other consistent responses occur in the body during the homeostatic challenge of stress. These include alterations in autonomic nervous system activity and in the circulating concentrations of a variety of other hormones, including norepinephrine (noradrenaline), prolactin, glucagon, opioids, vasopressin, growth hormone, gonadotropins, and the gonadal steroids (Rose and Sachar, 1981).

All stressors do not provoke the identical profile of hormonal and neural responses. Indeed, the way in which responses vary with each type of stressor has been a subject of considerable work and often debate. Nevertheless, there is still a striking consistency to the responses that the body activates, whether one is exposed to extreme heat or cold, whether one is a gazelle running from a lion in terror, or an adolescent facing the terror of one's first high school dance. Selye, viewing the consistency, termed these responses the "General Adaptation Syndrome." In so doing, he provided one of the intellectual cornerstones of the subject. The body mobilizes this *general* package of responses, he argued, because regardless of the stressor, certain adaptations are always needed to aid survival (Selye, 1971).

First among these responses is the increased availability of easily utilized energy to overcome such stressors. This shift of energy substrates from storage sites to the bloodstream is a hallmark of the stress-response. Glucose uptake, fatty-acid storage, and glycogen and protein synthesis are all inhibited at storage tissues, and the release of energy substrates (in the forms of glucose, amino acids, and free fatty acids) from muscle, fat, and liver is stimulated. Glucocorticoids, epinephrine, norepinephrine, and glucagon appear most responsible for these adaptations (Yates et al., 1980; Munck et al., 1984). Along with these changes in energy availability and utilization comes increased cardiovascular tone; blood pressure, heart rate, and breathing rate are stimulated by the sympathetic nervous system, glucocorticoids, and vasopressin (Yates et al., 1980).

Other anabolic processes are suppressed; in effect, the body is saying that this is an emergency and certain costly and slow building processes can be deferred until more auspicious times. For example, digestion is inhibited by a variety of mechanisms. Growth is slowed by direct inhibition of growth-hormone release as well as by inhibition of target-tissue sensitivity to growth hormone and other growth factors. Furthermore, as will be discussed throughout this chapter, reproduction is suppressed during stress—sperm and eggs and libido can wait until the crisis is over. Next, the immune system, responsible for surveillance for possible pathogens, is inhibited during stress by glucocorticoids and opiates (Munck et al., 1984).

Along with curtailed anabolism come a number of adaptations which keep the body functioning should there be an injury. Most of us are anecdotally familiar with the phenomenon of failing to note a painful injury during the heat of athletics or battle; recent work has implicated the release of opiates such as beta-endorphin in this "stress-induced analgesia" (Terman et al., 1984). Furthermore, the inflammatory response which would, for example, protect an injured joint by making it unusable, is inhibited during stress (Munck et al., 1984). That is, during an emergency, an injured but still usable knee is preferable to one which is protectively swollen but unusable; if one survives, there's time later to repair things. Finally, a number of hormones secreted during stress alter cognition and sensory thresholds, sharpening memory and sensation during the emergency (Bohus et al., 1982).

As a whole, these responses appear to play a critical role in surviving an *acute physical* stressor; they increase available energy substrates and increase cardiopulmonary tone, inhibit costly anabolism, keep the body functioning despite injury, and sharpen cognition. They aid the organism in attaining a stage of "adaptation." Selye characterized the first stage of a stress-response, where the stressor is perceived and responses mobilized, as the "alarm" stage. During an acute stressor, the second stage, adaptation, is usually reached, where the physiological responses just described restore homeostasis. However, with prolonged stress, adaptation fails, and we enter the realm of stress-induced disease. Selye termed this stage "exhaustion"; he theorized that the diseases of chronic stress occur because the organism loses its ability to mobilize a stress-response. In effect, reserves of glucocorticoids, epinephrine, and so on are depleted, and the organism becomes subject to the onslaughts of the stressor without protection. In actuality, research has shown that such "exhaustion" rarely occurs.

Chronic stress is pathogenic, not because the organism can no longer mobilize a stress-response, but because when mobilized chronically, the *stress-response itself* eventually becomes destructive. This is not surprising. All of the metabolic responses to stress described in the previous paragraphs are essentially catabolic in nature—costly, inefficient, even destructive, but necessary to survive the acute emergency. Activate them chronically and there is trouble. The shifting of energy substrates from stored to circulating sites is essentially a strategy of liquidating one's assets, and this is ultimately costly; myopathy, fatigue, and steroid diabetes are among the metabolic consequences of chronic stress or of chronic exposure to the hormones which mediate the metabolic responses to stress. Likewise, the increased cardiovascular tone which might be adaptive during an acute physical crisis can produce hypertension when provoked chronically. The consequences of prolonged inhibition of anabolism are obvious; growth and repair is compromised, digestion can be disrupted to the point of peptic ulceration, impotency and amenorrhea can result from the reproductive suppression, and numerous diseases can be more destructive in the face of chronic immunosuppression (Krieger, 1982). Finally, the very hormones which can alter cognition have been reported to be toxic to neurons and may play a role in the gradual loss of neurons in the aging brain (Sapolsky, 1985b).

Thus, stress provokes an array of integrated physiological responses which are critical for surviving a stressor. However, overstimulation of the stress-response can itself be highly destructive. Thus, it is as important to be able to terminate the stress-response appropriately as it is to initiate it.

INDIVIDUAL DIFFERENCES AND THE STRESS-RESPONSE

As discussed, 54% of the women in Theresienstadt ceased menstruating, and fully 60% of the amenorrhea occurred prior to malnutrition. Thus, this serves as a strong testimony to the power of stress to disrupt reproductive physiology. But one can interpret these data differently, and just as strongly. That is, *despite* stress, fear, hard labor, physical abuse, and malnutrition, nearly half of the women continued to menstruate. All individuals did not show equivalent stress pathologies. This is consistently observed whether individuals are exposed to sustained, major stressors or to the minor ones that fill our more fortunate lives. Pathologic responses occur, of course, but they are not universal or even the norm. We go through lives filled with challenges, periods of overwork and tension, close calls, unrequited loves, and disappointments, yet few of us collapse into puddles of stress-related disease. Certainly some of us are exposed to a higher frequency or severity of stressors than are others, but given the same stressors, we differ dramatically in our capacities to cope psychologically and physiologically.

It is easy to see that there are individual differences in the psychological mechanisms involved in coping with stress. We simply differ as to whether we perceive an event as being stressful; what might be a misery for you can be a neutral event or even recreational fun for someone else. Elegant studies in the last two decades have illuminated the psychological components of a stressful experience (Gray, 1982). First is the perception that an event is unpredictable. This was shown in an experiment in which two rats received identical electric shocks to their tails at the same time. Before each shock, the first rat would receive a signal, warning it that a shock was impending. The second rat received no such warning. Rats without warnings, presumably never certain when they were free of impending shocks, developed ulcers at a vastly higher rate than did rats receiving warnings. In other words, although the two treatments involved identical physical insults, they differed considerably in their psychological components, and the treatment with a larger component of unpredictability was more pathogenic. A similar pattern was observed in England during World War II. In London, air raids were inexorable, nightly, like clockwork. In contrast, in the suburbs, raids came less frequently but unpredictably. Peptic ulceration during the Blitz was much greater in the suburban population. A number of other somewhat overlapping factors contribute heavily to a perception of an event as being stressful, including loss of control, a sense of circumstances worsening, and a failure of expectations (Gray, 1982).

But given the same stressors, the same perceptions of them, two individuals may differ in their physiological responses to them. As obvious examples, we all differ in the concentrations of glucocorticoids in the blood at unstressful times, the speed at which we secrete increased amounts of the hormone during stress, the speed with which we terminate glucocorticoid secretion when it is all over with, and the sensitivity of our target tissues to the actions of the hormone. Such tremendous individual variation has differing physiological implications.

THE STRESS-RESPONSE AND SOCIAL RANK

Thus, individuals differ in their propensities towards stress-related diseases because of different rates of exposure to challenges and differing capacities to psychologically and physiologically cope. In my research, I have sought to understand how these differing capacities arise. I have studied the individual members of several troops of baboons living freely and undisturbed in a national park in East Africa. As social primates, they live in a sufficiently complex society so that some individuals have a more stressful life than do others. As particularly intelligent and individualistic primates, they differ among themselves in psychological and physiological makeup.

The question of primary interest is, Does the body of a high-ranking male baboon deal with stress differently than does that of a subordinate? Central to this question is a key feature of primate social behavior: dominance hierarchies. Primates spend a great deal of their time deciding how to deal with limited resources—there are never enough of the best things to eat, shady resting spots, desirable sexual partners, or safe sanctuaries from predators. Competition for any given disputed resource may be overt, violent, and clearly resolved by whoever pummels the other into acquiescence. But this is rarely observed; resources are usually seized by some individual without overt settlings of the matter with any and all comers; hubbubs are kept at a minimum. When a pair of animals violently contest a resource and one is soundly defeated, the odds are that a similar show of force will not have to be repeated the next time the pair comes to loggerheads. Instead, a more covert gesture by the former winner should be sufficient to remind the former loser of what happened last time. The logic of this is clear; each contest issue, each minor quibble, cannot be settled with bloody tooth and nail, and a series of conventionalized gestures that reinforce the assymetric strengths between a pair of animals slowly emerges. These features—that all individuals are not equally capable of gaining access to contested resources, and that one can save much energy and minimize risk by recognizing these differences without having to test them each time— combine to form dominance hierarchies. Depending on the species or the sex, these hierarchies can be inherited and static or may be extremely dynamic as animals test and overturn the status quo. The hierarchies may be extremely linear (i.e., there is a highest-ranking animal who supplants all others, followed by a second-ranking who supplants all but the first, . . .), circular (A supplants B who supplants C who supplants A . . .) or involve complex cooperative coalitions (A supplants C only when aided by B . . .) (Bernstein, 1981). Among male olive baboons (*Papio anubis*), the animals that I have studied, one's dominance rank determines enormously what essentials and luxuries in life are obtained and at what price.

In observing these baboons for long periods, one comes to view them as socially skilled and manipulative, living in vastly complex societies, filled with individuals utilizing different strategies to compete for high dominance rank with varying degrees of success. One can only look at these strikingly individualistic animals and wonder, what are the distinctive differences in physiology that lurk underneath their skins? This is what I set out to examine. I posed three classes of questions:

1. In a troop of wild baboons, do the bodies of high- and low-ranking males respond to stress differently? Are the stress-responses of one group more adaptive? What neuroendocrine mechanisms account for these differences?

2. Does social rank arise from these physiological differences and/or do physiological patterns arise from differences in social rank?

3. Do such physiological differences influence longevity, disease patterns, cumulative social status, or reproductive success?

WHY STUDY BABOONS IN THE WILD?

Behavior and its physiological underpinnings are exquisitely sensitive to social and ecological factors, and captivity is typically distorting in some manner. This is particularly so for social primates. The sex ratio or social structure of a captive group may differ significantly from what occurs in the wild. Housing area may be small, such that a subordinate who in the wild could retreat to the far end of the forest when a dominant animal threatened may now have only an uncomfortably close concrete corner in which to cower. Seasonal variation in reproduction and aggression may be altered with captivity in a temperate climate. Finally, captive primates are not exposed to their typical array of stressors and pathogens.

Thus, from the outset of my study, I resolved to research these issues in primates living relatively undisturbed in their natural environment. The baboon was an ideal study subject for a number of reasons.

In order to understand the relationship between the social behavior and physiology of primates, they must be habituated such that their behavior is not distorted by the presence of the observer. Observational techniques must be rigorous and unbiased, and animals must be observed for tremendous periods of time until you know individual histories, genealogies, and can spot a sideways glance or a nervous twitch from across a field. The olive baboon is big and easy to see (10–20 kg for an adult female, 20–35 kg for an adult male). It spends much of the day on the ground in bush or in open savannah in the woodland-grassland mosaics of East Africa. It lives in troops of 20–200 individuals. Females typically spend the 20–30 years of their lives in the same troop; males change troops at puberty and might change opportunistically after that but often remain in the same troop for years. Of the adult males and females still alive who were members of my main study troop when I began my work in 1978, the vast majority still reside in the same troop. Thus, there is a fair social cohesiveness in a troop that allows long-term study and intimate familiarity with individuals.

Once you understand the behavior of a particular baboon, know his dominance status, level of sexual activity, opponents and coalitional partners, the next task is to examine the workings of his body. It is necessary to capture him and conduct a number of physiological tests. For this, I dart my animals with a syringe filled with anesthetic, fired from a blowgun. All animals must be darted at the same time of year and of day, to control for rhythmic variations in physiology. Also, the anesthetic used cannot alter the variables being measured. Darting cannot occur if an animal has just had a fight, an injury, or a sexual interaction, as this will skew the normative data being collected. Animals have to be darted unawares, so there is no anticipatory stress; thus, miss an animal, explode a dart at his feet, and you are through with him for the day. Finally, drug dosage has to be guessed correctly so that the animal becomes unconscious quickly—a first blood sample must be obtained within a few minutes of darting, before hormone levels have changed in response to the stress of the darting. For all of these reasons, the baboon was also ideal. You are not trying to dart someone living 30 feet high in a forest canopy. They are big—an easier shot and easier for obtaining blood. Finally, their physiology is well known and similar to that of humans.

But one of the best reasons for studying olive baboons is the specifics of their social behavior. The variability in social organization in primates is extraordinary, with solitary prosimians, pair-bonding marmosets, harems of hamadryas females with a single male, and fluid chimpanzee societies. Competitive infanticide is observed in some species, tool use or organized hunting in others; in some, males care for infants as much as do females, while in others, male care is minimal (Jolly, 1972). Tremendous variation is seen in levels of aggression and in linearity and plasticity of dominance hierarchies. Among the primate species that would have been feasible study subjects for my project, baboons had highly stratified and overt dominance hierarchies, high levels of aggression, and high variability among males in reproductive activity. Most attractive of all was the complexity of the forms of competitive behaviors.

In a troop of some 60-odd individuals, there might be a dozen males who have reached sexual maturity and undergone the lengthy process of leaving their natal troop and slowly joining a new one. During stable periods, there is typically a single "alpha" male who is highest ranking, having primary access to disputed resources. However, he does not have exclusive access, as in age-graded species where, for example, there may be numerous males but only one who mates. Thus, males cannot be divided simply "alpha" and "others." Instead, there are hierarchies of access, where males of, say, ranks 3, 8, and 15 have qualitatively very different lives from the alpha male and from each other. As already noted, hierarchies are rarely strictly linear but will frequently have circularities imbedded within them. Furthermore, as one of the most potent wildcards available to a male baboon in his competitive strategies, cooperative reciprocal coalitions can form between or among males. Such coalitions are rare and typically unstable, as they require the mutual trust and delayed gratification for which male baboons are not particularly famous. However, when they do succeed, few dominant males, regardless of how forceful or confident, can withstand cooperating adversaries (Packer, 1977).

The fact that a male baboon, whether on his own or in a coalition, might challenge a higher-ranking male underlines another attractive feature of the species: ranks in the hierarchy shift. In other cases (female olive baboons, for example), rank is inherited in a fairly static manner from one's mother, such that daughters of high-ranking and low-ranking females have their relationships determined at remarkably early ages (Altmann, 1980). Male hierarchies, in contrast, are dramatically fluid. There will be periods of stasis and stability, where high-ranking individuals maintain their rank mostly out of covert intimidation, taking advantage of the status quo. This can be followed by periods of nervy subordinates challenging this status quo and, if succeeding, sending tremors of change throughout the hierarchy. In my own troops, an alpha male typically holds onto his position for less than a year. The capacity to compare high-ranking males who are stably entrenched with those in the midst of a revolution, or to compare a low-ranking adolescent years from his prime with a low-ranking elderly male years past his prime, added a tremendous richness to the study.

How dominance is expressed varies with the individual and circumstance. The extreme violence of male baboons has attracted considerable attention. Adults have sharpened canines longer than those of lions which, while useful for predation, are turned quite readily upon other baboons with frightful consequences. Canine slashes to the bone are common, and fatal fights have been observed. Furthermore, to compound the potential menace, such aggression is not limited merely to directly competing males, as "displaced aggression" occurs. Imagine a high-ranking male maintaining a close sexual consortship with a sexually receptive ("estrus") female. Throughout this consortship, he has been harassed by another high-ranking male. The two eye each other and bluff charge; the male in consortship tries to herd the female away while the harasser tries to intervene. Such tensions could continue for days, culminating, one might expect, in a fight between the two. However, approximately a quarter of the time, when the explosion finally comes, it is an innocent bystander who is attacked, perhaps the female herself, or a nearby subordinate male (Sapolsky, 1983b). Thus, the specter of injurious violence affects not only those who are voluntary participants in dominance competition.

Despite the drama of such bloody interactions, escalated aggression is relatively rare. Under stable conditions, an average male has a protracted fight perhaps once a month (Sapolsky, 1983a). As discussed, individuals cannot afford the energy and risk in violently testing the direction of a dyadic relationship with every confrontation. Thus, highest-ranking males do not necessarily initiate or even participate in the most fights. This has been a long-recognized feature of *stable* dominance hierarchies. The status quo of a high rank allows one to seize the benefit of the doubt much of the time and avoid violent confrontation.

Thus, baboons have evolved graded, conventionalized gestures such that a subordinate can be reminded of his subordinance with some element of subtlety. Most gestures involve a small, ritualized component of an aggressive act, such as a "threat yawn" (a directed display of his presumably intimidating canines) or a bluff charge. Subordinates, in turn, can ritualistically demonstrate their subordinance by glancing away, making an infantile vocalization, or "presenting"—crouching and presenting his buttocks in a submissive and vulnerable manner to the dominant male. These stereotyped gestures can reiterate directions of dominance when they are clear to both participants; gestural dominance interactions such as these occur at least an order of magnitude more frequently than does overt aggression.

What then are the rewards of success in this system? Access to limited resources is the answer, including food, particularly predated meat, safe spots from predators, comfortable resting spots, someone to groom you, a fertile sexual partner. It is not surprising that a correlation has been reported between a high rate of mating with estrous females and high rank in aggressive and gestural interactions (Hausfater, 1975; Seyfarth, 1976; Sapolsky, 1983a). Predictably, however, the issue is not so simple. Both observational studies and those examining the genetics of paternity have shown that the male most capable of defeating other males need not have the highest rates of reproduction (Smith, 1981; Dewsbury, 1982; Smuts, 1985). Obviously, females have some choice in the matter (although this possibility was often ignored by earlier generations of male primatologists). Thus, although a male may have vanquished all challengers and formed a consort-ship with an estrous female, the female might still slip away in dense bush and mate furtively with another (what primatologists call a "stolen copula-tion"). Furthermore, an uncompliant female might refuse to cooperate with the male when he tries to mate, or perhaps repeatedly lead the male to within close range of a challenging rival until the consorting male might voluntarily abandon the taxing consortship. Careful study has shown that females tend to choose males with whom they have formed long reciprocal relationships of grooming and who have cared for their prior offspring (Smuts, 1985). Thus, a variety of strategies are open to competing males, often involving subtle social skills in addition to outbursts of aggression.

For the male baboon, then, social life is filled with limited resources distributed unevenly, varied strategies available in pursuing these resources, the sorting out of allies and adversaries, the constant threat of displaced aggression involving you in someone else's problems, months of slowly building social affiliations with females, hours or days of relentless harass-ment of an opponent, and explosive moments of life-threatening violence. There are tremendous rewards and risks, where the successful male benefits from a good pair of canines, an optimal level of aggression, social intelli-gence, well-timed bravery, and well-timed cowardice. My studies have shown that such males also have bodies that respond to stress differently than do those of subordinates. In the remainder of this chapter, I will discuss one subset of these data, namely the effect of stress upon reproductive physiology in these animals.

STRESS AND SUPPRESSION OF TESTOSTERONE SECRETION

Primatologists have long known that stress inhibits reproduction. High-ranking marmoset monkeys can harass subordinates to the point of infertility (Epple, 1978). Not only is there a loss of fecundity in captive primates housed under crowded conditions, but many of us are plagued by loss of libido during times of sustained tension and anxiety.

Among male primates, one of the hallmarks of such reproductive suppression is decreased concentrations of testosterone (T) in the bloodstream. Testosterone is the principal androgenic steroid in primates and is secreted by the interstitial cells of the testes as the final step in a classical endocrine cascade: luteinizing-hormone-releasing hormone (LHRH) is secreted by the hypothalamus of the brain, which in turn stimulates secretion of luteinizing hormone (LH) by the pituitary, which stimulates testicular T secretion. Additional androgens can be secreted by the adrenal gland under the stimulation of pituitary adrenocorticotropic hormone (ACTH) and other, as yet unidentified factors. Once secreted, T has considerable effects throughout the body, supporting reproductive behavior and physiology, increasing aggression and muscle mass, and regulating cardiovascular physiology (Figure 11.1).

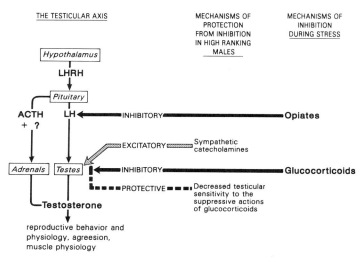

Figure 11.1. Far left: Schematic diagram of the testicular axis in the male primate. Center: Locus of actions of opiates and glucocorticoids in inhibiting the testicular axis during stress. Far right: Unique features of testicular axis of high-ranking males in buffering them from the suppressive actions of stress. These features include the relative protection of their testes from the suppressive actions of glucocorticoids, and the stimulation of testosterone release by catecholamines. Result is elevated testosterone concentrations during stress in high-ranking males.

Figure 11.2 demonstrates that, as with other primates, T concentrations in male baboons are suppressed by stress. The black bars show the remarkably consistent basal T levels in the males of my main study troops within the Masai Mara National Reserve (part of the Serengeti plain that spans Kenya and Tanzania near Lake Victoria), and in males from a troop living near the town of Gilgil (an agricultural region in the Rift Valley in central Kenya). The hatched bars on the right indicate occasions where T concentrations were suppressed. The first concerns a period of social

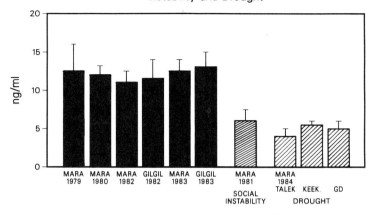

Figure 11.2. Basal testosterone concentrations in baboons of different troops living in varied social and ecological settings. "Mara" refers to baboons living in the Masai Mara National Reserve in the Serengeti Ecosystem in southwest Kenya. "Gilgil" refers to baboons living in a troop in the agricultural region of Rift Valley, Central Kenya, near the town of Gilgil. "Talek," "Keek," and "GD" refer to three different baboon troops living within Masai Mara. Data from Mara baboons in 1979–1983 derived from the single "Keek" troop.

instability among one troop of Mara baboons following the crippling of the alpha male and the disintegration of the coalition that had attacked him. As will be discussed below, this period, in which T concentrations were halved, was characterized by shifting dominance ranks and high rates of dominance interactions and aggression. The next three stippled bars indicate the suppression of T concentrations in baboons from three different troops in the Mara during the tragic East African drought of 1984.

These studies show that social or ecological stressors can be associated with suppressed T levels. Uncovering the mechanisms underlying this phenomenon is difficult, as drought or disintegration of a hierarchy are rare and unpredictable events. Figure 11.3 demonstrates suppression of the testicular axis by a far more readily studied stressor, namely the darting and capture process itself. As can be seen, concentrations of LH decline promptly and—as should be expected, given the organization of the testicular axis—T levels decline shortly thereafter (Sapolsky, 1986).

How does the stress of darting and capture suppress the testicular axis? Figure 11.3 demonstrates decreased circulating concentrations of LH and T in the blood following stress. Is this due to *decreased secretion* of, for example, T by the testes or *increased clearance* of T from the bloodstream by target tissues? One can conduct a T clearance test in which a miniscule quantity of radioactively tagged T is injected and the rate at which it is removed from the bloodstream is then monitored. Such studies indicate that the clearance rate is not the relevant variable, but rather than stress inhibits hormone secretion (Sapolsky, 1985a).

Beginning at the highest point in the axis at which a stress-effect is

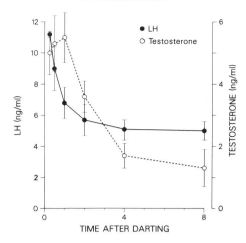

Figure 11.3. Time after darting and immobilization capture expressed in hours. LH expressed in ng of NICHD-rhesus monkey LH/ml. (From Sapolsky, 1986)

observed, what causes the decreased secretion of LH? As discussed, glucocorticoids, opiates (such as beta-endorphin), and the catecholamines of the sympathetic nervous system (epinephrine and norepinephrine) are all secreted into the bloodstream in increased quantities during stress. Laboratory studies have indicated that these hormones can all influence the gonadal axis in primates. Do LH concentrations decline because of the increased secretion of one or more of these hormones during stress?

To test this, I injected animals with drugs which selectively blocked these different hormonal components of the stress-response. Chlorisondamine, for example, is a sympathetic ganglionic blocker which prevents the release of epinephrine and norepinephrine during stress; the drug has been used clinically to lower blood pressure. Metyrapone blocks the glucocorticoid component of the stress-response by inhibiting the synthesis of the hormones in the adrenal cortex. Finally, naloxone is an opiate receptor antagonist which does not disrupt opiate release but blocks access of the hormones to target tissues, thus making them biologically ineffective.

These experiments have shown that the stress-induced decline in LH concentrations is due to the increased secretion of opiates during stress (Figure 11.4). In baboons simply darted but not treated with any drug, LH titers decline dramatically, as already shown. Chlorisondamine and metyrapone, neutralizing the sympathetic and glucocorticoid components of the stress-response, respectively, fail to prevent this decline in LH levels. Naloxone, in contrast, maintains LH levels above baseline, implicating the release of opiates in the suppression of LH.

How do opiates accomplish this? Studies with both humans and nonhuman primates suggest that the hormones do not act directly at the pituitary, but instead inhibit hypothalamic release of LHRH (Rasmussen et al., 1983). The decline in LH titers is thus secondary to the absence of LHRH stimulation. Unfortunately, it is not possible to determine whether

Figure 11.4. Role of stress-induced opiate release in suppression of LH concentrations. The figure presented is the LH concentrations two hours after darting; all drugs were administered during the first ten minutes following darting. Control animals were darted without any additional drugs. "Chloris." baboons received the sympathetic ganglionic blocker chlorisondamine. "Metyrap." baboons received the adrenocortical steroidogenesis inhibitor metyrapone. "Naloxone" animals received the opiate receptor antagonist naloxone.

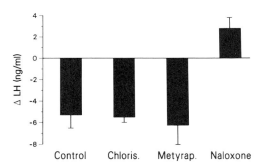

the opiates work at the level of the hypothalamus or pituitary in these baboons, because the primitive laboratory facilities in the field preclude the preservation and measurement of opioids.

Does the opiate effect upon LH secretion explain the entire suppression of the testicular axis? That is to say, do T concentrations decline during stress merely because LH concentrations decline first? This can be tested easily by determining if in males treated with naloxone and therefore having high LH titers, T levels are maintained. This is not the case (Figure 11.5); T titers decline in naloxone-treated baboons, even at the same time as LH titers remain high. Thus, there is more than one point of inhibition of the axis.

Luteinizing hormone is a peptide that can be enzymatically modified after secretion such that its biological potency is altered. Is the LH secreted during stress altered so as to be less capable of eliciting T secretion from the testes? A change in the "bioactivity" of LH or its capacity to release T in an in vitro tissue culture of interstitial cells turns out not to explain the declining T titers at a time when LH titers are still high (Sapolsky, 1985a). Clearly, stress not only inhibits LH release but also acts to inhibit testicular sensitivity to LH.

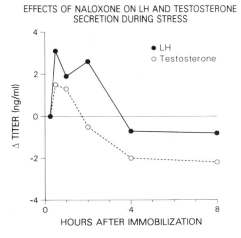

Figure 11.5. Administration of naloxone following darting stress prevents the typical decline in LH concentrations which occur under such circumstances, implicating stress-induced opiate release in this LH decline. Despite the elevation of LH titers following naloxone administration, testosterone concentrations decline as usual, demonstrating that there is an additional stress-induced decrease in testicular sensitivity to LH.

This effect turns out to be due to the release of glucocorticoids during stress. In one study, baboons were allowed to rest quietly, recovering over a number of hours from the stressful effects of the darting and capture. In half of them, glucocorticoid levels were then elevated again, as during stress, by infusion of a synthetic glucocorticoid, dexamethasone. All subjects were then injected with synthetic LHRH. As already demonstrated in Figure 11.4, glucocorticoids are not responsible for inhibiting LH secretion during stress. Thus, it is not surprising that in both the dexamethasone-treated and control baboons, LHRH elicits equivalent amounts of LH secretion (Figure 11.6A). However, the testicular sensitivity to LH is drastically inhibited by dexamethasone (Figure 11.6B); the glucocorticoid blocks the capacity of the testes to secrete T in response to LH stimulation (Sapolsky, 1985a). Laboratory studies suggest a number of ways in which this could occur, including glucocorticoids decreasing the number of receptors for LH in interstitial cells, or glucocorticoids interfering with the release of T itself, once an LH signal has been detected.

Thus, stress acts via the release of opiates to inhibit LH secretion, and via glucocorticoids to inhibit testicular sensitivity to LH (Figure 11.1B). Do high- and low-ranking baboons differ in their sensitivity to this suppression of their testicular axis during stress?

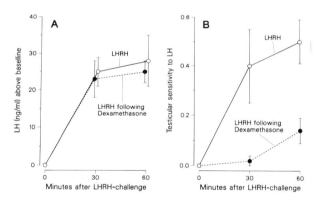

Figure 11.6. (A) Pituitary responsiveness to LHRH challenge, with or without prior dexamethasone treatment. The synthetic glucocorticoid failed to alter sensitivity of the pituitary to the releasing hormone. (B) Testicular responsiveness to LHRH-induced elevations of LH concentration, with or without prior dexamethasone administration. Testicular sensitivity was determined by dividing T concentrations at any given time by the LH concentration at the same timepoint. While dexamethasone did not influence the pituitary sensitivity to LHRH, testicular sensitivity to LH was greatly dampened.

RANK-RELATED DIFFERENCES IN TESTICULAR SUPPRESSION

There do appear to be rank-related differences in reproductive response to stress in male olive baboons. High-ranking males maintain their T concentrations or even elevate them during stress at times when titers plummet in subordinates. But before examining that, one must first ask whether males of differing ranks start at the same basal levels of T. That is, in the absence of stress, do high-ranking males have the highest T concentrations? Rose and colleagues (1971) reported just such a positive correlation in an all-male colony of captive rhesus monkeys during their first nine months together following group formation. However, study of mixed-sex groups living together for longer periods has never replicated this finding (Eaton and Resko, 1974; Gordon et al., 1976). As will be discussed below, during periods of social stability, high-ranking male primates are neither the most aggressive nor do they have the highest T concentrations. These correlations emerge only during times of group organization or reorganization. Thus, in all of the troops and years represented in black bars in Figure 11.2, there is no correlation between basal T concentrations and rank. Instead, the highest concentrations of T and rates of aggression tend to occur in low-ranking postpubescent males (Sapolsky, 1982, 1983a).

Thus, high-ranking males do not necessarily enter into a stressful situation with the highest T concentrations. However, they are uniquely capable of maintaining their T concentrations during stress. Figure 11.7A shows a representative example with the stress of darting causing a prompt decline in T titers in the five lowest-ranking males while titers actually rise in the five highest-ranking. What accounts for this unique protection of the testicular axis in dominant males?

One might speculate that T concentrations remain high (or elevate) in dominant males during stress because LH concentrations remain high. This is not the case; LH titers decline equally following darting in high-ranking and low-ranking males (Sapolsky, 1986) (Figure 11.7B). Furthermore, the bioactivity of the secreted LH does not differ by rank. Thus, the rank difference is mediated at the testicular level. Do high-ranking males secrete less glucocorticoids during stress, and thus induce less testicular inhibition? No; in fact, these males have a greater rise in glucocorticoid levels during stress than do subordinates (Sapolsky, 1982, 1983b). However, the testes of high-ranking males are less sensitive to these suppressive actions of glucocorticoids during stress. In subordinates, administration of dexamethasone is highly effective in blocking testicular sensitivity to LH; dominant males are less subject to this regulation. This could be due to fewer glucocorticoid receptors in the testes of high-ranking males or to a protective uncoupling of the glucocorticoid receptor system from the machinery that secretes T in response to LH.

This merely explains why T concentrations decline more slowly in high-ranking males. Yet Figure 11.7 demonstrated that there is even a transient rise in titers. What accounts for this? As shown in Figure 11.1, the adrenals are an alternative source of androgenic hormones, under control of a different hormonal trigger than the testes. Is the extra T of adrenal origin, stimulated by stress-induced release of ACTH? Administration of exogenous ACTH demonstrates that this is unlikely (Sapolsky, 1985a). Instead, dominant males have an additional and unique mechanism involving the sympathetic nervous system that allows for increased testic-

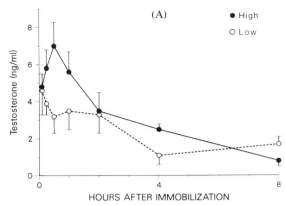

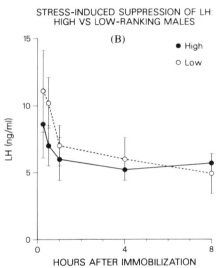

STRESS-INDUCED SUPPRESSION OF LH:
HIGH VS LOW-RANKING MALES

Figure 11.7. (A) Individual variation in testosterone concentrations following darting and immobilization. Low-ranking males (open circles) showed continuous declines in T concentrations throughout the 8-hour period. High-ranking males (closed circles) showed a transient elevation of T concentrations during the first poststress hour. In this and subsequent figures, rankings are based on reproductive activity which, in this troop, is highly correlated with high rank by approach-avoid and aggressive criteria. (B) Despite these rank differences in testosterone profile following immobilization, both high-ranking and low-ranking males had similar declines in LH concentrations during this period, suggesting that the rank difference arises at the testicular level. (From Sapolsky, 1986)

ular secretion of T during stress. Figure 11.8 demonstrates that neutralization of the sympathetic stress response (via administration of chlorisondamine to inhibit release of epinephrine and norepinephrine) fails to alter the decline in LH titers that occurs equally in all males. Furthermore, chlorisondamine fails to affect the declining T titers in low-ranking males. However, the drug completely eliminates the transient rise in T titers in high-ranking males (Sapolsky, 1986).

Laboratory studies suggest at least two ways in which this could occur. The sympathetic nervous system innervates the parenchymal blood vessels supplying the testes and can vasodilate them, increasing the blood flow into the testes. Thus, although systemic LH titers may decline, this mechanism could insure that more LH reaches the testes. Additionally, the sympathetic nervous system innervates interstitial cells in Old World monkeys and could directly stimulate the release of T, even in the absence of a stimulatory LH signal. Whichever mechanism or mechanisms occur in baboons, this sym-

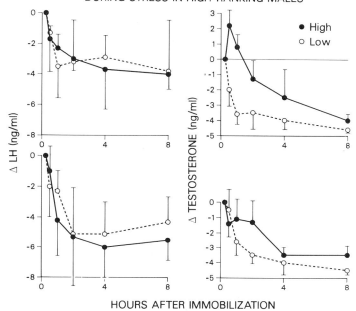

Figure 11.8. (Top left) LH concentrations following immobilization in high-ranking untreated males (closed circles) and high-ranking males administered chlorisondamine (**CHLOR**) (open circles). The response of the two groups did not differ significantly. (Bottom left) LH concentrations in low-ranking untreated males (closed circles) and low-ranking CHLOR-treated males (open circles). The response of the two groups did not differ significantly. (Top right) Testosterone concentrations in high-ranking untreated males (closed circles) and high-ranking CHLOR-treated males (open circles). CHLOR administration eliminated the transient rise in T concentrations seen in untreated high-ranking males. The two groups differed significantly in response during the first poststress hour. (Bottom right) Testosterone concentrations in low-ranking untreated males (closed circles) and low-ranking CHLOR-treated males (open circles). The response of the two groups did not differ significantly. (Sapolsky, 1986)

pathetic component is far more powerful in high-ranking males than in low-ranking males and accounts for their capacity to elevate T titers early in the poststress period.

Thus, the unique features of the testicular stress-response in dominant males can be attributed both to greater buffering from the inhibitory effects of glucocorticoids and to the unique sympathetically induced outflow of T (Figure 11.1C).

CHICKEN-AND-EGG QUESTIONS AND BEHAVIORAL ENDOCRINOLOGY

Do high-ranking males have these unique endocrine features because of their dominance, or is high rank conferred by their physiology? Is there, in fact, any causality in this relationship? Dominant males are generally prime-aged, in the best of health, with the best nutrition; does their stress-response depend merely on these factors and have nothing to do with social rank?

These questions plague behavioral endocrinologists. Studies with captive populations, where one can manipulate physiology (by injecting a hormone, for example) or behavior (by changing troop members) have indicated that physiology can affect the behavior, behavior affect the physiology, and sometimes both arise from other factors independently (Leshner, 1982). The strategy in my work has been to avoid any such manipulations, making it impossible to study the issue in that manner. Alternatively, one can follow the same individuals for years and note, for example, whether the behaviors of high-ranking males emerge shortly before or after the endocrine correlates. Obviously, however, such data are collected only very slowly.

A very informative time period with these baboons demonstrated at least one dramatic piece of causality in this behavior/endocrine relationship. In 1981, I returned to my troop to find the previous season's highest ranking male being heavily challenged by a coalition of six younger males. None was an obvious successor and capable of individually challenging him, but as a cooperative coalition, the six were more than he could withstand. Shortly into the season, he was badly crippled in a fight with the coalition and effectively dropped from the social scene. The coalition promptly disintegrated, and for the next three months a period of social instability ensued. While all six individuals were clearly dominant to the other males who made up the linear hierarchy of ranks 7 through 15, the rankings of the six shifted unpredictably, often more than once in a day. The number of dominance interactions and reversals rose, these males had the highest rates of aggression, and feeding and grooming were suppressed. During this period of instability, all of these individuals were clearly high-ranking (compared with the remaining males in the troop). All had the typical features of prime age, health, and good nutritional status. Yet, during that time, most of the psychological advantages commensurate with high rank during a stable period—predictability and control over contingencies in one's environment—were lost. If the endocrine profile of high-ranking males was identical in both stable seasons and the unstable one, then the unique physiology of dominance was unlikely to be sensitive to the behavioral features of dominance. Instead, an entirely different picture of dominance emerged (Table 11.1). In all other seasons, high-ranking males had the lowest levels of the glucocorticoid cortisol; at this time, their titers were significantly elevated and the capacity to turn on a cortisol stress-response was dampened. Basal T concentrations, only somewhat suppressed in these competing high-ranking males, were dramatically suppressed in the subordinates, who were subject to high rates of displaced aggression during this period. Out of these shifts came a correlation observed in no other season; high-ranking males were the most aggressive, initiating the most fights, and having the highest basal levels of T. Finally, the capacity to elevate T concentrations

TABLE 11.1. Effects of Social Instability Upon Cortisol and Testosterone Responses to the Stress of Darting

	Stable Season (1980)		Unstable Season (1981)	
	High-ranking	Low-ranking	High-ranking	Low-ranking
Basal cortisol titer (μg/100 ml)	20 ± 3	26 ± 2	25 ± 1	26 ± 3
Change in cortisol titer during first post-stress hour	+18 μg/ 100 ml	+12 μg/ 100 ml	+5 μg/ 100 ml	+13 μg/ 100 ml
Basal testosterone titer (ng/ml)	10 ± 3	20 ± 7	8 ± 1	2 ± 1
Change in testosterone titer during first post-stress hour	+11 ng/ml	−10 ng/ml	+1 ng/ml	−1 ng/ml

During the stable season, high-ranking males had significantly lower basal titers of cortisol than did subordinates; this difference disappeared during the unstable season. Furthermore, dominant males had the largest rises in cortisol titer stress in the stable season; this pattern was lost in the unstable season.

During the stable season, dominant males did not have the highest basal titers of testosterone, but were able to elevate titers during the first post-stress hour. During the unstable season, basal testosterone titers were sufficiently suppressed in subordinates such that dominant males now had the highest titers of testosterone. However, stress did not induce a rise in testosterone in these animals.

(Taken from a number of tables and figures from Sapolsky, 1983a)

during stress was lost in these dominant males during the unstable period (Sapolsky, 1983a).

These findings suggest two conclusions. First, the behavior/endocrine correlations presented in earlier pages might arise from causative relationships between the two, with the endocrine features of dominance being sensitive to the behavioral features. In these animals, when many of the psychological advantages of dominance are lost because high rank becomes the position of highest stress and instability, the unique endocrine features disappear. (Whether a change in the physiology also affects behavior is as yet untested in these animals.) A second conclusion is that the physiology of dominance varies depending on whether one sits atop a stable or an unstable hierarchy. During social instability, high rank is associated with high levels of aggression and high basal testosterone and glucocorticoid titers. This has also been observed in recently formed groups of rhesus, squirrel, and talapoin monkeys in captivity. During stable periods, neither high basal titers of T nor high levels of aggression appear relevant to dominance, as also shown with long-term studies of captive primates. Thus, there is no single picture of the physiology of social dominance in these complex intelligent animals, and one must take into consideration demography, group history, and social learning.

CONSEQUENCES

Does it matter that in a stable hierarchy, high-ranking males are protected from the suppression of T concentrations during acute stress? Imagine a male maintaining a consortship with an estrous female while he is harassed intermittently for days by another competing male. Assume that at the start of this harassment, both males have similar T concentrations; one is high-ranking, the other low. Most likely, during the first hour of each tense period of harassment, T concentrations will decline perhaps 80% in the low-ranking participant while rising perhaps 50% in the dominant individual (see Figure 11.7A). Is this advantageous for the latter? In determining this, it is necessary first to review the nature and time-course of the physiologic actions of T in primates.

Above all else, T promotes reproduction. The steroid acts at the Sertoli cells of the testes and/or at the spermatic germ cells themselves to stimulate the formation and maturation of sperm. Testosterone then indirectly provides the energy needed to maintain sperm sufficiently motile to fertilize an egg. This is accomplished via T-dependent seminal vesicle secretion, which provides the fructose which nourishes sperm. Similarly, T stimulates secretion of nutrients in the epididymis, the storage site for sperm. Finally, T increases the mass and contractility of the smooth muscles which surround the epididymal duct and which advance sperm toward the urethra during sexual arousal by contracting rhythmically (Goodman, 1980a).

Along with the promotion of reproductive potency, T also stimulates sexual behavior and interest. As correlative evidence, parallel increases in T concentration and sexual drive occur with puberty and during the breeding seasons of some primate species, and both typically (but not necessarily) decline during aging. A causal relationship between T secretion and sexual behavior is demonstrated by the declining libido which follows surgical castration or administration of antiandrogenic drugs. Furthermore, administration of T increases libido in castrates or in men with profoundly diminished T secretion due to endocrine dysfunction. When endocrinopathy occurs at the level of the hypothalamus (that is, where testicular and pituitary function are normal, but there is insufficient LHRH to stimulate the axis), LHRH can be administered to stimulate T secretion and raise libido. Interestingly, in such cases, sexual responsiveness begins to increase even before T concentrations rise significantly, suggesting that LHRH itself can promote sexual drive. This is supported by the presence of both LHRH and its receptors in parts of the brain which mediate sexual behavior.

These studies suggest the importance of T (and possibly LHRH) in promotion of sexual behavior and libido in the primate. However, in contrast to other species discussed in this volume, castration does not cause a prompt decline in primate sexual behavior; it can persist, albeit in a diminished and declining state, long after the surgery and disappearance of T from the blood. Furthermore, social history plays an important factor, as the greater the sexual experience of a primate prior to castration, the slower the postcastration decline in activity. Thus, sexual behavior is not abruptly stimulated or inhibited by the presence or absence of T and is sensitive to a variety of other regulatory influences (Rose and Sachar, 1981).

Testosterone can also influence aggressiveness in primates, and this effect is even more subtle than the role of T in sexual behavior just discussed. Again, a parallelism is noted between T concentrations and aggression between the sexes, over the course of puberty and senescence, breeding and nonbreeding seasons, and following manipulations such as castration or T replacement. However, T should not be considered the "cause" of primate aggression. Rather, it should best be viewed as a facilitator of aggression. For example, in one study, dominance rankings were established in a trio of castrated rhesus monkeys. Treatment of the number-two-ranking male with androgens (dihydrotestosterone, in this case) produced an increase in aggression and a rise in his rank to the number one position. However, the elevated aggression continued even after cessation of the androgen treatment (Dixson, 1980). This importance of social factors is also shown in a study of castrated tamarin monkeys. While the surgery lowered rates of aggression in some animals, *who* the castrated male was paired with was generally a more powerful factor in determining the level of aggression than were his own T concentrations (Epple, 1978). Perhaps the best demonstration of the subtlety of the effects of T on social aggression comes from a study of castrated talapoin monkeys by Dixson and Herbert (1977). Testosterone administration raised levels of aggression, but no male increased the rate of his aggressive challenges to a higher-ranking male. The increased aggression manifested itself entirely in greater rates of aggression directed toward subordinates, animals to whom the T-treated male could already be safely aggressive. Therefore, T influences aggression, but with a number of caveats: its action is typically to potentiate the severity of already existing patterns of aggression, and it is highly sensitive to social influences (Dixson, 1977).

The little that is known about the neurobiology of T modulation of aggression supports these caveats strongly. As discussed elsewhere in this volume, a number of sites in the limbic system, chiefly the septum, amygdala, and hypothalamus, have been implicated as regulators of aggression. Numerous studies have shown that electrical stimulation of the latter two sites can elicit spontaneous aggression in monkeys. The capacity for such electrically evoked aggression does not disappear with castration. However, the threshold of electrical current required rises; in other words, aggression is elicited less easily in the absence of T. Conversely, T administration to castrates reduces the threshold for stimulation of aggression (Perachio, 1978). Subsequent work provided a cellular mechanism for this observation. Stimulation of a neuron leads to depolarization of its charged membrane and consequent release of its neurotransmitters. Following this is a silent period where the neuron is unresponsive to stimulation and its membrane is being repolarized. Testosterone shortens the duration of this "refractory period" of neurons of the stria terminalis, a major anatomical projection from the amygdala to the hypothalamus (Kendrick and Drewett, 1979). Thus, research from the level of socially interacting primates to single neurons suggests that while T does not necessarily stimulate aggression in and of itself, it can increase the strength of an already established aggressive impulse.

In addition to this regulation of reproduction and aggression, T can alter metabolism and stimulate growth in target tissues. This can occur in highly androgen-sensitive, specialized tissues, resulting in the development of secondary sexual characteristics whose exact nature varies from species to species. Examples in primates include the blue skin pigmentation of the scrotum of vervet monkeys, the elongated canines and heavy capes of hair of the olive baboon, or the facial hair of the human male. These effects of T also extend to more generalized stimulation of growth of all skeletal muscle. This is accomplished by increases in nitrogen retention, sugar transport, and numbers and efficiency of the enzymes of intermediary metabolism in muscle. While these "anabolic" actions of T and other androgenic steroids are most dramatic at puberty, they can occur throughout the lifespan (Goodman, 1980a; Max and Toop, 1983).

To return to our example, with each new bout in the tense consortship harassment, T concentrations in the high-ranking male baboon have risen from 10 to 15 ng/ml; in the low-ranking male, declines from 10 to 2 ng/ml have occurred. Will this result in rank-related differences in reproductive physiology or behavior, aggression, or muscle metabolism? This is, in fact, two questions. First, does T have its effects within this rapid time-course? Second, are the T-influenced tissues sensitive enough to differentiate between 2 and 15 ng/ml of T in the blood?

It is unlikely that after one such stressor, there will be differences in the reproductive physiology of these two males. For example, sperm count will not rise in the dominant male because of the transient rise in T concentrations from 10 to 15 ng/ml. Such androgen effects are simply too slow to be sensitive to a rapid fluctuation such as this. Similarly, while T increases seminal fluid secretion by stimulating growth of the secretory epithelial cells of the seminal vesicle, this is a relatively slow process.

A single stressful incident of consortship harassment is also unlikely to influence reproductive behavior or libido in these two males. Although these effects of T on behavior occur somewhat faster than its effects upon reproductive physiology, they are still relatively slow. More importantly, the neural machinery which mediates sexual drive and behavior is relatively insensitive to small differences in T concentrations. For example, there has never been a convincing demonstration in a population of healthy humans of nonhuman primates that the level of sexual drive is well correlated with T concentrations. Furthermore, altering T concentrations *within the normal range* in an individual does not reliably alter sexual drive. Loss of sexual drive does not occur until there is a nearly complete loss of circulating T (due to profound endocrinopathy of the testicular axis, after castration, or after prolonged stress). Finally, relatively small amounts of exogenous T can restore sexual drive. Thus, the time-course and range of T fluctuation in our example of the single consortship harassment is probably insufficient to suppress libido in the subordinate or raise it in the dominant male.

The differing T concentrations in the two males are most likely to affect aggression and muscle metabolism. The facilitative action of T upon limbic electrophysiology is probably rapid and sensitive enough to fit within this scenario. Similarly, relatively small increments in T concentrations acutely stimulate glucose uptake into skeletal muscle (Max and Toop, 1983). Although more definitive studies are needed to answer the questions posed about these two hypothetical baboons (i.e., most of the studies just cited have utilized rodents instead of primates, and have not examined the dose-response relationship between T concentration and effects on neurons or muscle), they are suggestive. Over the course of the intermittent stress that typically characterizes coalitional challenges and consortship harassments among male baboons, the unique patterns of increased T secretion in high-ranking males is likely to increase the energy available to their muscles and accentuate their tendencies toward aggression, while the opposite is likely occurring in subordinates.

STRESS, RANK, AND REPRODUCTIVE SUPPRESSION IN FEMALE PRIMATES

As in the male, stress inhibits female reproductive physiology, and the severity of such suppression appears to be rank-related. This topic will be reviewed only briefly, as the focus of my research has been the male baboon. (This has been so for a number of reasons, including the static nature of female hierarchies compared to the fluid ones of males, the likely disruption of early-stage pregnancies by some of the experimental procedures described, and the unnerving habit of multiple generations of irate relatives of a female baboon to surround her as she becomes unconscious, in contrast to the studied indifference of baboons towards an unconscious [and usually unrelated] male.)

An extraordinary array of stressors, both somatic and psychogenic, severe and mild, will disrupt female reproduction and suppress libido. In the human, these stressors can include starvation and cachexia, death of a loved one, a large change in body weight or level of exercise, a major change in occupation or living situation. The adaptive logic of such a response is even clearer than in the male. In mammals, few events are more energetically demanding and evolutionarily critical than pregnancy. In primates with altricial young, the demands of pregnancy are compounded by the long period of infant care required. Thus, the female's reproductive axis is extremely sensitive to environmental perturbations which signal that it is not the most auspicious time for reproduction. A mathematical treatment of this reasoning can be found in Wasser and Barash (1983).

Stress-induced reproductive suppression can arise from decreased secretion of follicle-stimulating hormone (FSH), resulting in follicular immaturity. Failure of ovulation due to attenuation of the preovulatory surge of LH, FSH, and estrogen can also occur during stress. Furthermore, failure of implantation of or retention of the fertilized egg can occur because of stress-induced decreases in progesterone secretion during the luteal phase. These various changes occur during stress via some mechanisms similar to those already discussed in the male. These include opiate-mediated inhibition of LHRH release (with opiate secretion most likely triggered by secretion of corticotropin-releasing factor). Furthermore, the adrenocortical axis appears to suppress LH levels, predominantly through inhibition of pituitary sensitivity to LHRH. *In vitro* studies show this to be due to glucocorticoids, rather than to ACTH. The inhibition of testicular sensitivity to LH by glucocorticoids, which plays such a large role in reproductive suppression in the male, has not yet been reported to have a parallel in terms of glucocorticoid inhibition of ovarian responsiveness to LH (Goodman, 1980a; Ross et al., 1981).

Additional mechanisms for stress-induced reproductive suppression exist in the female. As mentioned, the pituitary hormone prolactin is secreted during stress, and it can inhibit the ovarian steroidogenic response to LH. Furthermore, prolactin can inhibit luteal phase progesterone secretion and thus compromise implantation and development of the fertilized egg. Interestingly, in addition to its role in mediating reproductive suppression during stress, prolactin secretion is stimulated by suckling and appears to mediate the similar reproductive inhibition that occurs during sustained nursing. As another mechanism, during the stress of undernutrition (such as during famine or with eating disorders), body fat is significantly reduced. In females, androgens are secreted by the adrenal glands, much as in males. Such adrenal androgens are typically aromatized to estrogen by enzymes found in peripheral fat pads of females. Thus, with diminished body fat, there is not only a drop in circulating estrogen, but an equivalent rise in circulating androgen levels. Both changes contribute to reproductive failure. Finally, there is some speculation that stress-induced ACTH secretion can elevate adrenal androgen secretion in females above what can normally be handled by fat cells, producing elevated and disruptive concentrations of androgens (Warren, 1983).

Numerous studies suggest that when reproductive failure occurs among social primates, it is the stressed and/or low-ranking females who are most afflicted. For example, in the rhesus and marmoset monkeys, sexual maturation is most often delayed in subordinate females, as is sexual receptivity. A similar rank bias is observed for ovulatory inhibition in gelada and papio species of baboons (see Wasser and Barash, 1983, for a review of this literature). These patterns could arise in a number of ways. Given the nepotistic inheritance of dominance in some (but not all) of these species, the increased rate of reproductive failure in the lower-ranking animals could represent genetic differences between dominant and subordinate lineages in fecundity. Furthermore, they could reflect the rank-related differences in nutritional status that occur in some species and locales. Many authors have interpreted these patterns as being stress-related. As part of this, reproduction in low-ranking females could be more sensitive to stress than in dominant females. This would be comparable to the data presented for males in this chapter and could reflect both the psychological and the genetic components of subordinance in females. No test of this hypothesis has as yet occurred. In addition, low-ranking females could be exposed to more frequent stress. This could be via poor nutrition and excessive exposure to predators or pathogens. It could also occur via high rates of social stress and harassment by dominant individuals. Most field studies suggest that considerable amounts of such harassment occur, and this appears to be the primary mechanism for infertility of low-ranking females in a number of species of marmosets and tamarins.

A detailed sociobiologic model of such reproductive suppression in social subordinates has been offered (Wasser and Barash, 1983). The authors reason that it is advantageous for a dominant female to harass a subordinate into infertility so long as the cost of the harassment does not outweigh the advantage in reproductive success arising from suppressing a competitor. Furthermore, in the model, the adaptiveness of deferring reproduction by the harassed subordinate until a more auspicious time is calculated in terms of her remaining reproductive potential. The authors also speculate that high-ranking females harass subordinates at specific times in the estrus cycles and pregnancies of the latter where vulnerability to stress-induced reproductive failure is greatest. While the broad features of this model are attractive and logical, the data on baboons presented by the authors are far too preliminary to allow any conclusions. Personally, I expect that the patterns of female harassment (whom, when, and how severely) will be most strongly influenced by individual relationships and personal histories of the animals involved. As is so often the case in primate studies, strict sociobiologic models fail to match closely what is observed in a society of strongly individualistic personalities.

The reproductive axis in the female primate is highly sensitive to stress, and numerous endocrine mechanisms mediate stress-induced reproductive suppression. Such suppression is most pronounced in subordinate females, who are typically subject to the highest rates of stressful harassment by conspecifics. Whether their reproductive axis is intrinsically more sensitive to suppression per stressor, as in the subordinate male baboon, is not known.

CONCLUSIONS

The research detailed in this chapter demonstrates that for a male baboon, social rank (and the changing psychologic baggage that is carried with his rank) is highly related to how well his reproductive system functions during stress. Laboratory studies and the fortuitous unstable season in the field suggest that the behavioral and physiological components of this correlation influence each other. In other studies of mine not detailed here, rank-related differences have also been found in these males in the functioning of their adrenocortical axes, the sympathetic nervous system, and cholesterol metabolism (Sapolsky, 1983b, 1986, in prep.). These studies show that in the highly stratified society of male baboons, the dramatic individual differences in social status have physiological underpinnings. Furthermore, an extensive literature in the pathophysiology of cholesterol metabolism, autonomic function, hyperadrenocorticism, and so on, lead one to tentatively conclude that the unique physiologic patterns of high-ranking males are more adaptive and less pathogenic.

The careful reader will realize, however, that the story presented here is only a crude beginning. This is shown anecdotally in Figure 11.9. On the left is Male 333 in 1980, when he was near the top of the hierarchy in a fiercely competitive, aggressive troop. He appears here to be a robust, healthy animal at his muscular prime. On the right is a picture of him four years later—aged, decrepit, with a limp, a recent canine puncture in his muzzle, and the bad fortune of being incessantly harassed by juveniles who outrank him. The ranks of male baboons change dramatically from year to year. The males currently reigning in my troops were in the throes of insecure puberty when I first met them in 1978; those who were intimidating terrors then are aged now. The findings in pathophysiology suggest that if a low-ranking male (with, as I have found, his readily suppressed T concentrations, elevated basal cortisol concentrations, and suppressed levels of high-density-lipoprotein-associated cholesterol) continues that way for years, he will pay a price in the forms of decreased fecundity, immunosuppression and disease risk, atherosclerosis, and so on. But most low-ranking males *will not* continue like this for years. The rankings change too frequently. Thus, the pictures I have presented in this chapter are mere snapshots at a particular stage of each animal's life. If one is interested in the long-term consequences of these behavior/physiology correlates, one must study successive snapshots sequentially, following these same individuals over their life cycle.

(A)   (B)

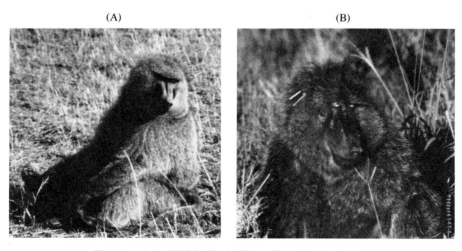

Figure 11.9. (A) Male 333 in 1980. (B) Male 333 in 1984.

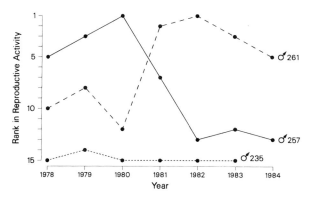

Figure 11.10. Individual differences in changing patterns of reproductive status over the years. A rank of "1" indicates the highest, most reproductively active position in the troop.

This is necessary not merely because rankings change yearly. Just as in any given season males compete with widely different strategies, the patterns of changing rank over time are also highly individualistic. A crude demonstration of this is shown in Figure 11.10, where reproductive rankings of three males are followed over the years. For one (Male 257), the rise to dominance was slow, the decline abrupt. This was the male crippled in the coalitional fight described earlier. For another (Male 261), an abrupt rise to dominance occurred; the same male voluntarily relinquished the alpha position and continues to decline slowly. Finally, a third male (235), not particularly aged, never rose from the bottom of the ranks and was never seen to mate or win a dominance interaction.

The hope then is to follow these same animals long enough to catch a glimmer as to what is truly happening with their behavior and physiology over their lifespans. For example, one goal is to collect sufficient data to compare the proximal physiology and cumulative social status, disease patterns, and reproductive activities of aged males who were once top-ranking with those males who never succeeded. Or to compare ex-alpha males who relinquished the position with those who had to be injured to be displaced. Or to compare males who never formed cooperative coalitions and close affiliations with those with a long history of such cooperation. Such studies will not be easy. But if accomplished, they will aid our understanding of the role of stress and behavior in disease susceptibility. Furthermore, they will hopefully also reaffirm the incredible richness of individuality which makes the study of these animals so pleasurable.

ACKNOWLEDGMENTS

This work was generously supported by the Harry Frank Guggenheim Foundation and the Life Sciences Research Foundation, of which the author was a Mathers Fellow. Research was approved by the Office of the President and the Ministry of Tourism and Wildlife, Republic of Kenya. Pamela Holland provided manuscript assistance, and field assistance for the studies described was provided by Richard Kimoso Kones, Josiah Masau, Francis Milili, Francis Onchiri, Hudson Oyaro, Dianne Rich, and Reed Sutherland.

REFERENCES

ALTMANN, J. (1980) *Baboon Mothers and Infants*. Harvard Univ. Press, Cambridge.

BERNSTEIN, I.S. (1981) Dominance: The baby and the bathwater. Behav. Brain Sci. *4*:419–457.

BOHUS, B., E. DE KLOET, and H. VELDHUIS (1983) Adrenal steroids and behavioral adaptation: relationships to brain corticoid receptors. In *Progress in Neuroendocrinology*, Vol. 2. R. Ganten and D. Pfaff, eds., pp. 1–23, Springer-Verlag, Berlin.

DEWSBURY, D. (1982) Dominance rank, copulatory behavior, and differential reproduction. Quart. Rev. Biol. *57*:135–159.

DIXSON, A. (1980) Androgens and aggressive behavior in primates: A review. Aggressive Behavior *6*:37–67.

DIXSON, A., and J. HERBERT (1977) Testosterone, aggressive behavior and dominance rank in captive adult male talapoin monkeys (*Miopithecus talapoin*). Physiol. Behav. *18*:539–543.

EATON, G., and J. RESKO (1974) Plasma testosterone and male dominance in a Japanese Macaque (*Macaca fuscata*) troop compared with repeated measures of testosterone in laboratory males. Horm. Behav. *5*:251–259.

EPPLE, G. (1978) Lack of effects of castration on scent marking displays and aggression in a South American primate (*Saguinus fuscicollis*). Horm. Behav. *11*:139–150.

GOODMAN, H. (1980a) Reproduction. In *Medical Physiology*, 14th ed. V. Mountcastle, ed., pp. 1602–1637, Mosby, St. Louis.

GOODMAN, H. (1980b) The pancreas and regulation of metabolism. In *Medical Physiology*, 14th ed. V. Mountcastle, ed., pp. 1638–1676, Mosby, St. Louis.

GORDON, T., R. ROSE, and I. BERNSTEIN (1976) Seasonal rhythm in plasma testosterone levels in the rhesus monkey (*Macaca mulatta*): A three year study. Horm. Behav. *7*:229–243.

GRAY, J. (1982) *The Neuropsychology of Anxiety*. Oxford Univ. Press, New York.

HAUSFATER, G. (1975) Dominance and reproduction in baboons: A quantitative analysis. *Contribs. Primatol.*, Vol. 7. Basel, Karger.

JOLLY, A. (1972) *The Evolution of Primate Behavior*. Macmillan, New York, p. 397.

KAPLAN, J., S. MANUCK, T. CLARKSON, F. LUSSO, and D. TAUB (1983) Social stress and atherosclerosis in normocholesterolemic monkeys. Science *220*:733–775.

KENDRICK, K., and R. DREWETT (1979) Testosterone reduces refractory period of stria terminalis neurons in the rat brain. Science *204*:877–879.

KRIEGER, D. (1982) *Cushing's syndrome*. Monographs in endocrinology, Vol. 22. Springer-Verlag, Berlin.

LESHNER, A. (1978) *An Introduction to Behavioral Endocrinology*. Oxford Univ. Press, New York.

MAX, S., and J. TOOP (1983) Androgens enhance *in vivo* 2-deoxyglucose uptake by rat striated muscle. Endocrin. *113*:119–126.

MUNCK, A., P. GUYRE, and N. HOLBROOK (1984) Physiological functions of glucocorticoids in stress and their relation to pharmacological actions. Endocrin. Rev. *5*:25–44.

PACKER, C. (1977) Reciprocal altruism in *Papio anubis*. Nature *265*:441–443.

PERACHIO, A. (1978) Hypothalamic regulation of behavioural and hormonal aspects of aggression and sexual performance. In *Recent Advances in Primatology*, D. Chivers and J. Herbert, eds., pp. 449–465, Academic Press, London.

REICHLIN, S. (1974) Neuroendocrinology. In *Textbook of Endocrinology*, 6th ed. R. Williams, ed., pp. 774–831, Saunders, Philadelphia.

RASSMUSSEN, D., J. LIU, P. WOLF, and S. YEN (1983) Endogenous opioid regulation of gonadotropin-releasing hormone release from the human fetal hypothalamus *in vitro*. J. Clin. Endo. Metab. *57*:881–885.

ROSE, R., J. HOLADAY, and I. BERNSTEIN (1971) Plasma testosterone, dominance rank and aggressive behaviour in male rhesus monkeys. Nature *231*:366–368.

ROSE, R., and E. SACHAR (1981) Psychoendocrinology. In *Textbook of Endocrinology*, 6th ed. R. Williams, ed., pp. 645–670. Saunders, Philadelphia.

ROSS, G., and R. VANDE WIELE (1981) The ovaries. In *Textbook of Endocrinology*, 6th ed. R. Williams, ed., pp. 355–399, Saunders, Philadelphia.

SAPOLSKY, R. (1982) The endocrine stress-response and social status in the wild baboon. Horm. Behav. *16*:279–292.

SAPOLSKY, R. (1983a) Endocrine aspects of social instability in the olive baboon (*Papio anubis*). Am. J. Primat. *5*:365–379.

SAPOLSKY, R. (1983b) Individual differences in cortisol secretory patterns in the wild baboon: Role of negative feedback sensitivity. Endocrinol. *113*:2263–2268.

SAPOLSKY, R. (1985a) Stress-induced suppression of testicular function in the wild baboon: Role of glucocorticoids. Endocrinol. *116*:2273–2277.

SAPOLSKY, R. (1985b) A mechanism for glucocorticoid toxicity in the hippocampus: Increased neuronal vulnerability to metabolic insults. J. Neurosci. *5*:1228–1231.

SAPOLSKY, R. (1986) Stress-induced elevation of testosterone concentrations in high-ranking baboons: Role of catecholamines. Endocrinol. *118*:1630–1635.

SAPOLSKY, R., and T. DONNELLY (1985) Vulnerability to stress-induced tumor growth increases with age in the rat: Role of glucocorticoids. Endocrinol. *117*:662–666.

SAPOLSKY, R., and W. PULSINELLI (1985) Glucocorticoids potentiate ischemic injury to neurons: Therapeutic implications. Science *229*:1397–1399.

SELYE, H. (1936) A syndrome produced by diverse nocuous agents. Nature *138*:32–34.

SELYE, H. (1971) *Hormones and Resistance*. Springer-Verlag, New York.

SELYE, H. (1979) *The Stress of My Life*. Van Nostrand-Reinhold, New York.

SEYFARTH, R. (1976) Social relationships among adult female baboons. Animal. Behav. *24*:917–938.

SMITH, D. (1981) The association between rank and reproductive success of male rhesus monkeys. Am. J. Primat. *1*:83–90.

SMUTS, B. (1985) *Sex and Friendship in Baboons*. Aldine Press, Hawthorne, NY.

TERMAN, G., Y. SHAVIT, J. LEWIS, J. CANNON, and J. LIEBESKIND (1984) Intrinsic mechanisms of pain inhibition: Activation by stress. Science *226*:1270–1276.

WARREN, M. (1983) Effects of undernutrition on reproductive function in the human. Endocrin. Rev. *4*:363–377.

WASSER, S., and D. BARASH (1983) Reproductive suppression among female mammals: Implications for biomedicine and sexual selection theory. Quart. Rev. Biol. *58*:513–538.

YATES, E., D. MARSH, and J. MARAN (1980) The adrenal cortex. In *Medical Physiology*, 14th ed. V. Mountcastle, ed., pp. 1558–1601, Mosby, St. Louis.

TWELVE
Human Sexology and Psychoneuroendocrinology

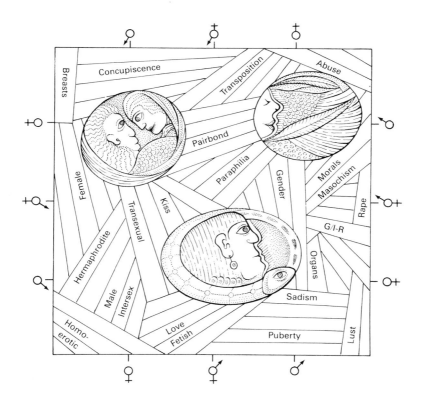

John Money
Department of Psychiatry and Behavioral Sciences
and Department of Pediatrics
The Johns Hopkins University and Hospital
Baltimore, Maryland

HISTORICAL ASPECTS OF HUMAN SEXOLOGY

Vital Fluid and Degeneracy Theory

The term hormone, from the Greek, *hormaein*, to set in motion, was first used in 1904 by Bayliss and Starling as the name for an internal or endocrine secretion. Virtually everything that is known about hormones is twentieth-century knowledge. Everything that is known about the hormonal governance of human eroticism, sexuality, and procreation is twentieth-century knowledge.

The antecedents of hormonal theory date back to Aristotle and Galen. Aristotle taught that the soul keeps in communication with the body by way of three vapors or spirits, natural, vital, and animal, which were, respectively, vegetative, sensitive, and rational.

Galen, in the second century, taught that natural humor or spirit from the liver ascends to the heart, where it is refined into vital spirit, which, in turn, ascends to the ventricles of the brain, where it is refined into animal, or animating, spirit. Galen's animal spirit supplied the soul with its faculties of sense, memory, and intellect. Vital spirit from the heart furnished the soul with emotions. Still today, in popular parlance love emanates from the heart, and its unbridled carnal passions are governed by the intellect.

In the eighteenth century, vitalism was given a new lease on life (Money, 1985). The old humors, vapors, or spirits were renamed vital sympathies, from which the contemporary term, sympathetic nervous system, is derived. There were also vital fluids. According to the eighteenth-century doctrine of the Swiss physician, Simon André Tissot (reprinted, 1974), the most powerful of the vital fluids was the semen, made from the most precious drops of the blood. Tissot's reasoning was that castration causes disappearance of the semen, which causes degeneration of virile strength, which causes all known forms of illness. Tissot lived too soon to know that the effect of castration was brought about, not by loss of semen, but by loss of male sex hormone from the Leydig cells of the testes.

On the basis of this epic error in reasoning, Tissot formulated his theory of degeneracy induced by concupiscence of the imagination and ideation, which brings about loss of semen in the disease of spermatorrhea (wet dreams), in the secret vice (masturbation), and in the social vice (promiscuity and whoring). After the discovery of germ theory, the first scientific theory of disease, by Pasteur and Koch at the end of the 1860s, degeneracy theory fell into disuse in all branches of medicine except sexual medicine. Degeneracy theory still lingers on; media and police attributions of paraphilic crimes and sex offenses are no longer attributed to masturbation but to commercial pornography. Pornography is the contemporary equivalent of concupiscence. It is feared with irrational superstition as a source of moral degeneracy. Thus, the serious science of sexology is still hindered and contaminated by the superstitious doctrines of prescientific sexosophy.

These superstitions covertly haunt the psychobiology of human sexuality and eroticism today by putting some aspects of research off limits—for example, the psychobiology of sexuoerotic development in childhood. Falling in love, or *limerence* (Tennov, 1979), is also widely considered too spiritual and sacred to be torn apart in research, and the anomalies of bizarre or kinky limerence, as in the paraphilias, are defined as sexual delinquencies and crime. Attributed to lust that has been morally depraved and degenerated by pornography, paraphilias are socially defined as the raw materials of, chiefly, the police and punishment industry, and rarely of scientific investigation. Scientists are afraid of contaminating their own names and careers if they deal with paraphilic sexuality. In many respects their fear is justified, for the antisexual power of society to enforce its ancient sexual taboo is insidious and far-reaching in its extent.

PSYCHOENDOCRINE ASPECTS OF HUMAN SEXOLOGY

Both normophilic and paraphilic limerence or falling in love are experienced or rehearsed, no matter how briefly or protractedly, as fantasies, images, thoughts, or ideas in the mind before they are implemented in action. That is to say, they are initially part of the *proceptive* phase (Beach, 1976), which is preparatory to the *acceptive* phase, which in turn is prerequisite to the *conceptive* phase of mating and procreation.

Proceptive Phase

The proceptive phase is known variously, and in different species, as the phase of courtship, solicitation, the mating dance, flirting, teasing, seduction, and foreplay. In human beings, proception may extend over either months of courtship, hours of flirting, or minutes of foreplay. What happens in the beginning of a courting or flirting relationship between two people of either sex, heterosexual or homosexual, is to some degree programed by the dictates of a specific time and place, and of local customs of dress, perfume, and adornment. To a remarkable extent, however, the proceptive program is *phyletically* dictated. In other words, it is shared by all members of the species cross-culturally, as demonstrated by Eibl-Eibesfeld (Donahue, 1985).

The defining characteristics of this program are establishing eye contact, squinting with a slight smile, and holding the gaze; talking inconsequentially but animatedly (by reason of vocal inflection, exclamation, exaggeration, laughing, heightened pitch, loudness, and accelerated speed); progressively rotating so as to face each other; moving closer together; moistening the lips and smiling; revealing or displaying partially covered parts of the body; being brushed or lightly touched one by the other, as if inadvertently, without recoiling; exaggeratively mirroring one another's postures, gestures, and facial expressions; and jointly synchronizing (Perper, 1985) actions and movements. Individuals engage in this program of proceptive behavior without training, without prior practice, and without being systematically aware that what they are doing is participating in a phyletic ritual, not an ontogenetic, personalized one. Some people are proceptively proficient far more than others—confidence tricksters, for example, as compared with the excessively shy or partially autistic population.

There is no known evidence that the neurobiology or neurochemistry of the phyletic program of human proception is sex-hormonally preordained or governed, nor that it is male-female dimorphic. There is, however, evidence that the threshold for the activation of the program is lowered by the sex hormones of puberty and adulthood. Nonetheless, most if not all of the components are observable in the proceptive rehearsals of childhood between the ages of three and eight. The youngest age of a pair-bonded love affair that may endure through puberty into adulthood, and that includes genital stimulation, would appear to be age eight (Money, 1980b, pp. 148–9). Further systematic observations are needed, however.

In nonprimate male mammals, as compared with primates, the nose rather than the eye is the organ of proception, and the stimulus that initiates proception is an odor or pheromone. The female's vagina releases the pheromone at the time of estrus and ovulation. Estrus itself is hormonally governed by a biological clock in synchrony with the seasons or some other periodic rhythm. In many mammalian species there is also a biological clock that governs the periodic rhythm of sex-hormonal secretion in males and, with it, spermatogenesis and readiness to respond to proceptive signals.

In nonhuman primates, or at least among those studied in the wild, the nose and pheromonal governance of mating take second place to the eyes and visual signals. In some species, female visual signaling is under hormonal governance, and is cyclic in synchrony with ovulation and estrus. The signal is swelling and bright coloration of the sexual parts. In some primate species living in the wild, estrus may be loosely synchronized with the seasons and seasonal fluctuations in the photoperiod or in the food supply, whereas in the laboratory such periodicity is masked. Among human beings, there is no seasonal or climatic fluctuation in the release of sex hormones, in ovulation, or in the prevalence or frequency of proceptivity.

The question of whether or not women's proceptivity fluctuates in synchrony with the menstrual cycle is a vexed one, for which no adequate answer is forthcoming. The first vexation is that, because proception is a relatively new concept (Beach, 1976), there have been no studies addressing human proception, per se. Rather, the few studies that may be relevant have addressed instead the issue of cyclic fluctuations either in desire or in copulatory frequency.

Desire is an inferential construct about a motivational state that cannot be observed or measured directly. All motivational states are notoriously slithery, for there is no absolute zero or criterion standard, invariant from person to person, against which to measure them. In addition, there is no agreed-upon, operational definition of desire. It may mean desire to take the initiative, or desire to be taken, sexually. Both may be experienced, but at different hormonal phases of the menstrual cycle. To complicate matters further, it is necessary to allow for the possibility that men may be differently responsive to subliminal stimuli or signals that fluctuate in synchrony with the hormonal phases of the female's menstrual cycle. Should a couple fluctuate in synchrony, then there is no point in using copulatory frequency as an index of desire in either partner alone.

As an index of desire, the frequency of copulation is also pointless if in either the male or the female copulatory desire should be not implemented by reason of adherence to customary superstitions and restrictions on copulation during the menstrual period. Irrespective of menstrual bleeding, the copulation of a sizeable, though unspecified, proportion of women and men is further restricted by a phobia of genital penetration which prevents the translation of desire into copulatory action.

Should female proceptivity fluctuate cyclically in synchrony with hormonal fluctuations of the menstrual cycle, then manipulation of hormonal fluctuation, as when women take the contraceptive pill, may be expected to yield data on proceptive fluctuation. There are no conclusive findings, however, because the hormonal contents of the different brands of pill are not uniform, and because of great individual variation in side effects of the pill on mood, sense of well-being, and proceptive arousal. Conversely, the pill may have the beneficial side effect of suppressing or ameliorating premenstrual tension which otherwise may interfere with proceptive arousal. The same applies also to menstrual cramping.

As in the case of menstrual cyclicity, hormonal changes at the menopause show no consistency of synchronization with changes in proceptivity. Some women become proceptively inert, postmenopausally, whereas others do not change, and still others become proceptive more readily. Postmenopausally, there is a possibility that, without estrogenic and progestinic competition, low-level androgen normally circulating in the bloodstream lowers the threshold for proceptive arousal.

There is some human clinical evidence (Money, 1961), and some primate experimental evidence that androgen is the hormone of proceptive arousal not only in men, but in women also. However, the evidence is not final and conclusive. One source of confusion has been the discovery that in males, both prenatally and postnatally, certain cells in the brain's pathways underlying sexual processes utilize testosterone by first converting it, intracellularly, to estradiol. In both sexes, there is much still to be learned about the intracellular metamorphosis of the sex steroids in the governance of both proceptive and acceptive erotosexual responsivity. In the meantime, the least speculative generality is that, in either sex, though proceptivity is possible irrespective of hormonal level, its threshold of arousal is lowered and its expression facilitated by having an optimal level of androgen. Androgen in excess of the optimal level does not increase proceptivity, or the subjective sense of sexual drive or desire. Contrary to folk reasoning, so-called erotomania or hypersexuality in men or women is not a function of elevated sex hormonal levels—nor is violent and assaultive paraphilic sex, as in rape and lust murder. Conversely, erotic inertia or apathy is not a function of low sex-hormonal level, except at the very low level of castration.

Perhaps because of the age-old evidence of the effects of castration on male animals, including boys and men, it has been widely taken for granted that the sex steroids, named male and female hormones, respectively, are solely responsible for proceptive arousal and genital performance. The possibility of either a direct, or a synergistic, or an antagonistic influence of other hormones, and in particular the pituitary peptides, has been little investigated. One exception was the discovery of a negative influence of hyperprolactinemia* (Ambrosi et al., 1980) on proceptive arousability and erectile potency in males. The corresponding effect in females has suffered the fate of much else in female sexology, namely, neglect.

The era of neurohormones, neurotransmitters, and neuromodulators is still too new for a comprehensive body of knowledge and theory to have been developed regarding the function of these substances in relation to either proceptivity or genital sexuality.

Acceptive Phase

Ordinarily, though not always, the proceptivity of flirting and courtship culminates, sooner or later, in erotic foreplay and the genital attainment of orgasm. In a masturbation fantasy, the partner may be represented in absentia. When the two partners are together, proception usually leads to acception, that is to say to the union of body parts, one body accepting the other, reciprocally. For procreation, the penis and the vagina accept or receive one another. The vagina receives the penetrating penis, and the penis receives the engulfing vagina. For conception to occur, ejaculation of semen through the penis is a prerequisite. Only in extremely rare instances does ejaculation occur without the subjectively experienced sensation of orgasm, whereas the vagina and vulva do not need to orgasm as a prerequisite of ovulation and fertilization. Anorgasmia is more prevalent in women than in men. There is no hormonal explanation of this inequality, nor any other explanation that is satisfactorily complete and comprehensive.

The role of hormones in not only orgasm and anorgasmia, but all the genital functions of copulation, is a story not yet fully told. Gonadal and pituitary hormones have an essential and undisputed role in the maintenance

---

* Selected terms are defined in the end-of-chapter glossary.

of fertility in both sexes. Apart from fertility, the copulatory function of the sex hormones may be said to be facilitatory rather than essential to the act of copulation.

In the female, estrogen is responsible for vaginal lubrication. Vaginal dryness is a complaint of hormonally untreated hypogonadal or agonadal women, and also of postmenopausal women. There is no definitive evidence, one way or the other, as to whether vaginal lubrication may occur in prepubertal girls. Engorgement of the vulva rather than vaginal lubrication is probably the equivalent, in girls, of prepubertal erection in boys. Erection occurs in utero, as evidenced by sonogram, and throughout postnatal life from infancy on. Nocturnal penile tumescence (NPT) occurs, on the average, three times a night while sleeping, for an average of 2½ to 3 hours total. Whether or not castration, either prepubertally or postpubertally, will abolish erection, either in NPT or from stimulation while awake, is individually variable. The effect of castration on copulation is also variable across species. One invariant effect is the loss of the testosterone-dependent fluid of ejaculation from the prostate and seminal vesicles, one consequence of which is that orgasm, when it occurs, is dry.

The disorders and malfunctions of the copulatory organs are vascular and neural in origin more often than they are hormonal. The differential etiology includes, in addition to vascular and neural pathology at the periphery, epileptic or other pathology affecting the neural circuits involved in sex; birth defect of the sex organs; genital trauma, including surgical trauma; tumor; neurochemical toxic side effect, including that of medications prescribed for hypertension and psychosis; infection; hormonal deficit at the periphery or in the brain; and the amorphous entity generally known as psychogenic. A psychogenic etiology is usually ascribed by exclusion of the others. It carries the implication of being reversible, though not invariably so. The disability may be situation specific, or it may be a persistent residual of abusive punishment and adversive neglect of sexual learning and species-typical sexual rehearsal play during infantile and juvenile development.

In addition to anorgasmia, erectile impotence, and vaginal dryness, the disabilities of genital functioning in the acceptive phase include genital insertion phobia or revulsion; genital anesthesia; dyspareunia; premature ejaculation; and vaginismus.

The three sex steroids are present in both sexes, but in different ratios. In men, an excess of either estrogenic or progestinic hormone has an androgen-suppressant effect. The effect is reversible, but while it lasts it reduces or suppresses erection and ejaculation. Exogenous estrogen induces breast enlargement, which is positive for male-to-female transsexuals. The androgen-suppressant effect of exogenous progestin is utilized in the treatment of male paraphilic sex offenders. It is an aid to their gaining greater self-governance of genital functioning without dependence on paraphilic imagery and/or behavior.

In women, exogenous androgen, as in the treatment of female-to-male transsexuals, suppresses ovarian hormone secretion, with consequent suppression of menstruation. Other morphologic effects are like those of male puberty. The feeling of orgasm, if it changes, is enhanced in intensity.

The cross-sex hormonal treatment of transexuals is based on their history of already having a transexual gender identity and role. Hormonal treatment does not induce a cross-over of masculine and feminine gender status. The same applies in those clinical syndromes in which adolescent boys get gynecomastia, and girls virilize and become hirsute. Typically, in these instances the hormonal error and its effects are personally mortifying. They do not induce feminization of the gender identity/role [G-I/R] (Money and Lewis, 1982) in boys, nor its masculinization in girls.

Conceptive Phase

Once the egg and sperm have united, the progress of gestation from implantation to delivery is heavily under the influence of hormonal programing—the mother's hormones and those of the fetus, too. Apart from being relatively autonomous, the hormonal programing of pregnancy takes place whether or not the mother is paired with a partner. Proception and acception, by contrast, are phyletically programed as an interaction between partners. For this reason, the conceptive phase, usually classified not as sexuality, but reproductive physiology, is not included in this chapter.

Whether or not the hormones of pregnancy have an effect on either proceptivity or acceptivity is arguable. Perhaps the effect, if any, is idiosyncratic, affecting different women in different ways. The same applies to the hormones of the postpartum and lactating period. Traditions around the world regarding abstinence during pregnancy and the postpartum are ethnically too divergent to be attributed to folk wisdom consistently derived from hormonally induced changes in either proceptivity or acceptivity.

DEVELOPMENTAL ASPECTS OF HUMAN SEXOLOGY

Heterosexual, Bisexual, Homosexual

Ever since the sex steroids were synthesized in the 1930s, some people have reasoned from analogy that if androgen is male sex hormone, then more of it will masculinize effeminate, homosexual males and make them heterosexual. The counterpart, as applied to lesbians, has not been so popular.

The search for a deficiency or anomaly of male sex hormones in homosexual men has yielded equivocal and contradictory results except for two studies (Parks et al., 1974; Sanders et al., 1985). These studies also happen to be the only two that are faultless in their sample selection, experimental design, and statistical methodology. The findings in each of these studies showed no difference in the circulating levels of various pituitary and gonadal sex-hormonal levels in the bloodstreams of homosexual men and their heterosexual controls.

A new approach to homosexual hormonal studies addresses itself not only to circulating levels of gonadal and pituitary hormones, but to the feedback effect of an injection of conjugated estrogens (Premarin) on the release of luteinizing hormone (LH). From the initial study by Dörner and colleagues (reviewed in Money, 1980a), it was reported that the feedback effect in homosexual males resembled that of heterosexual females, and differed from that of both heterosexual and bisexual males. In homosexuals, serum LH level initially decreased, and then rebounded to a level higher than the level before the estrogen injection. In a recent replication study, Gladue et al. (1984) obtained similar findings (Figure 12.1). However, in a still more recent replication study, Gooren (1986) in Amsterdam not only

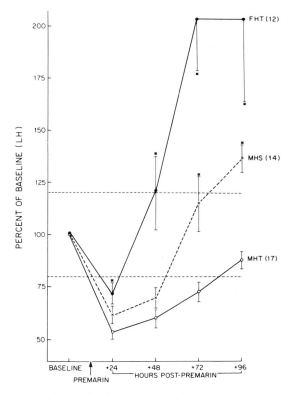

Figure 12.1. Changes in luteinizing hormone (LH) in response to a single injection of the estrogen preparation Premarin®. Values indicate percentage of baseline LH (baseline calculated as average of two daily samples taken on two days prior to administration of Premarin®). FHT: female heterosexuals; MHT: male heterosexuals; MHS: male homosexuals. Vertical bars indicate standard error of the mean. Dashed lines indicate the 95% confidence interval range of baseline values for all groups. Group comparisons: ∗ indicates FHT significantly different from MHT and MHS at all times (P < 0.05). MHS is also significantly different from MHT at +72 and +96 hrs (p < 0.05). Note that all groups show a decrease from baseline at +24 hrs post-Premarin®. N of subjects indicated in parentheses. Homosexual men, as a group, show a response pattern intermediate to and significantly different from those of heterosexual men and women.

failed to get confirmatory findings but showed that the elevation of LH was due to a hitherto neglected variable, namely, the steroidal responsivity of the Leydig cells to gonadotropic stimulation (Figure 12.2). Some homosexuals and some heterosexuals as well showed a poor Leydig-cell response to the gonadotropin test, which accounted for the anomalous LH rebound effect. An additional group of male-to-female transexual applicants not on hormone therapy, noteworthy for their feminine gender identity, did not show either the Leydig-cell effect or the LH rebound.

It is to be concluded, as of the present, that the difference between homosexual and heterosexual men cannot be attributed to the sex-hormonal levels of adulthood. That does not rule out the possibility of difference that might be back-dated to the period in prenatal or neonatal life when sex steroids are known, on the basis of many animal studies, to imprint a sexually dimorphic template in the developing pathways of the neural circuits involved in sex as either masculinized or nonmasculinized—or, presumably, in some instances, partially masculinized. This is the Adam/ Eve principle at work, for in mammals Nature's first template is to

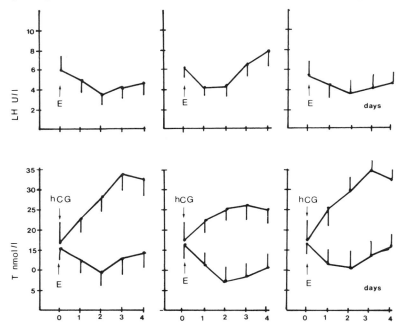

Figure 12.2. The different response of LH to estrogens (E) and of testosterone (T) to E and hCG stimulation in males. Some males (5 of 15 heterosexuals and 11 of 23 homosexuals) displayed a female type of LH response to E (middle panels). In these males T fell deeper upon E administration and T rose less to hCG stimulation (middle panels). In other males (10 of 15 heterosexuals and 12 of 23 homosexuals) not displaying this type of response the fall of T to E was smaller and the rise of T to hCG stimulation was greater (left panel). A female type of response of LH to E administration was not found in 6 transexual males (right panels) in whom the pattern of response was similar to that of the males in the left panels. Apparently the testicular steroidogenesis determines the type of response of LH to E.

differentiate a female. Something has to be added to make a male. In embryonic life, the something is androgen, plus müllerian-inhibiting hormone. Once the template has been formed, it can subsequently be activated in adult life by either androgen or estrogen.

The converse of masculinization is not feminization but nonmasculinization (or demasculinization). Likewise, the converse of feminization is defeminization. Thus an individual brain may be masculinized without being defeminized; or feminized without being demasculinized (see Ward, 1972; Baum, 1979).

Nordeen and Yahr (1982) produced in rats an intriguing finding that may or may not have human relevance. They placed estrogen pellets in either the right or left hypothalamus of neonatal female rats, exposing only one side at a time. Estrogen in the left hypothalamus had a defeminizing effect on development. In the right hypothalamus it had a masculinizing effect.

Prenatal Hormonalization: The Adrenogenital Syndrome (Congenital Virilizing Adrenal Hyperplasia)

In the human species, the Adam/Eve principle at work in prenatal life does not set an absolute seal that preordains masculinization or feminization, but rather sets a threshold that will either facilitate or hinder the postnatal overlay.

The joint significance of the postnatal, nonhormonal overlay, together with the prenatal hormonal underlay in the male/female differentiation of G-I/R, is exemplified in the matched-pair method of hermaphrodite study. In some hermaphroditic syndromes in which individuals are concordant for prenatal etiology and development, some are assigned and reared as boys and some as girls, the two groups thus being discordant for postnatal history. This discordancy has been studied in cases of the adrenogenital syndrome, also known as congenital virilizing adrenal hyperplasia (CVAH). The condition is genetically recessive in origin. The excess of prenatal androgen is erroneously produced from the fetus's own adrenocortices.

In extreme CVAH prenatal virilization, a 46,XX baby with two ovaries, uterus, and tubes is born with a penis and empty scrotum in place of a clitoris and vulva (Figure 12.3). In less extreme cases, the clitoris is hypertrophied, but without a penile urethra (Figure 12.4).

If a 46,XX baby with a penis is assigned as a boy, all of the clinical management, hormonal, surgical, and psychological, is designed for habilitation as a boy. Except for infertility, the boy grows up to be a typically masculine adult, distinguishable from other men only by his clinical history (Money and Daléry, 1976). He marries as a man and has the heterosexual life of a man.

The matched-pair counterpart of this man is a woman whose clinical management from birth onward is feminizing (Figure 12.5). She feminizes at puberty with breasts, menstruation, and fertility. In adulthood her romantic and sexual life may be that of a heterosexual woman. Alternatively

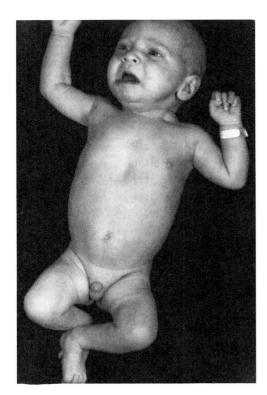

Figure 12.3. Newborn baby with the 46,XX syndrome of congenital virilizing adrenal hyperplasia (CVAH), with complete masculinization of the external genitalia. The internal genitalia are female.

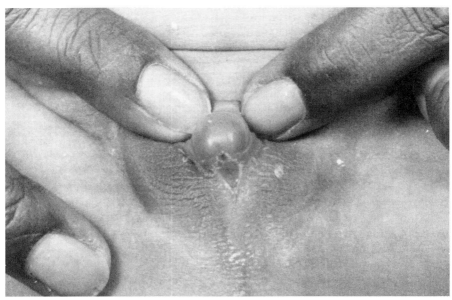

Figure 12.4. Newborn 46,XX CVAH baby with the external genitalia incompletely masculinized.

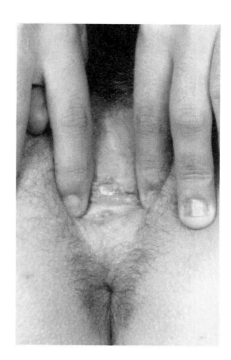

Figure 12.5. Genitalia of the same patient as in Figure 12.4 after surgical feminization.

she may have fantasies and/or experiences that are either bisexual or exclusively lesbian. She may be able to fall in love only with a woman.

Thirty cases of CVAH women who were born not with a penis but a greatly hypertrophied clitoris have been followed to maturity (Money, Schwartz, and Lewis, 1984). Each has been assigned, reared, and habilitated as a girl (Figure 12.6). As a group, they differed from their teenage mates in having an undeveloped romantic and dating life. Also they were unable to talk about their own sexuoerotic imagery or experience. Later, in their middle to late twenties, they were able to make more intimate personal disclosures. As shown in Table 12.1, 11 of the 30 (37%) disclosed themselves to have had bisexual imagery and/or practice; 5 (17%) of the 11 in the group rated themselves as exclusively ($N = 2$) or predominantly ($N = 3$) lesbian. Only 12 (40%) of the 30 claimed to be exclusively heterosexual. The remaining 7 (23%) were noncommittal. These percentages were statistically dissimilar ($p < .001$) from those obtained from a clinical comparison or control group.

The control group was composed of 27 women with the androgen-insensitivity syndrome (AIS; $N = 15$), and the Mayer-Rokitansky-Küster syndrome (MRKS; $N = 12$). The two syndromes were combined because behaviorally they were indistinguishable from one another (Lewis and Money, 1983; Money and Lewis, 1983). In both syndromes the body morphology and hormonalization are female, the vagina is shallow and blind, the uterus is cordlike, and there is no menstruation (Figure 12.7). Gonadally and chromosomally the two syndromes are divergent, namely, testicular and

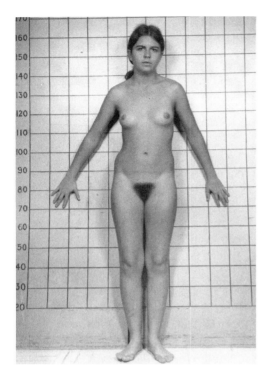

Figure 12.6. The same patient (deceased) as in Figures 12.4 and 12.5, pubertally feminized by her own ovarian hormones while constantly regulated on adrenocortical hormonal replacement therapy.

46,XY in the AIS, and ovarian and 46,XX in the MRKS—which demonstrates that the sex chromosomes and gonadal histology do not, per se, program sexuoeroticism.

Table 12.2 compares the percentages of the present CVAH sample

TABLE 12.1.   46,XX Adrenogenital Syndrome (CVAH) Female Rearing: Present Self-Ratings of Erotosexual Status (Imagery ± Activity)

Rating	CVAH ($N = 30$)	Controls ($N = 27$)*
Noncommittal	7 (23%)	0 (0%)
Heterosexual only	12 (40%)	25 (93%)
Bisexual	6 (20%)	2 (7%)
Homosexual only or predominantly	5 (17%)	0 (0%)
	Chi square = 18.5; $p < .001$†	

Legend

CVAH: syndrome of congenital virilizing adrenal hyperplasia
AIS: androgen-insensitivity syndrome
MRKS: Mayer-Rokitansky-Küster syndrome
*Androgen-insensitivity syndrome ($N = 15$); Mayer-Rokitansky-Küster syndrome ($N = 12$).
†Omitting the noncommittal line so that N (CVAH) = 23, and N (Control) = 27, and combining bisexual and homosexual ratings, then chi square = 10.5; $p < .01$.

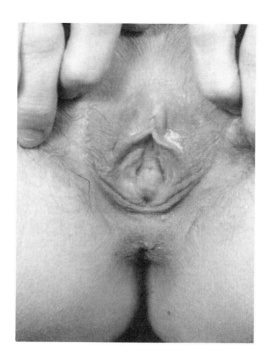

Figure 12.7. Normal female external genitalia of a patient with the 46,XY androgen-insensitivity syndrome. Note the typical sparseness of pubic hair, growth of which requires androgen.

(with and without the seven who were too reticent to be intimately self-revelatory), with those of the control sample and with those obtained by Kinsey in his large survey sample (Kinsey, Pomeroy, Martin, and Gebhard, 1953). Despite their age, the Kinsey data have not been superseded by a more modern survey. They indicate that the CVAH percentages are unlikely to have been an artifact of sampling.

The most likely explanation of these CVAH percentages, and the extremely divergent ones of the control sample, is that prenatal and/or

TABLE 12.2. Comparison of Homoerotic Incidence in CVAH, AIS/MRKS, and Kinsey's Sample

	Kinsey's Sample	CVAH $N = 30$	CVAH $N = 23*$	AIS/MRKS $N = 27$
Homoerotic arousal imagery by age 20	15%	37%	48%	7%
Homoerotic partner contact by age 20	10%	17%	22%	4%

Legend
CVAH: syndrome of congenital virilizing adrenal hyperplasia
AIS: androgen-insensitivity syndrome
MRKS: Mayer-Rokitansky-Küster syndrome
Kinsey sample: see Kinsey et al., 1953
*$N = 30 - 7$ (who were noncommittal) $= 23$.

neonatal hormonal masculinization did make a difference. It masculinized not only the genitalia, but presumably the sexual dimorphism of the brain, also. Conversely, in the control sample, the corresponding hormonal demasculinization made a difference in favor of feminization.

In the CVAH group, the prenatal masculinization effect was not sufficient to preordain transexualism in the quest for sex reassignment in childhood or later. Whatever the degree of masculinization, it was incorporated into a G-I/R that in adulthood was socially recognized as acceptably feminine, or a variant thereof. Those who declared themselves as predominantly or exclusively lesbian did so because they could fall in love only with a woman, not with a man. Thus it may prove to be a general rule that there is a crucial period of prenatal hormonal masculinization, which leaves its imprint on subsequent erotic life by way of the response to the visual gender image of a partner with whom a pairbonded, limerent relationship may be established.

Lovemaps

Examples such as those from the adrenogenital syndrome need a name for that which differentiates as homosexual, bisexual, or heterosexual. This name, a new term, is *lovemap*. A lovemap is defined as a personal developmental representation or template in the mind and in the brain depicting the idealized lover and the idealized program of sexuoerotic activity projected in imagery or actually engaged in with that lover (Money, 1986).

Whatever the prenatal hormonal contribution to the ultimate design of one's personal lovemap, the postnatal contribution is of undisputed significance in filling in the details. The analogy is with native language which requires, initially, a healthy human brain with subsequent social input of language through the senses, normally hearing and sight.

In early childhood development, social input to the lovemap is assimilated according to the principles of identification and complementation— identifying with those of one's own sex, copying their ways, and applying them so as to complement or reciprocate the responses of the other sex.

In the first phase of lovemap development, social input is through the skin senses, in cuddling, stroking, and rubbing, or lack thereof. During the first year of life, there is also the social response to an infant's self-discovery of the sensuousness of the genitals in response to rhythmic pressure, squeezing, rubbing, touching, and thrusting. By age three or four, at nap time or bed time, if children are in close proximity, side by side, rhythmic pelvic thrusting may be observed, perhaps in association with rhythmic thumb sucking. A boy who suckles naked at the mother's breast until this age may be seen to have an erection of the penis, and to pay it no heed.

Three or four is also the age at which children may be seen to engage in play rehearsal of flirtatiousness and proceptivity. The little girl plays coquette, and the little boy plays escort. A parent, older child, or other person of the opposite sex is the recipient of their flirtatious attention, which is fairly obviously patterned after models in the social environment, including those seen on television.

By age five or thereabouts, as the number of agemates increases in the yard, or at kindergarten or school, flirtatious play becomes boyfriend-girlfriend playmate romance. This also is the age when pelvic rocking or thrusting movements against the body of a partner while lying side by side give way to the rehearsal play of coital positioning (Money, et al., 1970).

The extent to which the positioning of coitus conforms to local traditions by being transmitted down the age ladder from older to younger children remains to be ascertained. It will be necessary to collect information from ethnic groups that do not veto sexual rehearsal play in their own children. In our own society some children assimilate erroneous information about what goes where, in sexual intercourse. Some children, indeed, equate coitus with kissing. For many children, sexual rehearsal play is equated with playing doctors and nurses, that being the full extent of their knowledge and experience of genital contact.

At around the age of eight, two partners in sexual rehearsal play may become pairbonded in a love affair that might be defined as a pairbonding rehearsal. However, it is scarcely a rehearsal when, as happens in some cases (see above), the couple remain intensely bonded through adolescence and into adulthood and beyond.

Because the moral climate of the times makes it virtually impossible to undertake systematic, real-life investigations of sexuoerotic rehearsal play in young human beings, one turns to studies of other primates, in particular, rhesus monkeys. In this species, sexuoerotic rehearsal play has proven to be an essential precursor of male-female breeding in adulthood. The play of juveniles includes sexual rehearsal play with agemates. It begins at around three months of age, as presenting and mounting, but in a jumble of confused positioning, front, side, and rear, irrespective of whether the playmates are boys or girls. In the ensuing three to six months, the positioning of the female presenting on all fours, and the male mounting from the rear, becomes perfected. Finally the male achieves the adult positioning of his feet, not on the floor, but grasping the legs of the female above the ankles (Figure 12.8).

Monkeys deprived of playmates by being isolation-reared grow up unable to present or mount, even when paired with a gentle and experienced mate. Therefore, they do not copulate. Thus, they do not reproduce their kind.

Even so short a playtime as half an hour a day proved sufficient to allow some monkeys to achieve the mating position. It was not sufficient for two-thirds of the group, however, and the remaining third were slow achievers. They were between 18 and 24 months of age when they finally succeeded. Even so, in adulthood they were poor breeders and had a low birthrate (Goldfoot, 1977).

Monkeys allowed unrestricted playtime, but only in all-male or all-female groups, engage in presenting and mounting play with one another when they become adolescent. Though normally reared partners of the opposite sex find

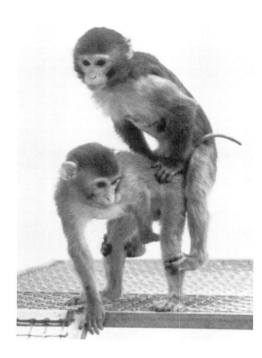

Figure 12.8. Sexual rehearsal play in juvenile rhesus monkeys, with the male showing the double footclasp mount. (Courtesy of David A. Goldfoot)

them sexually attractive, they cower and are scared. A male does not mount a female, even though he inspects and touches her genitalia with curiosity. A female resists the approach of a male partner, who succeeds in copulating only if he is exceptionally gentle and skilled at not making her more scared. When back with their same-sexed friends with whom they played as juveniles, males continue to mount males, and females to mount females, with a frequency unrecorded in males and females that grew up and engaged in sexual rehearsal play together as juveniles (Goldfoot and Wallen, 1978; Goldfoot and Neff, 1987; Goldfoot et al., 1984).

In individual monkeys, the prevalence of mounting versus presenting in rehearsal play may be dependent on the degree of exposure to male sex hormones in prenatal life, according to the evidence of females hermaphroditically masculinized by prenatal injections of testosterone into the mother. So far as is known, however, in monkeys, and in human beings, also, the activation of prepubertal sexuoerotic rehearsal play is not dependent on either gonadal or pituitary hormones.

Thwarting, delay, or precocious initiation of sexuoerotic rehearsal play in children in some, if not all instances, has a deleterious effect on lovemap formation. According to the available clinical and anthropological evidence, still awaiting systematic confirmation in prospective studies, normal sexuoerotic play in childhood leads to a normophilic and typically heterosexual lovemap which becomes fully activated by the hormones of adolescence and adulthood. Correspondingly, the same hormones activate a lovemap that has been disrupted or vandalized so as to become paraphilic or, in colloquial parlance, kinky or bizarre. The value of an antiandrogenic hormone (in Europe, cyproterone acetate, and in the United States, medroxyprogesterone acetate) in the treatment of paraphilias is that it returns plasma testosterone to the level of prepuberty. This change enhances the possibility of redesigning the lovemap to become sufficiently normophilic to allow the individual to live free from social and police accusation of being deviant or criminal. There is more information on the paraphilias in Money (1986).

SUMMARY

The superstitions of prescientific degeneracy theory still impede psychoendocrine research, especially with respect to the developmental sexuality and eroticism of prepuberty and early adolescence, in health and disease. The three phases of sexuoeroticism are proceptive, acceptive, and conceptive. Proceptivity is rehearsed in imagery and ideation, as well as being put into practice. The threshold for its appearance is hormonally regulated, but its content is not. The threshold for genital acceptivity also is hormonally regulated, but not in toto. The complete story of hormones in relationship to both proceptive and acceptive dysfunction, cyclicity, and menopausal change has not yet been discovered. Relatively more is known regarding the hormonal governance of the conceptive phase. At puberty and subsequently, the sex hormones do not determine heterosexual, bisexual, or homosexual status. In prenatal or neonatal life, however, they may leave a sexually dimorphic imprint in the brain that is activated at puberty. The hermaphroditic, 46,XX adrenogenital syndrome offers substantiating evidence. Lovemaps are developmental brain/mind templates that owe something to prenatal hormones, and more to postnatal socialization. Normophilic lovemap development may become pathologized into paraphilic. Rhesus monkeys provide an animal model. Antiandrogenic treatment combined with sexological counseling helps paraphilic men, including sex offenders, gain improved sexual self-governance.

ACKNOWLEDGMENTS

This work was supported by USPHS Grant HD00325 and the William T. Grant Foundation Grant #83086900.

GLOSSARY

Androgen-insensitivity syndrome (*also called* **testicular-feminizing syndrome**). A congenital condition identified by a 46,XY chromosomal karyotype in girls or women who appear externally to be not sexually different from normal females, except in some cases for a swelling or lump in each groin, or for the absence of pubic hair after puberty. The cells of the body are unable to respond to the male sex hormone, which is made in the testes in normal amounts for a male. They respond instead to the small amount of female sex hormone, estrogen, which is normally made in the testes. The effect before birth is that masculine internal development commences but is not completed. It goes far enough, however, to prevent internal female development. Externally, the genitalia differentiate as female, except for a blind vagina, which is usually not deep enough for satisfactory intercourse and needs either dilation or surgical lengthening in or after middle teenage. There is no menstruation and no fertility. Breasts develop normally.

Anorgasmia. A hypophilic condition or syndrome, variable in etiology, of being unable to attain orgasm under normally conducive modes of stimulation.

CVAH (congenital virilizing adrenal hyperplasia). A syndrome produced by a genetically transmitted enzymatic defect in the functioning of the adrenal cortices of males and females, which induces varying degrees of insufficiency of cortisol and aldosterone and excesses of adrenal androgen and pituitary adrenocorticotropin (ACTH). Abnormal function of the adrenal cortex starts in fetal life and, unless treated, persists chronically after birth. Females born with the syndrome have ambiguous genitalia and, if they survive without salt loss and dehydration, undergo severe virilization. Males are usually not recognized at birth but, if they survive, will prematurely develop sexually during the first years of life. In the severe form of the disease, untreated, mortality rate is almost 100% for both sexes. Treatment with glucocorticoids and in some cases also with salt-retaining hormone is life-saving and prevents untimely and, in girls, incongruous postnatal virilization. Plastic surgery is needed to feminize the genitalia. With appropriate therapy, prognosis for survival and good physical and mental health is excellent.

Dyspareunia. A hypophilic condition or syndrome of difficult or painful coitus, of variable etiology, in men and women (from Greek, *dyspareunos*, badly mated). The term is used chiefly in reference to women, but applies equally well to men.

Gynecomastia. Enlargement of the breasts in males, particularly during puberty and early adolescence, usually transiently, but in some instances persistently.

Hyperprolactinemia. An endocrine condition characterized by excessive secretion of the hormone, prolactin, from the pituitary gland, in some cases associated with a pituitary tumor. In males impotence may be one of its symptoms.

Hypogonadal (*noun*, **hypogonadism**). Deficient functioning of the gonads (testes or ovaries), particularly of hormonal functioning, with consequent failure in young people of the onset of puberty; and, if the onset is postpubertal, failure to maintain adult hormonal masculinization in males, or feminization in females.

Mayer-Rokitansky-Küster syndrome. A sexual birth defect characterized by impaired differentiation of the müllerian ducts so that the uterus is rudimentary and cordlike. The deep or inner part of the vagina is absent and the outer part is shallow or in the form of a dimple. The fallopian tubes may be defective, and there may be other, sporadic congenital anomalies. The ovaries are normal and induce normal feminizing puberty, except for lack of menstruation secondary to the defective uterus. Psychosexual differentiation is as a female.

REFERENCES

AMBROSI, B., M. GAGGINI, P. MORIONDO, and G. FAGLIA (1980) Prolactin and sexual function. JAMA *244*:2608.

BAUM, M.J. (1979) Differentiation of coital behavior in mammals: A comparative analysis. Neurosci. Biobehav. Rev. *3*:265–284.

BEACH, F.A. (1976) Sexual attractivity, proceptivity, and receptivity in female mammals. Horm. Behav. 7:105–138.

DONAHUE, P. (1985) *The Human Animal: Who are we? Why do we behave the way we do? Can we change?* Simon and Schuster, New York.

GLADUE, B.A., R. GREEN, AND R.E. HELLMAN (1984) Neuroendocrine response to estrogen and sexual orientation. Science 225:1496–1498.

GOLDFOOT, D.A. (1977) Sociosexual behaviors of nonhuman primates during development and maturity: Social and hormonal relationships. In *Behavioral Primatology, Advances in Research and Theory*, Vol. 1. A.M. Schrier, ed., Lawrence Erlbaum, Hillsdale, NJ.

GOLDFOOT, D.A., and D.A. NEFF (1987) On measuring behavioral sex differences in social contexts. In *Masculinity/Femininity: Basic Perspectives*. J.M. Reinisch, L.A. Rosenblum, and S.A. Sanders, eds., Oxford University Press, New York.

GOLDFOOT, D.A., and K. WALLEN (1978) Development of gender role behaviors in heterosexual and isosexual groups of infant rhesus monkeys. In *Recent Advances in Primatology*, Vol. 1, *Behavior*. D.J. Chivers and J. Herbert, eds., Academic Press, London.

GOLDFOOT, D.A., K. WALLEN, D.A. NEFF, M.C. McBRAIR, and R.W. GOY (1984) Social influences upon the display of sexually dimorphic behavior in rhesus monkeys: Isosexual rearing. Arch. Sex. Behav. 13:395–412.

GOOREN, L.J.G. (1986) Estrogen positive feedback effect in heterosexuals, homosexuals, and transsexuals. J. Clin. Endocrinol. Metab. (In press).

KINSEY, A.C., W.B. POMEROY, C.E. MARTIN, and P.H. GEBHARD (1953) *Sexual Behavior in the Human Female*. Saunders, Philadelphia.

LEWIS, V.G., and J. MONEY (1983) Gender-identity/role: G-I/R Part A: XY (androgen-insensitivity syndrome) and XX (Rokitansky syndrome) vaginal atresia compared. In *Handbook of Psychosomatic Obstetrics and Gynaecology*. L. Dennerstein and G. Burrows, eds., Elsevier Biomedical Press, Amsterdam-New York-London.

MONEY, J. (1961) The sex hormones and other variables in human eroticism. In *Sex and Internal Secretions*, 3rd ed. W.C. Young, ed., Williams and Wilkins, Baltimore.

MONEY, J. (1980a) Endocrine influences and psychosexual status spanning the life cycle. In *Handbook of Biological Psychiatry*, Part III. H.M. van Praag, ed., Marcel Dekker, New York.

MONEY, J. (1980b) *Love and Love Sickness: The Science of Sex, Gender Difference, and Pair-Bonding*. Johns Hopkins University Press, Baltimore.

MONEY, J. (1985) *The Destroying Angel: Sex, Fitness and Food in the Legacy of Degeneracy Theory, Graham Crackers, Kellogg's Corn Flakes and American Health History*. Prometheus Books, Buffalo.

MONEY, J. (1986) *Lovemaps: Clinical Concepts of Sexual/Erotic Health and Pathology, Paraphilia, and Gender Transposition in Childhood, Adolescence, and Maturity*. Irvington, New York.

MONEY, J., J.E. CAWTE, G.N. BIANCHI, and B. NURCOMBE (1970) Sex training and traditions in Arnhem Land. Br. J. Med. Psychol. 43:383–399.

MONEY, J., and J. DALÉRY (1976) Iatrogenic homosexuality: Gender identity in seven 46,XX chromosomal females with hyperadrenocortical hermaphroditism born with a penis, three reared as boys, four reared as girls. J. Homosex. *1*:357–371.

MONEY, J., and V. LEWIS (1982) Homosexual/heterosexual status in boys at puberty: Idiopathic adolescent gynecomastia and congenital virilizing adrenocorticism compared. Psychoneuroendocrinology 7:339–346.

MONEY, J., and V.G. LEWIS (1983) Gender-identity/role: G-I/R Part B: A multiple sequential model of differentiation. In *Handbook of Psychosomatic Obstetrics and Gynaecology*. L. Dennerstein and G. Burrows, eds., Elsevier Biomedical Press, Amsterdam-New York-London.

MONEY, J., M. SCHWARTZ, and V.G. LEWIS (1984) Adult erotosexual status and fetal hormonal masculinization and demasculinization: 46,XX congenital virilizing adrenal hyperplasia and 46,XY androgen-insensitivity syndrome compared. Psychoneuroendocrinology 9:405–414.

NORDEEN, E.J., and P. YAHR (1982) Hemispheric asymmetries in the behavioral and hormonal effects of sexually differentiating mammalian brain. Science *218*:391–393.

PARKS, G.A., S. KORTH-SCHUTZ, R. PENNY, R.F. HILDING, K.W. DUMARS, S.D. FRASIER, and M.I. NEW (1974) Variation in pituitary-gonadal function in adolescent male homosexuals and heterosexuals. J. Clin. Endocrinol. Metabl. *39*:796–801.

PERPER, T. (1985) *Sex Signals: The Biology of Love*. ISI Press, Philadelphia.

SANDERS, R.M., J. BAIN, and R. LANGEVIN (1985) Peripheral sex hormones, homosexuality, and gender identity. In *Erotic Preference, Gender Identity and Aggression in Men: New Research Studies*. R. Langevin, ed., Lawrence Erlbaum, Hillsdale, NJ.

TENNOV, D. (1979) *Love and Limerence: The Experience of Being in Love*. Stein and Day, New York.

TISSOT, S.A. (1974) *A Treatise on the Disease Produced by Onanism*. Translated from a New Edition of the French, with Notes and Appendix by an American Physician. New York, 1832. Facsimile reprint edition in *The Secret Vice Exposed! Some Arguments Against Masturbation*. C. Rosenberg and C. Smith-Rosenberg, advisory eds., Arno Press, New York.

WARD, I.L. (1972) Prenatal stress feminizes and demasculinizes the behavior of males. Science *175*:82–84.

Index

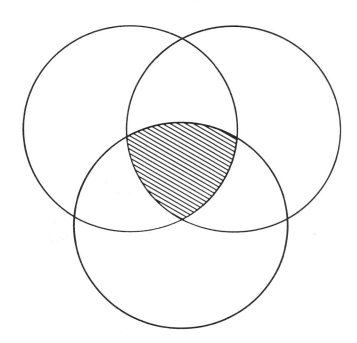

Arginine vasotocin (AVT) *(cont.)*
  behavioral effects of, 42, 63–69,
    77
  brain content, 66, 75
  distribution in vertebrates, 62
  neuroanatomical distribution,
    74–76
Aromatase, 240
Arousal versus stress, 223
Artificial selection, 217
Associated reproductive pattern, 93
Avian sexual behavior, 124–28,
  151–72

B

Behavior:
  aggressive, 10–11, 13, 149, 153,
    156, 159–61, 163, 164, 166,
    167, 172
  agonistic, 149, 155, 156, 159, 161,
    162
  courtship, 3–22, 29–56, 153, 156,
    164, 165
  mate-guarding, 149, 154–56, 166,
    167, 171
  parental, 132–36, 163–67, 169,
    171
  territorial, 149, 153–56, 159–61,
    163, 167, 169, 171, 172
Beta-endorphin, 79, 294, 304
Birth cycle, 182, 196–97
Bisexual behavior, 14, 40, 105–14
Body size, 211, 215
Brain, 39, 43–45, 53–54
Brain content of neuropeptides, 66,
  72, 75
Brain mechanisms for fish reproduction (fish brain), 3–5, 14,
  16–22, 24, 54
Brain stimulation (in sea bass),
  16–22
Breeding rhythms, 121–26, 131,
  133, 136, 207, 215

Breeding season, 149, 150, 154,
  156, 170, 262, 272, 276, 277,
  279, 281, 284
Brooding, 124, 125, 128

C

Castration, 44–45, 94, 98, 324, 328,
  329
Chlorisodamine, 304, 308
Circadian clock, 122, 127, 137
Circadian rythms, 121–23, 126, 131,
  133, 137, 139–43
Clitoris, 260, 262, 263, 273
Conceptive phase, 325, 330, 341
Conditioned-avoidance response, 71
Congenital virilizing adrenal hyper-
  plasia (CVAH), 333–38, 342
Constant reproductive pattern, 100
Copulation, 92, 105, 153–56, 164,
  166, 167, 171, 267–70, 272, 274,
  279, 280, 286
Cortisol, 310
Cost of reproduction, 90
Critical period, 235

D

Degeneracy theory, 324, 325, 341
Delayed implantation, 260, 266,
  268, 269, 271, 272, 274, 282
Developmental effects of
  hormones, 197–98, 234, 246
Development, 102
Dexamethasone, 306, 307
Diestrus (-ous), 279, 282, 283, 286
Differentiation, 233, 250
Dissociated reproductive pattern, 96
Diversity of reproduction, 100
Dominance, 179, 184, 296, 306
Dyspareunia, 329, 342

E

Eggs (ovulated), 33–35, 38
Egg trading (in sea bass), 14–15, 24

Ejaculation, 328, 329
Emotional state, 223
Encephalic photoreceptors, 138, 139
Energetics, 210
Entrainment, 123, 124, 127, 131, 137, 138–41
Epinephrine (adrenaline), 221, 293, 294, 304
Erection, 329
Estradiol (*see also* Estrogen), 30–31, 35, 45, 56, 164, 165, 264, 266–68, 270, 271, 282–86
Estrogen (*see also* Estradiol), 124, 125, 131, 185–86, 197, 264, 266–68, 270, 271, 282–86
Estrous cycle, 181–83, 195, 198
Estrous synchrony, 181–83
Estrus (-ous), 265–71, 279–86
Evolution of behavioral regulators, 78–82
Evolution of hormonal regulation, 78–82, 105
Evolution of hormone structures, 62
Experience, 30–31, 102

F

Facilitation of reproduction, 107, 178
Feminization, 233
Fertilization mode (internal versus external), 29, 35, 43, 57
Fish sexual behaviors, 2–58, 67–68, 77
5 α reduction (5 α reductase), 240
Follicle-stimulating hormone (FSH), 151, 221, 315
Foraging, 211
Free-running rythms, 123, 124, 126, 127, 138, 140

G

Gamete release (in fishes):

egg release (oviposition), 3–5, 16, 18–20, 22
sperm release, 3–5, 16, 18–20, 22
General Adaptation Syndrome, 294
Glucagon, 294
Glucocorticoids, 293, 294, 307, 310, 316
Gonadal hormones (steroid hormones, *see also* Androgen, Estradiol, Estrogen, Progesterone, Testosterone), 125, 130–38
Gonadal steroids, 65, 78–82
Gonadotropic hormone (GTH) LH, FSH, 132–38
Gonadotropin, 32, 35–36, 38, 46–48
Gonadotropin-releasing hormone (GnRH, *see also* Luteinizing-hormone releasing hormone), 54, 73, 79, 81, 132, 133, 135–37, 151
control of sex in fishes, 5, 20–21, 24
Gonads (testes, ovaries), 124, 125, 131–35, 137, 138, 140, 151, 157, 163, 165, 167
Gynecomastia, 330, 342

H

Hermaphrodites, 40
Hermaphroditism (in fishes):
acquired, 2–5, 23
self-fertilizing, 2, 22–23, 24
sequential protandrous, 2, 5
sequential protogynous, 2, 5–14, 23–24
simultaneous, 2, 14–22, 24
Heterosexual, 330, 332, 333, 335–38, 340, 341
Homeostasis, 293
Homosexual, 330–32, 335, 338, 341
Hormone receptors, 242
Hyperprolactinemia, 328, 342

Organization, 234, 250
Oscillator, 122–24, 126, 128, 131, 134, 137, 139–43
Oviposition (effects of vasotocin), 68
Ovotestis (in sea bass), 15–16
Ovulation, 31–35, 37–38, 40–43, 46, 50–52, 55–57, 179–84, 192, 194–195, 221
  induced, 260, 266, 268, 269, 271, 272, 274, 282
  spontaneous, 265, 267–69, 274, 282
Oxytocin:
  distribution in vertebrates, 62
  mammal behaviors, 69–71, 73
  neuroanatomical distribution, 74–76

P

Panogamy, 193
Paraphilia, 325, 329, 340–44
Paraventricular nucleus (PVN), 132, 136
Parental behavior, 44, 125, 126
Parthenogenesis, 106
Parturition, effects of vasotocin, 68
Passive-avoidance situation, 71
Penile spines, 272, 273
Pharmacological effects on behaviors, 72–73
Pheromones, 3, 20, 49–57, 178, 180–87, 221, 326
  snakes, 104
Photoperiod, 123, 127, 129, 133–35, 137–42, 156–59, 165, 182, 183, 186, 217, 263, 264, 281
Photoperiod cue, 91
Photorefractoriness, 157, 158, 168, 169
Physical environment, 177, 183, 186–92, 195–96
Pineal gland, 132, 137–39, 140–42
Pituitary, 125, 132–37, 151
Plant predictors, 219
Polyestrus (-ous), 265, 266, 268

Polygyny (-ous), 277, 286
Postpartum estrus, 190–91, 196–97
Predictability, 90
Pregnancy (-ant), 182, 190, 197, 265–67, 282, 283
Preoptic area (fishes), 5, 20–21
Preoptic area (POA), 132, 136, 137
Proceptive behavior, 248
Proceptive phase, 325–28, 338, 341
Proestrus (-ous), 260, 265, 266, 269–72, 279, 282, 284
Progesterone, 124, 125, 131, 264–68, 271, 282–84
Prolactin, 124, 125, 167–69, 221, 316
Prostaglandins, 30, 35–43, 56–57
  role in female sex behavior in fishes, 18, 21
Proximate factors, 89, 91, 150, 215
Pseudopregnancy (-ant), 265–67, 282

R

Rainfall, 211
Receptive behavior, 246
Receptivity, 30–31, 42–43
Receptors for neurohypophysial peptides, 76
Release calls in frogs, 64–65
Reproductive pattern:
  associated, 93
  constant, 100
  dissociated, 96
Reproductive suppression, 178, 180, 182, 184, 187, 196–97
Reptile sexual behaviors, 93–100, 104–14

S

Scent-marking, 272
Seasonal breeding, 90, 121, 131, 132, 134, 137, 141, 206, 261, 264, 265, 277, 281
Seasonal prediction, 216